J. Landon and T. Chard (Eds)

Therapeutic Antibodies

With 17 Figures

Springer-Verlag
London Berlin Heidelberg New York
Paris Tokyo Hong Kong
Barcelona Budapest

John Landon, MD, FRCP
Department of Chemical Pathology, St Bartholomew's Hospital Medical College, Charterhouse Square, London EC1M 7BQ, UK

Tim Chard, MD, FRCOG
Joint Academic Unit of Obstetrics, Gynaecology and Reproductive Physiology, St Bartholomew's Hospital Medical College, West Smithfield, London EC1A 7BE, UK

Cover illustration: Ch. 2, Fig. 2. The structure of IgM.

ISBN-13: 978-1-4471-1939-5 e-ISBN-13: 978-1-4471-1937-1
DOI: 10.1007/978-1-4471-1937-1

British Library Cataloguing in Publication Data
A catalogue record for this book is available from the British Library

Softcover reprint of the hardcover in 1st edition 1995

Typeset by the Electronic Book Factory, Fife, Scotland.
28/3830–543210 Printed on acid-free paper

Contents

Preface

We live in an era of unprecedented technical and scientific advance and nowhere is this more evident than in the production and use of antibodies for diagnostic and therapeutic purposes. Thus the past 20 years have witnessed the use of ovine antibody fragments for the treatment of drug overdose; the production of murine monoclonal antibodies by means of hybridoma technology; the exploitation of molecular biology to provide chimeric antibodies; and the design of immunogens which result in specific antibodies with catalytic activity.

Many scientists are expert at marketing their newest ideas to their commercial colleagues. Every statement has the ring of sincerity; problems are non-existent or easy to surmount; production will cause no problems; costs can soon be markedly curtailed; and large fortunes wait merely to be claimed. Success remains certain until, with happy abandon, they change their minds and move to an even more innovative and questionable approach, leaving the investing public with massive losses and the business executives to seek new posts. This is a particular problem in some companies in which to question an accepted course of action may be regarded as unacceptable pessimism, disloyalty, heresy or worse. Many companies must even now be planning to introduce molecular-engineered synthetic antibodies to replace their recently discarded monoclonal products or urging an increasingly reluctant public to invest in the distant haven of catalytic antibodies.

Several recent books and monographs have been devoted to monoclonal and related antibodies and there is no doubt that, in appropriate situations, they have much to offer clinically. Furthermore, their present disadvantages (such as high cost and frequent lack of efficacy) will be overcome eventually. While this book covers some new topics, such as catalytic antibodies, it is unique in focusing attention on the successful therapeutic application of polyclonal antibodies and their fragments. Such products, although seemingly old-fashioned, offer the advantages of several million years' natural evolutionary development and can be produced with a fraction of the effort and at a fraction of the cost of their monoclonal counterparts. Another attribute is that such products are usually effective, in keeping with the observation that the body invariably mounts a polyclonal humoral immune response.

J. Landon
T. Chard

Contributors

Dr Gordon R. Bernard, Center for Lung Research, School of Medicine, Vanderbilt University, Nashville, Tennessee 37231-2650, USA

Dr K. L. Brigham, Division of Pulmonary Care and Critical Medicine, Department of Medicine, Vanderbilt University, Nashville, Tennessee 37232, USA

Professor Tim Chard, Department of Reproductive Physiology, St Bartholomew's Hospital Medical College, West Smithfield, London EC1A 7BE, UK

Miss Ruth E. Coxon, Department of Chemical Pathology, St Bartholomew's Hospital Medical College, West Smithfield, London EC1M 7BQ, UK

Dr Gerry Gallacher, Division of Chemistry, Department of Pharmacy, University of Brighton, Cockroft Building, Lewes Road, Moulsecoomb, Brighton BN2 4GJ, UK

Professor Frank Hay, Division of Immunology, Department of Cellular and Molecular Sciences, St George's Hospital Medical School, Cranmer Terrace, London SW17 0RE, UK

Dr Andrew J. Heath, 50 Otis Street, Westborough, MA 01581-4500, USA

Dr P. A. Knight, Wellcome Biotech, Langley Court, Beckenham, Kent BR3 3BS, UK

Professor J. Landon, Department of Chemical Pathology, St Bartholomew's Hospital Medical College, Charterhouse Square, London EC1M 7BQ, UK

Dr J. A. Ledermann, Department of Oncology, The Courtauld Institute of Biochemistry, 9 Ridinghouse Street, London W1P 9BT, UK

Dr Charles McLean, Department of Chemical Pathology, St Bartholomew's Hospital Medical College, Charterhouse Square, London EC1M 7BQ, UK

Dr T. Poulton, Division of Immunology, Department of Cellular and Molecular Sciences, St George's Hospital Medical School, Cranmer Terrace, London SW17 0RE, UK

Dr Damon C. Smith, Therapeutic Antibodies Ltd, Department of Chemical Pathology, St Bartholomew's Hospital Medical College, Charterhouse Square, London EC1M 7BQ, UK

Dr R. D. G. Theakston, Liverpool School of Tropical Medicine, Pembroke Place, Liverpool, UK

Dr A. P. Wheeler, Division of Pulmonary and Critical Care Medicine, Department of Medicine, Vanderbilt University, Nashville, Tennessee 37232, USA

Miss J. A. Woolley, Department of Chemical Pathology, St Bartholomew's Hospital Medical College, Charterhouse Square, London EC1M 7BQ, UK

Dr Peng Lee Yap, Department of Transfusion Medicine, Royal Infirmary, Edinburgh EH3 9HB, UK

1 An Introduction to the Clinical Applications of Antibodies

J. Landon, T. Chard and R.E. Coxon

History

It is now over 100 years since von Behring and Kitasato conducted the investigations that led to the use of foreign antibodies for treatment. Biologically inactive toxoids prepared from tetanus and diphtheria toxins were used to immunize small animals. The recipients were protected against many times the usual lethal dose of the respective toxin (i.e. active immunity). Furthermore, serum from an immunized rabbit could neutralize the toxin and, when injected systemically, protect mice or guinea-pigs (i.e. passive immunity). Recognizing the clinical implications of these studies, von Behring was able to reduce morbidity and mortality in children with diphtheria by use of serum from horses that had been hyperimmunized with the appropriate toxoid. This approach was soon extended by Calmette to the use of equine antisera for the treatment of snake and scorpion envenomation. As discussed in Chapter 6, horses have remained the preferred species for antivenom production because of their ease of handling and the large volumes of blood (up to 10 litres) that can be collected.

The dangers associated with the systemic administration of unrefined equine serum were quickly recognized. Most patients developed serum sickness after about 8 days while a few, who had been exposed previously to horse proteins, experienced acute and sometimes fatal anaphylaxis. The incidence of deleterious effects was reduced by use of an immunoglobulin fraction of the serum. Further improvement followed the use of pepsin to cleave immunoglobulins into Fc and $F(ab')_2$ and administration of only the latter for treatment. There have been few further improvements in antivenom production during the past 50 years. Currently, about 60 centres worldwide prepare equine immunoglobulin concentrates or equine $F(ab')_2$ for the treatment of envenomation, despite the fact that they cause allergic side-effects in about 60% and 10% of subjects respectively. This is unsatisfactory, as indicated by the statement in the British National Formulary of 1981 that "The adder bite itself may be less dangerous than the so-called specific snake bite antiserum . . .". The high incidence of allergic effects may be due to high levels of IgG(T) in immunized horses; this is a very immunogenic form of immunoglobulin. Because of the risk of causing such effects, many clinicians are reluctant to administer antivenoms or to use foreign antibodies in other situations. Fortunately, antibodies of human origin are not allergenic and, as discussed in Chapter 8, are used extensively for the prevention and/or treatment of infectious diseases. Orally administered antibodies are also relatively free of allergic effects and, as reviewed in Chapter 3, hens' eggs provide an inexpensive source of natural antibodies for use in the treatment of gastrointestinal infections in both clinical and veterinary practice.

Since the pioneering research of Landsteiner in the 1930s, it has been common practice to raise antibodies directed against small molecules (referred to as haptens), such as drugs. Although not themselves immunogenic (i.e. capable of eliciting a humoral immune response), haptens can be made so by covalently coupling them to a large carrier molecule, such as albumin or keyhole limpet haemocyanin. During the late 1960s a group in Boston succeeded in producing antibodies directed against digoxin and other cardiac glycosides, which they used to develop a sensitive and specific radioimmunoassay. Subsequently these antibodies were shown to reverse the hyperkalaemia and other clinical manifestations of digoxin overdose. Three important innovations were incorporated into the development of this therapeutic agent. First, sheep (which are widely available, inexpensive, lack IgG(T) and produce higher antibody levels) were preferred to horses; second, the immunoglobulins were cleaved with papain to produce Fab fragments with a single binding site; and third, only Fab fragments directed specifically against the cardiac glycosides were used therapeutically, being separated from the much larger amounts of non-specific Fab by affinity chromatography. At the present time, two such ovine-specific Fab products are available commercially and, as discussed in Chapter 5, have been given to several thousand patients. These products have an enviable reputation as regards both safety and efficacy.

As their name implies, natural polyclonal antibodies (PcAb) of avian or mammalian origin are derived from a large number of different clones. As a result, they are directed against many epitopes [1] to which they bind with a range of affinities [2]. It might have been expected that the advent of safe, effective, polyclonal antibody products for the treatment of digoxin toxicity would have rekindled interest in this approach to immunotherapy. However, it has failed to do so, perhaps because it took place at the same time as the introduction of monoclonal antibodies (McAb). Thus in 1975 Kohler and Milstein first reported their epic research, which has led to the production of an immense range of monoclonal products.

Unlike their polyclonal counterparts, McAb are derived from a single clone of B lymphocytes. All molecules of a given McAb bind to a single epitope with the same affinity. Most are the product of hybridomas comprising a mouse myeloma cell fused to a lymphocyte from a mouse previously immunized with the antigen. Hybridomas can be stored indefinitely at low temperature

---

1. Also termed antigenic determinants, which are that part of the antigen to which binding occurs.
2. The term used to denote the strength of binding between an epitope and the binding site of an antibody.

and can provide large amounts of product. Murine McAb are ideal for the development of two-site immunoassays using labelled antibodies. They also offer great potential for in vivo imaging procedures. Given their undoubted diagnostic success, it is not surprising that the academic and pharmaceutical communities have examined the use of McAb for therapy. Some murine monoclonal products, such as OKT3, have proved of value in this respect, although, as would be expected, their systemic administration usually induces a human anti-mouse antibody (HAMA) response. This problem has been partly overcome by the production of chimeric antibodies in which all but the variable regions of the murine heavy and light chains (or even all but the complementarity determining regions) are replaced by human domains. Another important development, described in Chapter 4, has been the production of PcAb and, especially, McAb with catalytic activity. The availability of antibodies capable of, for example, cleaving cocaine has immense therapeutic potential, although it may be several years before such products reach clinical trial.

Given recent advances in McAb production, it is legitimate to question the need for a book that includes the therapeutic applications of PcAb and their fragments. Several reasons can be advanced for returning to this seemingly old-fashioned topic. First, in recent years numerous books, monographs and symposia have been devoted to McAb but none to their polyclonal equivalents. Second, the relative complexity of monoclonal and, especially, chimeric antibody production has limited these techniques to a small number of centres. It has also limited study of the value of combinations of antibodies directed, for example, against the initiators, mediators and effectors of septic shock. A third and increasingly important consideration is cost. The expense of producing McAb limits the amounts that can be given; usually prevents detailed dose–response studies; threatens to impose an unacceptable burden on healthcare costs in the developed world; and places their use beyond the reach of developing countries. Finally, and most important, McAb are often disappointing in terms of efficacy, for example in septic shock (Chapters 9 and 10). In contrast, it is relatively simple to raise and purify PcAb and their fragments and thereby study combination antibody therapy; PcAb production costs are a fraction of those for monoclonal antibodies; and, for reasons discussed later, they are more likely to be effective in many situations.

Types and Sources of Antibodies

Antibodies are usually classified according to their class and subclass, as discussed in Chapter 2. All have the same basic structure of two light and two heavy chains held together by interchain disulphide bonds and non-covalent forces. Interestingly, the interchain bridges are not essential to normal function and it is the intrachain disulphide links between opposing beta sheets within each domain that are important. Thus ". . . the repetitive intradomain [disulphide bridges] are so highly conserved that their presence is required for a protein to be considered a member of the immunoglobulin superfamily." (Steiner 1985). Human antibodies belong to one of five classes

(IgA, IgD, IgE, IgG and IgM). All are bifunctional in that their variable regions are responsible for binding to a specific epitope, for example on the surface of a microbe, while the Fc component has an effector role, being able to bind phagocytes and complement and activate the latter. Such bifunctionality is ideally suited to bringing innate protective mechanisms into juxtaposition with invading microorganisms.

Antibody preparations can be discussed according to their source and whether they are monoclonal or polyclonal (Table 1.1). In general, antibodies of the IgG class are preferred for diagnostic use because of their high circulating levels, excellent affinity and stability. Because only minute amounts are required, PcAb for this purpose can be raised in guinea-pigs or rabbits. During recent years, increasing use has been made of murine McAb for diagnostic application. Their high cost poses no problem because only small quantities are needed and there is no advantage in moving to chimeric antibodies other than for in vivo imaging. Antibodies used for therapeutic purposes are also usually of the IgG class, although several McAb directed against lipopolysaccharides are IgM. The main attributes of IgM as compared with IgG (to agglutinate microorganisms, enhance their phagocytosis and activate complement) are probably irrelevant in this context.

As discussed in Chapter 8, human immunoglobulins are often used to treat infectious diseases, especially in immunocompromised patients. Unrefined plasma, collected by venepuncture or plasmapheresis, can be infused with little risk of inducing a humoral immune response. However, supplies of

Table 1.1. A classification of the sources and types of antibodies for therapeutic use

Polyclonal antibodies	
Intact:	
Human IgG	Given as plasma or an immunoglobulin concentrate: the latter may be enriched with IgM
Animal IgG	Usually an equine immunoglobulin concentrate
IgA	Given orally and usually from bovine milk
Avian IgY	Given orally as whole egg, egg yolk or purified IgY
Fragments:	
$F(ab')_2$	Usually equine
Fab	Usually ovine
Fv	
Monoclonal antibodies[a]	
Normal or activated human B lymphocytes	
Activated primate B lymphocytes	
Human myeloma cells	
Hybridomas	Homogeneous, usually murine:murine
	Heterogeneous, usually human:murine
Quadromas	
Transfectomas	
Transgenic animals	

[a] May be chimeric (i.e. murine Fab or Fv with the remainder of the molecule being human), composite (i.e. the molecule is human except for murine complementarity determinant regions), or bifunctional (with binding sites directed against different epitopes).

human plasma are limited; it is unethical to immunize subjects with infectious agents, tumour products or drugs; the affinities and titres of specific antibodies in human plasma tend to be low; and there is a risk of transferring infections such as hepatitis. These problems are all overcome by the use of other mammalian immunoglobulins, but are then replaced by the more serious risk of an allergic response. Therapy usually demands large amounts of antibody. Polyclonal immunoglobulins for this purpose are therefore normally produced in sheep or horses and administered in the form of purified concentrates. Avian antibodies, derived from hens' eggs, may well prove to be ideal for oral use, but the risk of causing severe allergic reactions will prohibit their systemic administration.

Polyclonal Antibody Fragments

In 1939 Pope used the proteolytic enzyme pepsin to cleave immunoglobulins into $F(ab')_2$ and Fc. The incidence and severity of allergic side-effects were considerably reduced by the use of equine $F(ab')_2$ in preference to intact equine immunoglobulins. The reasons for this will be discussed later, as will the virtual freedom from allergic side-effects associated with the intravenous infusion of therapeutic products based on ovine Fab.

Frequent mention is made in this book of the therapeutic use of ovine Fab and it is relevant, therefore, to consider its structure in more detail. Each Fab has a molecular weight of about 50 000 Da and comprises four separate domains, which are globular in structure and consist of 110–120 amino acids. The two N-terminal domains include the variable parts of the light (V_L) and heavy (V_H) chains and contain a single binding site. The other two comprise the constant domain of the light chain (C_L) and the first constant domain of the heavy chain (C_H1), which is normally attached to the other constant domains of this chain by the hinge region. Each domain has one three-stranded and one four-stranded beta sheet joined by a single disulphide bond, while an interchain disulphide bond covalently couples C_H1 to C_L. Padlan et al. (1986) studied the association of C_H1 and C_L. Irrespective of the class or subclass of immunoglobulin or of their species of origin, the same arrangement is apparent. Thus the four-stranded part of each of the two domains is in apposition over an area of 50–60 nm^2. Several highly conserved hydrophobic amino acids within this area, together with a variable number of interacting residues at its periphery, ensure that the two remain firmly joined by means of non-covalent forces.

The close juxtaposition of C_H1 and C_L facilitates the association of V_H and V_L, upon which antibody binding depends. The V_H and V_L each have three complementarity-determining regions (CDRs) flanked by four relatively conserved framework regions (FRs), which form the bulk of the beta sheets. The carbon atoms of the three CDRs are clustered at the tip of V_H and V_L, where they provide a cleft in which the antigen is bound, while the FRs act as a simple scaffold on which new binding sites (i.e. CDRs) can be built. C_H1 and C_L are not essential for antibody binding. Thus, in 1973 Hochman et al. purified a mouse myeloma immunoglobulin of the IgA class that bound 2, 4-dinitrophenol (DNP). They cleaved this with pepsin to obtain a product of molecular weight 25 000 Da, which they termed Fv, because it comprises only the variable parts of the H and L chains. Its affinity for DNP was similar to that of the original IgA. Furthermore, after dissociating the two components of Fv they could reassociate spontaneously to give a product that retained more than 85% of the affinity for DNP of the original Fv and IgA. There are no intrachain disulphide bridges between V_L and V_H and this reassociation demonstrates the great importance of non-covalent forces in ensuring realignment of the CDRs within the two domains.

Fv should offer similar advantages to Fab for therapeutic use. However, there has been no comparison of the clinical efficacy and safety of the two. Furthermore, it may be difficult to obtain Fv in high yield at minimal expense from a polyclonal source.

Monoclonal Antibodies

"At present there are dozens of monoclonal antibody products being tested clinically for a variety of indications . . ." (DiPiro et al. 1992). The majority are the products of mouse lymphocytes fused to mouse myeloma cells. Immunization, fusion, assessment and cloning techniques have now been developed to the stage at which murine McAb can be produced that are specific for virtually any analyte or surface epitope. Many hundreds of laboratories have established the necessary expertise and, using hollow-fibre and similar automated systems, can provide gram amounts of highly purified product. However, such techniques are complex and time consuming; in vitro culture is expensive; the affinity and stability of such antibodies tend to be lower than that of their polyclonal counterparts; and, when given systemically to patients, they may induce a humoral immune response which curtails their biological half-life. In order to avoid the latter, considerable effort has been expended on attempts to produce human McAb. However, none of the McAb synthesized by human myeloma cell lines has proved of clinical value, while attempts to immortalize human B lymphocytes, for example with Epstein-Barr virus, have met with limited success. It is difficult to select cells that are secreting antibodies of the desired affinity and specificity, and yields tend to be small. Efforts to produce human hybridomas have also been unavailing because of the lack of suitable human myeloma cell partners. Some success has been achieved with heterohybridomas comprising human B lymphocytes and mouse myeloma cells, but the amounts of antibody produced are small and the hybridomas unstable.

Various groups, notably Winter and his colleagues in Cambridge, have adopted an alternative approach based on molecular engineering. Murine V_L and V_H genes can be linked to the genes responsible for human constant domains of any class required. This process is termed "interspecies isotype switching". The new genetic material can then be inserted into yeast cells, *Escherichia coli* or mouse myeloma cells for expression of chimeric McAb. Such "transfectomas" are relatively stable and produce large amounts of antibodies which are less immunogenic in patients than murine McAb. In a further extension of this approach only the three CDRs from the V_H of a mouse antibody were substituted for the corresponding CDRs of V_H in a human myeloma protein. Indeed, "Such 'CDR replacement' may offer a means of constructing human monoclonal antibodies from the corresponding mouse monoclonal antibodies." (Jones et al. 1986). A final possibility is the use of transgenic sheep or cows to provide large amounts of a human McAb, especially if this is released into their milk.

However, a word of caution is necessary. These are immensely difficult, expensive and time-consuming techniques. Furthermore, as discussed later, there may be situations in which McAb, irrespective of their source, are likely to be ineffective.

Diagnostic Applications

A brief consideration of the diagnostic merits of PcAb and McAb, while not strictly relevant to this book, helps in arriving at an understanding of their relative therapeutic roles.

Immunoassays

All immunoassays depend on the reversible, non-covalent binding of the analyte (the antigen) by the binding sites of specific antibodies in a reaction that obeys the Law of Mass Action. They can be categorized into those requiring no labelled reactant, those using labelled antigen and those based on the use of labelled specific antibodies.

Non-labelled Immunoassays

Many immunoassays are based on the detection of large antigen–antibody complexes, either as a precipitation line in a gel or by turbidometric or nephelometric means. Such assays lack sensitivity and are applicable only to molecules with multiple epitopes. They use relatively large amounts of PcAb and are totally unsuited to the use of McAb. Thus the latter are directed against a single epitope and are unable to form large antigen–antibody complexes unless several different McAb are mixed together.

Immunoassays Using Labelled Antibodies

The development of immunometric assays by Miles and Hales in 1968 ranks in importance with the introduction of radioimmunoassay, over which they offer considerable advantages. Such assays, especially of the two-site type, seem certain to prevail for macromolecules with more than one epitope when sensitivity, specificity, precision and speed are requisites. Immunometric assays employ a reagent excess and the affinity of the antibodies seldom poses a problem.

The specificity of McAb makes them ideal for this purpose, as illustrated in Fig. 1.1. The analyte is represented as a globular macromolecule with six distinct epitopes. The link antibody, which is coupled to a solid phase support,

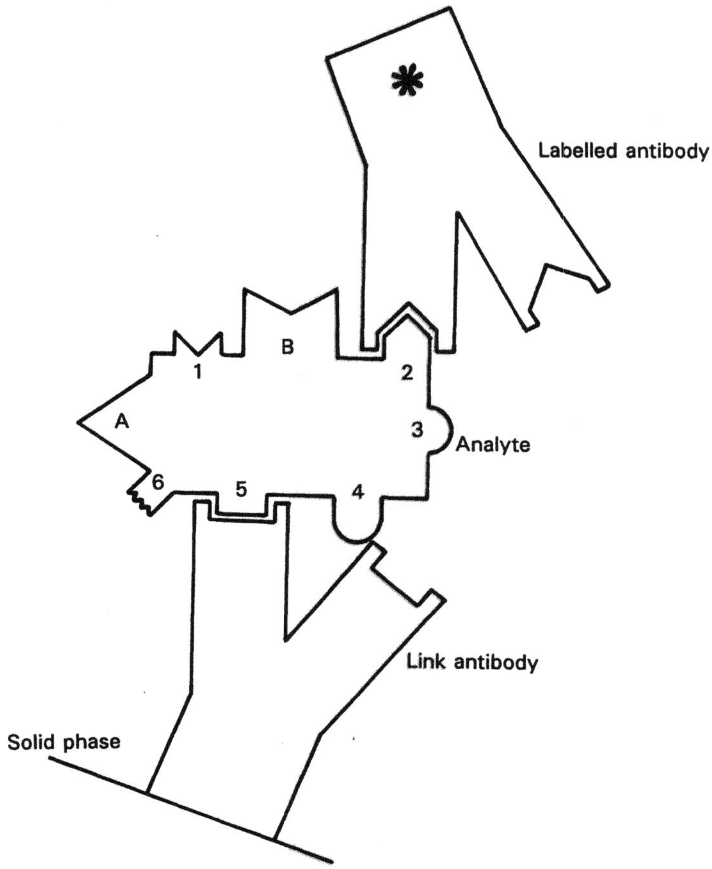

Fig. 1.1. The two-site immunometric assay.

binds to epitope 5 and clearly it would sterically prevent another antibody from binding to epitope 4. This could cause problems if PcAb were used, but in this instance a second labelled McAb has been chosen that binds to epitope 2 so that steric hindrance is avoided. Assay kits using matched pairs of McAb or (because of patent protection) a monoclonal and a polyclonal antibody now dominate the market. This may explain why most groups have concentrated their efforts on the production of McAb for therapy. The analyte in Fig. 1.1 is depicted as having two active sites (A and B), each of which exerts its biological effects by binding to a specific cell receptor. We will return to this example later to explain why a McAb that is well suited to a diagnostic role may be ineffective therapeutically.

Immunoassays Using Labelled Antigens

This type of immunoassay, introduced by Yalow and Berson in 1960, differs in a number of respects from immunometric assays. Thus they are of the limited reagent type, in which labelled and unlabelled analyte compete for a fixed number of binding sites. They are applicable to haptens as well as macromolecules and their ultimate sensitivity depends on the affinity of the antibodies used.

McAb do not offer the advantages to this type of assay that they do to immunoassays using labelled antibodies. For example, they may be too specific and measure only a drug and not its active metabolite. More important, they have a lower affinity than their polyclonal counterparts. Thus we expect routinely to raise antibodies in sheep with an affinity in excess of 1×10^{10} l/mol for haptens, such as the tricyclic antidepressants, and in excess of 1×10^{11} l/mol for macromolecules. It is difficult to obtain McAb with affinities in excess of 1×10^{9} and 1×10^{10} l/mol for haptens and macromolecules respectively.

Immunohistochemistry and Immunocytochemistry

The determination of serum levels of alphafetoprotein (AFP), human chorionic gonadotrophin (hCG), carcinoembryonic antigen (CEA) and other tumour-associated antigens may help to diagnose the presence of some neoplasms and enable an assessment of likely tumour load. Both McAb and PcAb are suitable for such purposes. However, the exquisite specificity of a McAb comes into its own when antibodies are used in immunohistochemistry and immunocytochemistry to detect cell surface antigens. Thus, for example, they can facilitate the detection of tumour cells that have metastasized to lymph nodes and help to identify their likely primary source. They have also been used to quantify oestrogen and progesterone receptors in reproductive tissue cancers and thereby predict prognosis and likely response to hormonal manipulation (Greene 1988). In addition, panels of McAb have been used to differentiate between the various kinds of lymphoma and other haematological neoplasms.

Certain generalizations can be made with regard to the diagnostic applications of McAb in oncology. There is probably no such thing as a "tumour-specific" antibody defined as an antibody to a product or epitope unique to cancer cells. Thus ". . . it may be futile to search for truly tumour-specific Mabs." (Hellström and Hellström 1990). The term tumour-associated antigen (TAA) is better than tumour-specific antigen and, when applied to cell surface antigens, reflects quantitative rather than qualitative differences. For example, there is a protein associated with human melanomas (p97). Each melanoma cell has on its surface 50 000 to 500 000 molecules of p97, whereas hepatic cells have about 8000 and most other cells only a few hundred. TAAs include proteins such as p97, AFP and homologues of receptors for various growth factors; mucins such as the one defined by McAb OC125 on ovarian neoplasms; and glycolipids, such as some blood group antigens, which may be expressed at high levels by cancer cells (Hellström and Hellström 1990). Cancer cells are very heterogeneous with regard to expressing a particular TAA. Thus while most cells may express a surface antigen, some cells or even clumps of cells may not and others may have internalized the TAA. This does not matter in terms of diagnosis, provided sufficient numbers of the cancer cells express the TAA. However, it may be important in terms of therapy.

McAb have also proved of considerable diagnostic value in areas other than oncology. For example, panels of McAb are used for tissue typing, blood grouping and the differentiation of T helper cells (with CD4) from T cytotoxic and suppressor cells (with CD8). Their great specificity also enables them to detect subtle antigenic differences between strains of microorganisms and has, for example, facilitated studies of antigenic drift in influenza viruses. There is no doubt that the use of panels of McAb, together with DNA fingerprinting, will provide the basis for future classifications of microorganisms.

In Vivo Imaging

Radioimmunoscintigraphy (RIS), using a radionuclide coupled to an antibody, is of considerable value in some clinical situations. The need is to generate a large signal over a relatively short period: technetium-99m (^{99m}Tc), with a half-life of about 6 h, is an ideal radiolabel. Only about 500 μg of specific antibody is required, which minimizes both cost and the risk of inducing a humoral immune response in the recipient. Applications include the use of ^{99m}Tc-labelled antibodies directed against myosin to diagnose and assess the extent of a myocardial infarction; labelled McAb directed against fibrin to locate the site of a thrombosis; and labelled human PcAb from normal donors to diffuse into, and thereby demonstrate, areas of inflammation.

Labelled McAb are used increasingly in RIS to detect colorectal, ovarian and other cancers. They are of particular value in detecting plaques of neoplastic tissue that are not visualized by computed tomography (CT) and in differentiating between a pelvic mass due to fibrosis and one due to neoplastic tissue. For example in a recent study by Granowska et al. (1993), a ^{99m}Tc-labelled McAb directed against an epithelial mucin glycoprotein core antigen had an overall accuracy of 93% in the detection of ovarian cancers; this was superior to that achieved by CT scanning. RIS can also be used to detect bone and hepatic metastases and new McAb may identify squamous cell carcinomas of the head and neck.

Therapeutic Applications

There is virtually no limit to the potential of antibody-based products for therapeutic purposes provided that they are safe (*primum non nocere*). Clinical applications are listed in Table 1.2 and many are discussed in detail in later chapters of this book. At the present time McAb have not enjoyed the same success when used therapeutically that they have for diagnosis. Many believe that such lack of success is only temporary and will be corrected by the replacement of murine McAb by their humanized or human equivalents. Others, including the authors, are less certain and consider that the choice between a McAb and a PcAb for a particular

Table 1.2. Some therapeutic applications of exogenous antibodies

For extracorporeal use	
With blood (to remove apo B, etc.)	
With bone marrow (to remove T lymphocytes or neoplastic cells)	
For oral use	
To prevent and/or treat gastrointestinal infections	
To prevent absorption of drugs and other potentially toxic compounds	
For systemic use as therapy	
For replacement in immunodeficiency states	
To bind to and thereby neutralize the biological effects of:	
haptens	cardiac glycosides, steroid hormones, etc.
macromolecules	toxic constituents of snake, scorpion and spider venoms
	microbial endotoxins and exotoxins
	mediators of septic shock
	platelet-derived and other growth factors
	human chorionic gonadotrophin for fertility control
	autoantibodies in idiopathic thrombocytopenic purpura, etc.
To bind and thereby block cell surface epitopes:	
receptors	such as that for IL-1 or the Fc part of immunoglobulins
adhesin molecules	
glycoproteins	such as those necessary for platelet aggregation
To bind to cell surface epitopes and thereby help to destroy the cell:	
examples include	CD3 on T lymphocytes
	Rh(D) on neonatal red cells
	tumour-associated antigens on haematologically derived and solid tumours
	IgE-bearing cells
	microorganisms including parasites, bacteria and viruses
Catalytic antibodies	
For systemic use to deliver therapy	
Antibodies attached covalently or non-covalently to:	
radionuclides (yttrium-90, etc.)	
foreign toxins (ricin A chain, diphtheria toxin, etc.)	
enzymes (to convert prodrugs to drugs or bring tPA or urokinase to the site of thrombus)	
drugs (adriamycin, etc.)	
natural protective molecules (TNF, IL-2, etc.)	
cytotoxic cells, using bifunctional antibodies	
For use as vaccines	

clinical situation will depend in large part on the mechanisms involved. This section will confine itself largely to applications not considered later and to a consideration of the relative merits of McAb and PcAb in various situations.

Extracorporeal Use

It is not always necessary to administer exogenous antibodies systemically for them to exert their effects. For example, blood can be circulated through an affinity column comprising antibodies directed against apolipoprotein B covalently coupled to insoluble and inert beads. These columns are used to remove low-density lipoproteins from the blood of patients with severe forms of familial hypercholesterolaemia, which, if not treated, may result in death due to cardiovascular disease before the age of 20 years. Considerable success has been achieved, with the disappearance of cholesterol deposits in the skin and elsewhere and improved life expectancy. In another example, antibodies directed against human IgG are used to cause transient hypogammaglobulinaemia prior to transplantation. Clearly, PcAb will be preferred to remove specific proteins from blood because of their higher affinity, more general specificity and lower cost.

Antibodies coupled to an insoluble matrix are also used to "cleanse" bone marrow prior to its transplantation. Such antibodies may remove T lymphocytes from the marrow and thereby minimize the risk of graft-versus-host reactions. Antibodies have also been used to remove neoplastic cells. This is seldom successful because there are few, if any, totally specific antigens on the surface of such cells. Furthermore, because of their heterogeneity, there are few occasions on which every neoplastic cell will display such an antigen.

Oral Use

As discussed in Chapter 3, antibodies taken by mouth can help in the prevention and/or treatment of gastrointestinal infections caused by viruses or bacteria. They have also been used to prevent dental plaque and caries and could be employed to bind toxic chemicals or drugs within the gastrointestinal tract and thereby minimize absorption. However, antibody binding is prevented by the extremes of pH in the stomach. Thus it would be necessary to block hydrogen ion secretion (or neutralize it with bicarbonate) if antibodies were to be used in the treatment of peptic ulceration by preventing *Helicobacter pylori* from colonizing the gastric antrum. It is also necessary to prevent enzymatic degradation of antibodies in the stomach if they are to be active in the small intestine, which is the main site of gastroenteritis. This can be achieved by increasing the gastric pH to values above that at which pepsin acts. Avian IgY and especially immunoglobulins of the IgA class are more resistant than IgG or IgM to proteolytic cleavage.

For Systemic Use as Therapy

For Replacement in Immunodeficiency States

Patients with primary immunodeficiency syndromes, such as congenital agammaglobulinaemia, require repeated infusions of human immunoglobulins and especially IgG. These are prepared from pools of plasma collected from several thousand donors and therefore contain a range of relevant antibodies. Amounts from 200 to 400 mg of IgG per kilogram body weight need to be infused intravenously at monthly intervals to ensure the minimum serum IgG levels required to prevent infection.

To Bind to and Thereby Neutralize the Biological Effects of Haptens

As discussed in Chapter 5, foreign antibodies are used to treat drug overdose. Antibodies have been raised against many toxic haptens, such as the herbicides paraquat and diquat, the carcinogenic polycyclic aromatic hydrocarbons and various environmental pollutants, including the chlorinated biphenyls. Will exogenous antibodies be effective in the treatment of poisoning by all these molecules? Such therapy is likely to be of value when the toxic hapten is present in relatively small amounts and initiates its deleterious effects by binding to cell surface receptors. Antibody-based products are not effective if the product has been internalized prior to treatment. For example, we have found that high-affinity antibodies protected mice against a lethal dose of paraquat only if given before, or simultaneously with, this herbicide. Delaying administration for 60 min (the usual clinical situation) yielded no benefit because the drug had already been taken up into alveolar

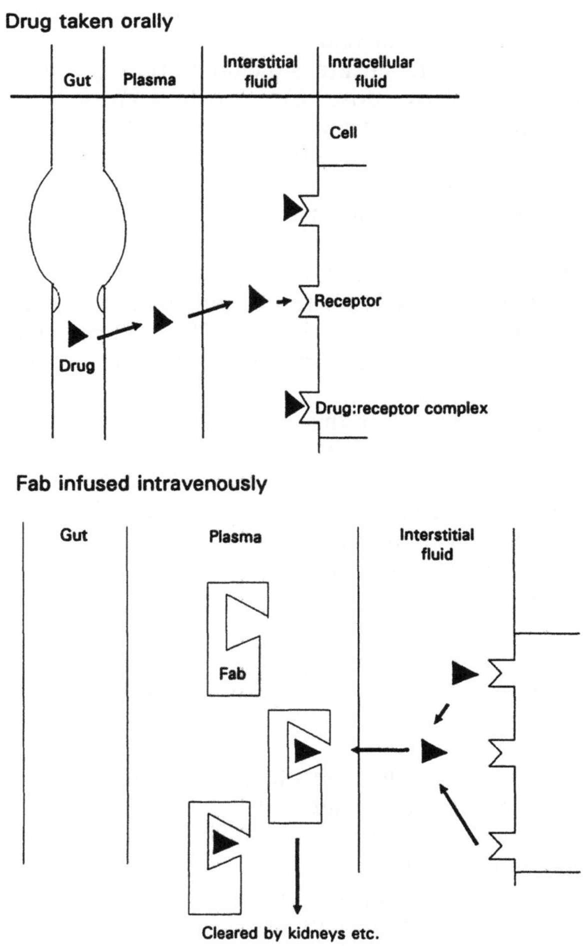

Fig. 1.2. Reversal of drug toxicity by specific Fab fragments.

and other cells. It is also possible for antibodies to enhance the toxicity of some poisons, such as the amatoxins, by delaying their clearance (Piqueras 1989).

The mechanism whereby antibodies reverse drug toxicity is illustrated in Fig. 1.2. Following ingestion, the drug is absorbed via the small intestine into the circulation, where some is bound loosely by a plasma-binding protein (such as albumin) while the rest remains free. Free drug diffuses into the interstitial fluid and is bound by specific receptors on the cells and tissues. This results, in the case of digoxin, in myocardial levels some 50- to 200-fold those in blood. Following an intravenous infusion of specific ovine anti-digoxin Fab, virtually all the circulating digoxin becomes antibody bound and the concentration gradient is reversed. The drug dissociates from its receptors and diffuses into the extracellular fluid compartment for as long as free antibody binding sites remain. Clearly, the success of such therapy depends on sufficient antibodies being available, with an affinity higher than that of the drug receptor(s). The latter is not a problem because typical antibody affinities range from 10^9 to 10^{11} l/mol, while those for cell receptors seldom exceed a value of 1×10^6 l/mol.

Digoxin is ideal in this context. The small toxic dose and relatively large molecular weight mean that only small amounts of ovine Fab (200–1000 mg) are adequate to ensure stoichiometric equivalence and reversal of all manifestations of overdose. Coupled to a carrier protein, digoxin is an excellent immunogen that yields high concentrations (greater than 6 g/l) of specific high-affinity antibodies in the serum of most immunized sheep. A few other drugs, such as colchicine, are equally appropriate. However, most drugs that commonly cause toxicity pose considerable problems and, in particular, require large amounts of antibody. For example, the low molecular weight of the tricyclic antidepressants combined with the large number of tablets intentionally taken by many patients prohibits the use of a stoichiometric amount of antibody, because 200 g or more might be required. Fortunately, it is unnecessary to bind all the drug and only 10–20 g may be needed.

All of the clinical successes in this area have been achieved using ovine Fab despite the fact that murine McAb to digoxin with affinities of 10^9 l/mol or more have been available for several years (Mudgett-Hunter et al. 1985). Why have the PcAb fragments not been replaced by their monoclonal counterparts? One possibility is that the regulatory requirements involved in such a change are too onerous, but the most likely explanation is that the cost differential is too high.

To Bind to and Thereby Neutralize the Biological Effects of Macromolecules

The dimensions of a digoxin molecule approximate to those of the cleft in an antibody combining site, while most haptens will occupy only part of such a site. It should also be noted that the dissociation rate constant for an antibody:hapten complex is relatively rapid with a half-life ranging from about 1 to 30 min, depending on the size of the hapten. In contrast, the proteins and other macromolecules listed in Table 1.2 are many times the size of the binding site and the dissociation rate constant is measured in days, weeks or even months.

Most macromolecules exert their biological effects by means of an active site that binds to a specific receptor on the surface of cells. For example, some of the most toxic components in snake venoms act by binding to pre- or post-synaptic receptors and thereby inhibit neuronal conduction and/or neuromuscular transmission, with resultant paralysis. It is likely that some of the antibody populations in an effective antivenom provide protection by binding to the toxic component, thereby preventing the active site from contact with its receptor. Herein lies the potential fallacy of using a single population of McAb to neutralize the biological actions of a macromolecule.

At this stage it is appropriate to return to Fig. 1.1, which illustrated the benefits of using a pair of matched McAb for a two-site immunometric assay. From a therapeutic standpoint, the McAb shown binding to epitope 5 (and McAb directed against epitopes 3 and 4) will bind to the macromolecule, but is unlikely to hinder either of the two active sites (A and B). The antibody shown binding to epitope 2 might block the biological effects initiated by the B but not the A active site, while a McAb directed against epitope 6 should have the reverse effect. Finally, it is possible that a McAb that binds to epitope 1 may block the biological effects of both active sites. Based on this very simple picture (which does not, for example, take note of the fact that antibody binding may influence the tertiary structure of the entire analyte), the binding of a macromolecule by a single McAb may:

1. Not neutralize any of the biological effects of the analyte; or
2. Neutralize only some of its biological effects; or
3. Neutralize all its biological actions.

Failure of a McAb to neutralize the effects of a macromolecule is more likely the larger the analyte and the greater the number and diversity of its epitopes. The risk of such failure is enhanced if the analyte has more than one active site, if not enough of the McAb is infused or if the McAb has a low affinity. Lipopolysaccharides are large macromolecules with molecular weights ranging from 400 to 4000 kDa (Brock-Utne and Gaffin 1989).

By contrast, immunization of animals with the macromolecule shown in Fig. 1.1 will yield populations of antibodies directed against each of the six epitopes. Thus, both active sites can be blocked. Clearly, use of a carefully selected cocktail of McAb will have the same effect and provide a product as effective as its polyclonal equivalent, albeit at considerable cost. Alternatively, it might be possible to select a McAb directed against epitope 1; clone selection should always be based on the role for which the McAb is intended (Campbell 1985). Unfortunately, assessment of clones that secrete antibodies is already one of the most time-consuming factors in producing a McAb and the need to include several bioassays to demonstrate neutralization may impose an impossible load.

Most of the examples cited in Table 1.2 are considered in detail later in the book. These include the use of antivenoms for the treatment of snake, spider and scorpion envenomation (Chapter 6) and of antibodies to improve the prognosis in septic shock (Chapters 9 and 10). Amongst other applications are the infusion of human immunoglobulins (400 mg/kg/day for 5 days followed by further less frequent infusions) to raise and then maintain the platelet count in children and adults with acute or chronic idiopathic thrombocytopenic purpura. This autoimmune disease reflects accelerated platelet destruction mediated by endogenous antibodies. Foreign antibodies and antibody-derived products can prevent excessive bleeding, delay the need for splenectomy and prepare the patient for surgery. Antibodies directed against hCG may be of value in fertility control, while the use of antibodies to platelet-derived and other growth factors may prevent accelerated atherosclerosis following coronary angioplasty or bypass surgery.

To Bind to and Thereby Block Cell Surface Epitopes

There are two mechanisms by which a foreign antibody, $F(ab')_2$ or Fab can prevent a soluble antigen, such as tumour necrosis factor, exerting its biological effect on a cell. One is to bind to an epitope on the macromolecule that is close to its active site. The second is to bind to the surface receptor on the cell. Both operate by steric hindrance. Blocking of the interleukin-1 receptor has been used in an attempt to ameliorate septic shock (Chapter 10) and a McAb directed against the receptor might have a similar effect. Clearly, the Fc part of an immunoglobulin is not relevant and two Fab fragments should be more effective than a single IgG. However, there is evidence that the large numbers of receptors found on some cells and the many different types of cell bearing such receptors may limit this approach.

There is need for an innovative approach to the treatment of systemic viral infections because of the lack of suitable drugs. When considering the use of exogenous antibodies for this purpose, it is important to understand the various mechanisms whereby they act. For example, if it is to enhance complement-mediated and antibody-mediated cell cytotoxicity then intact antibodies would be required. However, if they depend on steric hindrance for their effect then Fab (including ovine Fab) may be appropriate.

Wunner et al. (1988) found that McAb directed against nucleocapsid proteins were ineffective in neutralizing rabies virus. However, McAb directed against one of the surface glycoproteins (glycoprotein G) were effective. They speculated that antibodies might inhibit viral attachment to the cell surface or cause release once attached; might prevent fusion between the virus and cell surface or internalization of the virus; or, once internalized, might inhibit the pH-dependent fusion of the viral membrane with those intracellular components that remove the viral coat and nucleocapsids to initiate replication. They concluded that ". . . the antibody-mediated neutralization of rabies virus is most likely the result of several different mechanisms, including inhibition of virus attachment, release of cell-bound virus, and inhibition of intraendosomal fusion." Antibodies have been raised to cytomegalovirus, influenza virus and many others, but it remains to be determined if antibody fragments are as effective as intact PcAb and McAb. In our experience, ovine Fab can prevent rotavirus infections in piglets, possibly by inhibiting penetration of the epithelial cells of the small intestine.

To Bind to Cell Surface Epitopes and Facilitate Cell Destruction

There are several mechanisms whereby the binding of a McAb or a PcAb to a normal or cancer cell or a microorganism can lead to its destruction. It can be directly cytotoxic; bind to surface receptors and thereby interfere with cellular metabolism; or prevent interaction of the cell with essential growth factors, such as epidermal growth factor and interleukin-2. Alternatively it can act indirectly to cause complement-mediated cytotoxicity or antibody-dependent cell-mediated cytotoxicity involving T lymphocytes or macrophages (Dillman 1989).

Antibodies to CD3

All mature T lymphocytes have a surface CD3 complex. Initially, antithymocyte (antilymphocyte) globulins were produced by immunizing rabbits and horses with intact lymphocytes; more recently a murine McAb against CD3 has been commercially available. At an intravenous dose of 5 mg daily for 10–14 days, this antibody, called OKT3, is highly effective in preventing acute rejection following renal, hepatic and cardiac transplantation. At circulating levels of about 1000 μg/l, OKT3 results in the rapid disappearance of nearly all mature T lymphocytes (Hooks et al. 1991). Despite a high incidence of side-effects on first administration, this McAb has an established position in the prevention of allograft rejection.

Antibodies to Human Rh(D)

A woman lacking Rh(D) red cell antigen who has a Rhesus-positive child may be immunized at birth when small numbers of the child's red cells enter her circulation. The resultant anti-Rh(D) immunoglobulins of the IgG class cause no problems until she has a further pregnancy involving a Rhesus-positive fetus. The specific IgG can then cross the placenta and bind to and destroy fetal red cells, leading to haemolytic disease of the newborn. This risk can be prevented by administration of exogenous anti-Rh(D), which destroys fetal red cells before they can induce an immune response. PcAb obtained from human volunteers are extremely effective and relatively inexpensive. Alternatively, human McAb have been introduced. They are synthesized by B lymphocytes immortalized with Epstein-Barr virus; only 100–300 μg is required. It will be interesting to see if they replace their less expensive PcAb equivalents.

Antibodies to Human Tumour-Associated Antigens

In general, PcAb lack the required specificity and contain populations of antibodies directed against normal cell surface antigens as well as populations specific to tumour-associated antigens. Conversely, many hundreds of McAb have been produced that are directed solely against TAA. The amounts of such antibodies recommended for therapy are large (about 400 mg/m^2) and the cost is high. Some success has been achieved in the treatment of haematologically derived cancers, such as the lymphomas. This reflects the ready accessibility of the cancer cells, the presence of recognized cell

Table 1.3. Difficulties encountered in the treatment of cancer with foreign antibodies

- No truly tumour-specific antigen
- Tumour-associated antigens are usually present on some normal cells so that the relevant foreign antibodies may bind in part to normal tissues
- Tumour-associated antigens are often released into the circulation where they bind to some foreign antibodies before they come into contact with tumour cells
- Characteristically, tumour cells are heterogeneous and therefore individual cells or even clumps of cells may not express the relevant tumour-associated antigen. In other instances the antigen may be internalized or capped
- Characteristically, solid tumours are poorly vascularized. Their blood supply passes from the periphery inwards and the centres of large tumours tend to receive little blood and therefore may not be in contact with foreign antibodies
- Tumour cells may be present in "sanctuary sites" where they are not accessible to foreign antibodies
- In time, the humoral immune response elicited by the foreign antibodies in the recipient may block the biological effects of the exogenous antibodies, potentiate their clearance and/or prevent them from binding to tumour cells
- Treatment with foreign antibodies and immunoconjugates is usually a last resort when the tumours are large and have metastasized widely.

surface determinants and a relative degree of homogeneity, which ensures that virtually all cells express the chosen antigen.

The use of McAb for the treatment of solid tumours has been disappointing. Some of the reasons for this are listed in Table 1.3, but the authors agree with the statement by Dillman (1989) that "Those who feel that the efforts of the past ten years indicate that this approach is a failure are overlooking the complexities of the challenge and the progress which has been made." The heterogeneity of tumour cells and the fact that not all express a given TAA is a major problem, which might be overcome by the use of a mixture of McAb to different surface antigens. Nonetheless, it is difficult to envisage a major success as long as treatment with foreign antibodies is regarded as a terminal measure used only when the tumour is large and has metastasized.

Antibodies to Microorganisms

Some features of the use of antibodies for treating cancer are relevant to their use in infectious diseases. In particular, a single McAb may be too specific and bind to an epitope not present on all the microbes. Even if only a few lack this determinant, their rapid replication will ensure that they quickly replace those that have been destroyed. Some microorganisms may spontaneously cease to express a particular epitope, while others may find "sanctuary sites" in which they are inaccessible to foreign proteins.

The advantage of human PcAb and humanized or human McAb is that the Fc part of the molecule can bind macrophages and activate complement. Thus complement-mediated cytotoxicity, the formation of membrane attack complexes, antibody-mediated cell cytotoxicity and phagocytosis are all enhanced. Again, cocktails of human McAb directed against different epitopes would be ideal, while ovine Fab would probably be ineffective in the destruction of parasites, bacteria or viruses.

For Systemic Use to Deliver Therapy

Immunoconjugates have received considerable attention as "magic bullets", designed to target therapy to a specific site. Alas, "Bullets there are a plenty, but magic there is not." (Britton et al. 1991). Some examples of different types of immunoconjugates are listed in Table 1.2, and the number of choices reflects their great promise but singular lack of success.

Radioimmunoconjugates

As a generalization, radioimmunoscintigraphy (RIS) for diagnostic purposes has proved to be reasonably successful, whereas radioimmunotherapy (RIT) has not. The two are often combined, with RIS (using a short-lived radionuclide) being used to locate the tumour followed by RIT. The larger the amount of McAb injected, the more will reach the deepest parts of a solid tumour, so that it is usual to give about 40 mg in RIT as compared with 0.2–2 mg in RIS. The degree of irradiation experienced by the tumour cells will relate to the amount of radioimmunoconjugate taken up, the residence time and the half-life of the radionuclide. The residence time is prolonged by the slow dissociation rate of an antibody:protein complex and a McAb may remain bound to its tumour-associated antigen for many weeks. Isotopes such as yttrium-90 or phosphorus-32 are used because of their long half-life and their penetrating, high-energy beta particles. Phosphorus-32 offers the potential advantage that it may be internalized, incorporated into DNA and thereby directly irradiate the cell nucleus.

The main problem of RIT is to ensure maximum irradiation of tumour cells while minimizing the irradiation of normal tissues and especially the bone marrow. It is probably impossible to achieve an adequate tumour to normal tissue ratio by infusing radionuclide coupled directly to McAb and various alternative strategies are being studied (Britton et al. 1991). Regional administration into the peritoneal or pleural cavity has proved disappointing, although some success has followed intrathecal injections. Two- and three-step approaches seem a logical development. For example, a bifunctional McAb can be used with one of its binding sites directed against a TAA and the other against a ^{32}P ligand. Following infusion, a small fraction will bind to the tumour cells while the remainder will be cleared by the reticuloendothelial system. After a delay of 3 days or more the ^{32}P ligand is injected: some will bind to the McAb in the immediate vicinity of the tumour cells, while the rest will be cleared rapidly via the kidneys.

Other Immunoconjugates

Considerable ingenuity has been displayed in the design of immunoconjugates for the treatment of cancer. Immunotoxins have been used that target diphtheria toxin or the A chain of ricin to the surface of cancer cells. Once the A chain has been internalized it inhibits protein synthesis, but with a molecular weight of about 32 000 it may induce a humoral immune response in the recipient which eventually neutralizes its effectiveness. Chemoimmunoconjugates are also available in which a drug, such as adriamycin, is covalently coupled to an appropriate McAb. In theory this will ensure site-specific delivery, stabilize the drug, delay its metabolic clearance and reduce the incidence of side-effects. In practice, coupling the drug may neutralize its cytotoxic effects by inhibiting internalization. Furthermore, it is difficult to deliver sufficient drug to an adequate number of tumour cells, and the use of a single cytotoxic drug is seldom effective in oncology (Reisfeld and Schrappe 1990). An alternative is to couple an enzyme to the McAb that converts a non-toxic prodrug to a cytotoxic drug in the immediate vicinity of tumour cells.

Antibodies, and especially those of the bifunctional type, can bring other therapeutic agents into the appropriate locality. These include cytotoxic T lymphocytes and phagocytic cells as well as macromolecules such as tumour necrosis factor, gamma interferon and interleukin-2. It may eventually prove most effective to use a cocktail of McAb directed against several different TAA to implement several different therapies. However, this is easy to suggest but difficult and costly to achieve.

Immunoconjugates should not be considered solely as a means of targeting therapy to cancer cells. For example, Haber et al. (1988) have suggested a novel approach by which to retain the benefits of thrombolytic agents (such as streptokinase) following a myocardial infarction while avoiding the risk of severe bleeding or a cerebral haemorrhage. They produced McAb to epitopes exposed on molecules of fibrin but hidden in the precursor fibrinogen. These were covalently coupled to urokinase or tissue plasminogen activator (tPA) and shown to be effective both in vitro and in vivo in a rabbit model. They further suggested that a conjugate of a McAb to fibrin with another directed against tPA would concentrate endogenous tPA (which normally circulates at levels of about 5 ng/ml) in the immediate vicinity of a thrombus.

For Use as Vaccines

Active immunization has had a dramatic impact on the incidence and severity of several important human and animal diseases. It has resulted in the eradication of smallpox worldwide, while poliomyelitis, diphtheria and some other infections are now uncommon in developed countries. Active immunization is much preferred to passive protection, and a goal of many oncologists (which may never be realized) is to develop vaccines against cancer. A vaccine should be a well-defined molecular species that is free from contaminants and easy to prepare.

The use of McAb as vaccines is the subject of intense study. It is relatively straightforward to produce a murine McAb directed against an epitope on the surface of a microorganism or tumour cell. The V_H and V_L domains of such an antibody (which will be referred to as McAb1) will mirror the structure of the epitope. McAb1 can then be used as an immunogen to immunize, for example, human B lymphocytes immortalized with Epstein-Barr virus. Some of these cells will generate antibodies (referred to as McAb2) directed against the combining site of McAb1. The combining site is also termed the idiotype and the resultant antibodies are therefore called anti-idiotypic. Not surprisingly, McAb2 will usually be able to prevent McAb1 from binding to its specific epitope.

McAb2 has in its Fv region a structure that mimics that of the initial epitope. Thus McAb2 can be used as a vaccine when sufficient amounts of the initial epitope are not available. Steinitz et al. (1990) noted that "Induction of an anti-tumor immune response in tumor hosts by intervention through vaccination with anti-idiotypic antibodies may be an effective therapeutic approach." However, they also comment that ". . . the induction of anti-tumor antibodies by vaccination with anti-idiotypic antibodies does not necessarily correlate with anti-tumor immunity."

Potential Side-Effects

Any form of treatment may be associated with undesirable side-effects and the systemic administration of foreign antibodies or their fragments is no exception (Table 1.4). The benefits of therapy must outweigh any risks involved and every effort must be made to reduce the incidence and severity of side-effects to a minimum. This can be achieved only if all deleterious effects are recognized and the mechanisms are fully understood. The risks of passive immunization will be considered under three headings: those that are an inevitable consequence of specific binding by the therapeutic product; those of an allergic nature; and finally a range of non-specific effects.

Risks Due to Specific Antibody Binding

The systemic administration of ovine and bovine McAb to gonadal steroids can activate the hypothalamic–pituitary axis by reducing circulating levels of free steroid, releasing excess gonadotrophins, and thereby improving fecundity (Groves and Morris 1988). However, such effects are not always beneficial. One of the few deleterious effects of ovine anti-digoxin Fab is that removal of this steroid from its myocardial receptors may precipitate recurrence of the cardiac failure or arrhythmia for which the drug had been prescribed. Thus it is standard practice to attempt to calculate a dose that will correct the manifestations of toxicity but not bind all the cardiac glycoside. Another example of a deleterious effect is the haemolytic anaemia that may follow administration of large amounts of human immunoglobulins containing antibodies directed against A, B and/or Rh red cell antigens.

Most transplant patients treated with OKT3 or polyclonal antithymocyte globulin develop fever, myalgia, headache and several other symptoms (Debets et al. 1989; Hooks et al. 1991). These side-effects probably reflect the destruction of large numbers of lymphocytes, leading to a rapid increase in circulating levels of tumour necrosis factor and other cytokines (Abramowicz et al. 1989). More worrying is the report of an increased incidence of lymphoproliferative disorders, such as immunoblastic lymphomas, in patients receiving OKT3, with an incidence related directly to the amounts given (Swinnen et al. 1990). Such observations emphasize the need for great care in introducing new antibody-based therapeutic regimens, especially when these are directed against endogenous cells or products.

Table 1.4. Some potential side-effects associated with the systemic administration of exogenous antibodies

Due to specific effects of the exogenous antibodies

Potentially beneficial
- Increased gonadotrophin secretion due to binding of sex steroids

Detrimental
- Recurrence of cardiac problems, with excess anti-digoxin Fab
- Characteristic symptom complex following first administration of antilymphocyte globulin and OKT3 due to T lymphocyte destruction
- Increased incidence of lymphoproliferative disorders following use of OKT3
- Potential deleterious effects due to blocking biologically important molecules

Allergic response

To exogenous antibodies (or contaminating proteins)
- Type I anaphylactic hypersensitivity
- Type III immune-complex-mediated hypersensitivity
  - primary (delayed) serum sickness
  - secondary (accelerated) serum sickness
- Humoral immune response blocking or enhancing clearance of exogenous antibodies
- Possible immunomodulation

By exogenous antibodies
- Type III immune-complex-mediated hypersensitivity
  - involving foreign antibodies as the binding reagent
  - with infusion of antibody aggregates, including idiotype:anti-idiotype complexes

Non-specific side-effects

Microbial contaminants
- endotoxins
- bacteria
- mycoplasma and fungi
- conventional human, rodent and bovine viruses
- slow viruses

Other contaminants

Potential tumorigenicity

Cardiac

Renal

Allergic Responses

Administration of any foreign protein can evoke an immune response; this is the main area of concern with passive immunization. Hypersensitivity reactions range from a mild rash to severe, sometimes fatal anaphylactic shock; all are examples of an inappropriate immune response that may lead to tissue damage. In general, the less pure the protein, the more foreign its nature and the larger the amount given, the greater is the risk of an allergic reaction. Some examples are listed in Table 1.4 and discussed below.

Type I Anaphylactic Hypersensitivity

There is a familial predisposition to allergic disorders such as eczema; this type of sensitivity requires prior exposure to the foreign antibody (or contaminating

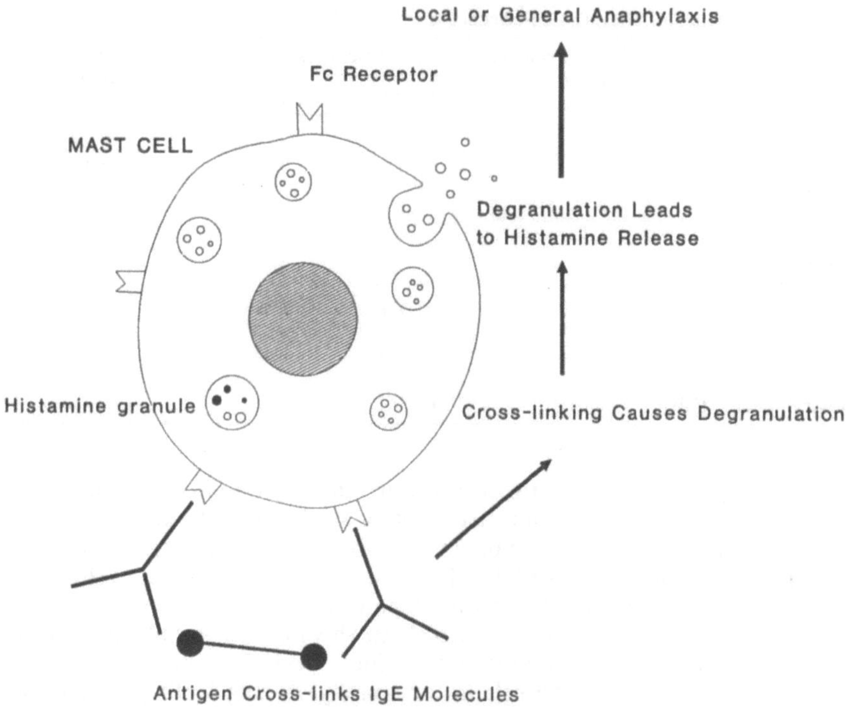

Fig. 1.3. Course of type I hypersensitivity.

protein) and it is mediated by IgE. Specific IgE secretion is stimulated by the first exposure. Some becomes attached to Fc receptors on mast cells. A second exposure to even small amounts of the protein leads to bridging between two IgE, with degranulation of mast cells and release of histamine and other vasoactive molecules (Fig. 1.3). Clinical manifestations occur within minutes of re-exposure and can include tachycardia, hypotension, bronchospasm and angioneurotic oedema.

Type I hypersensitivity reactions were common with equine-based products due, for example, to prior exposure to tetanus antitoxin derived from horses. Reactions of this type may also be seen in patients given repeated infusions of human plasma or immunoglobulins. This is because a significant number of individuals are deficient in IgA and respond to the first infusion by synthesizing IgE directed against this molecule (Schifferli 1992). The incidence of this and other allergic effects resulting from systemic administration of exogenous antibodies is shown in Table 1.5. Fortunately, anaphylactic hypersensitivity is unlikely with murine or human McAb or with ovine PcAb because prior exposure is rare.

Type III Immune-Complex-Mediated Hypersensitivity

This is more common than type 1 reactions and is mediated by IgG. Each IgG molecule or its $F(ab')_2$ has two binding sites which permit "cross-linking"

Table 1.5. Incidence of allergic side-effects expected with various types of antibodies

	Anaphylactic sensitivity	Serum sickness		Exogenous antibodies
		Primary	Secondary	
Monoclonal				
Murine		+		(+)
Humanized		(+)		(+)
Human				(+)
Polyclonal				
Human	+	+	+	+
Equine	+++	+++	+++	+
Equine $F(ab')_2$	+	+	+	+
Avian	+++	+++	+++	+
Ovine total Fab		+		
Ovine specific Fab		(+)		

to occur (Fig. 1.4) if the antigen has more than one epitope. Thus immune complexes can be formed comprising many antibody and antigen molecules. Some immune complexes remain in solution in the circulation; others precipitate out or become fixed to the wall of a blood vessel. All immune complexes can cause platelets to aggregate and release vasoactive amines, such as serotonin. Macrophages attach to the Fc and initiate phagocytosis and release interleukin-1 and other cytokines. Complement also binds to the Fc and is activated with the release of anaphylatoxins (split products of C3 and C5), which are chemotactic for polymorphonuclear cells and cause mast cells to release their vasoactive mediators.

By what mechanisms do immune complexes form during and/or after the systemic administration of foreign antibodies? The simplest example is when exogenous antibodies bind macromolecules (such as the constituents of a snake venom) already present in the patient. Much more common are primary (delayed) and accelerated serum sickness, in which the patient's own antibodies are involved.

Primary (Delayed) Serum Sickness. This occurs in patients not previously exposed to the foreign protein. The exogenous antibodies act as an immunogen and the extent of the immune response depends on their immunogenicity and the amount given. After about 8 days the patient secretes specific IgG, which can form immune complexes with what still remains of the foreign antibodies in the body. The more that remains the more is available to form such complexes; if none remains then no complexes can form. The amount remaining relates directly to the initial amount injected and to the rate of clearance. Primary serum sickness is usually manifested by fever, rashes and generalized lymphadenopathy. The kidneys, cardiovascular system and joints may also be involved.

Primary serum sickness is common after treatment with equine products, in part because horses have high blood levels of an extremely immunogenic form of immunoglobulin, termed IgG(T). Avian antibodies might also be troublesome if given systemically because they are larger and more immunogenic than mammalian IgG (see Chapter 3). The administration of murine McAb might cause serum sickness because, as discussed later, a HAMA response is virtually invariable. In practice, serum sickness is not encountered because only small amounts (up to 200 mg) of McAb are given. Ovine Fab is even safer because it is less immunogenic and is cleared much faster than intact IgG. This reflects its small molecular weight. For example, ovine Fab has a clearance rate of about 9h in the baboon as compared with 61 h for ovine IgG.

Secondary (Acclerated) Serum Sickness. This is similar to the primary form of serum sickness except that the patient has been previously exposed to the foreign antibodies and as a result has circulating specific antibodies of the IgG class and/or specific memory cells. In general, the more recent the prior exposure the sooner will clinical manifestations become apparent; they are usually more severe and last for longer than in the primary type. Sometimes the initial exposure may have evoked both an IgE and an IgG response. Under these circumstances, re-exposure may precipitate a type I anaphylactic reaction within minutes and a type III response within a few hours or days.

Immune Complexes with Foreign Antibodies as the Binding Reagent

Immune complexes may form during the time when exogenous antibodies are being infused if sufficient antigen is already present. For example, a large

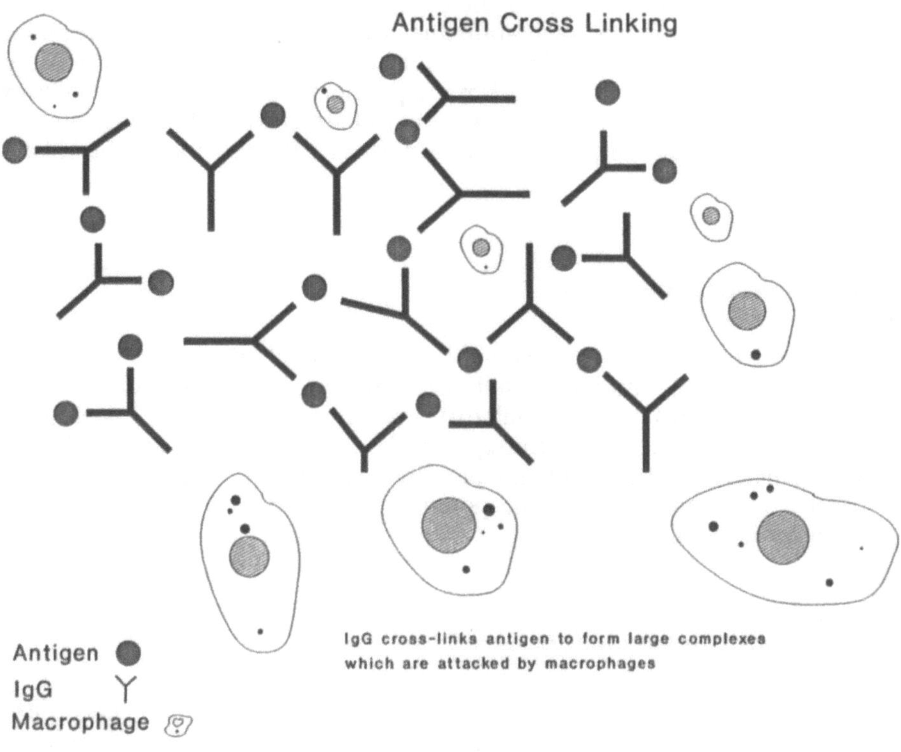

Fig. 1.4. Cross-linking.

snake may introduce several hundred milligrams of toxic proteins during envenomation. These may form immune complexes with the antibodies in the antivenom. Removal of the Fc part of IgG and the use of $F(ab')_2$ minimizes fixation and activation of macrophages and complement. Treatment based on Fab is even better: Fab does not form immune complexes because of the single binding site. Infusions of intact human immunoglobulins can also activate complement by forming immune complexes. This can occur if insufficient time is allowed for freeze-dried IgG to dissolve so that aggregates are given. IgG dimers may also form as the result of idiotype–anti-idiotype binding. Patients with hypogammaglobulinaemia are at particular risk during their first treatment with human products.

Other Immune Responses

The systemic administration of small amounts of an exogenous antibody may not cause an allergic response. However, repeated injections of even microgram amounts will inevitably provoke a humoral immune response. The resulting endogenous antibodies bind to the foreign antibodies and greatly increase their rate of clearance. Furthermore, the beneficial effects are blocked. This is well illustrated by the HAMA response to murine McAb and is often, but probably incorrectly, advanced to explain their lack of efficacy. The use of humanized and especially human McAb might overcome this problem. However, such antibodies will all have an identical combining site which may be recognized as "non-self" and lead to an anti-idiotype response by the recipient. This is not a problem with their human polyclonal counterparts, which have a large number of structurally different combining sites directed against a particular antigen because they are the product of many different clones.

Non-Specific Side-Effects

Table 1.4 lists some of the non-specific side-effects that may be associated with the use of antibody-based therapeutic products. McAb cause considerable concern to the regulatory authorities because ". . . hybridomas being used as the manufacturing vehicle could transmit pathogenic active oncogenes, microbial contaminants and particularly viruses . . ." (Brown 1990). Such problems may be potential rather than real and will only be considered briefly.

Microbial Contamination

Use of a sterilizing filter will ensure the removal of any bacteria but will not remove bacterial components, such as lipopolysaccharides and peptidoglycans, from the cell walls. Filtration is also ineffective at removing viruses, and human plasma and immunoglobulin concentrates are assessed for the presence of several viruses. Hepatitis non-A non-B and human immunodeficiency virus (HIV) are of considerable concern. Serological and polymerase chain reaction (PCR) techniques are now available for the former, while there is no recorded instance of the transfer of HIV by such products. It is difficult to envisage a more complex regulatory situation than that which exists when human McAb are produced by human B lymphocytes that have been transformed with Epstein-Barr virus, fused with murine myeloma cells and cultured in a medium containing bovine or fetal calf serum. There is a requirement to test for a minimum of 16 human, 10 rodent and several bovine viruses by techniques such as in vitro serology, reverse transcriptase assays, in vivo culture and transmission electron microscopy. The manufacturing steps should also be validated for their ability to remove viruses of the type responsible for bovine spongiform encephalopathy in cows and scrapie in sheep; the end-point is injection into hamster cerebral tissue and a delay of 6–12 months before electron microscopy.

Other Contaminants

These may include other proteins present in plasma (such as albumin) or culture medium or contaminants that have been introduced during manufacture (such as pepsin or papain).

Potential Tumorigenicity

There is a slight risk that oncogenes, intact viruses and viral DNA or RNA may be tumorigenic if administered systemically. Thus there is concern with the use of McAb produced in virus-transformed cells and/or myeloma and other neoplastic cells. Extensive testing is recommended, including identification of human oncogenic sequences; a search for active oncogenes in DNA extracted from producer cells by transformation studies in NIH 3T3 cells; assessment of chromosomal aberrations in at least 500 metaphase cells from the producer line; and comparisons with a known tumorigen in nude mice.

Renal

Intravenously administered ovine Fab may impair renal function. A single bolus injection of only 2 mg/kg body weight of digoxin-specific Fab into rats caused a transient decrease in urine volume and creatinine clearance, attributed to a reduction in glomerular filtration (Timsina and Hewick 1992). However, the decrease in creatinine clearance lasts for only a few days even when massive amounts of ovine Fab (3.2–5.3 g/kg body weight) are given to dogs (Keyler et al. 1991). The infusion of large amounts of human immunoglobulin into patients with renal disease also causes an increase in plasma creatinine and a decrease in clearance. However, these effects are transient and are unlikely to reflect permanent glomerular impairment. There is no rise in blood urea and the inulin clearance rate (the best measure of glomerular filtration rate) is unaffected. Schifferli (1992) concluded that the transient renal effects are limited to the active secretion of creatinine by the tubules and should not discourage use of foreign antibodies.

Anticipated Developments and Conclusions

Antibody-based products have immense therapeutic potential in both human and veterinary healthcare. The potential market for such products in oncology alone exceeds $3 billion. Other important areas include the treatment of infectious diseases (especially those due to viruses for which there are few suitable drugs) and septic shock, transplantation rejection and autoimmune diseases (including rheumatoid arthritis). Many other diseases, such as accelerated atherosclerosis following bypass surgery or angioplasty, are good targets for foreign antibodies. However, at the present rate of progress, it will be several years before such products are accepted as safe and have a significant impact on disease statistics.

A review in *Scientific American* (July 1993) recalled a 1980 headline in the *New York Times* that "Cloned antibodies promise medical revolution." The reviewer went on to comment on the present lack of success achieved by biotechnology companies preparing murine McAb. Despite many years of intense effort and many hundred million dollars of investment, only one therapeutic product, OKT3, has obtained FDA approval. Finally the review suggested that many more products will be introduced now that some companies have perfected the complex techniques necessary to manufacture humanized and fully human McAb. Such products avoid the risk of inducing a HAMA response and the Fc part of the molecule is more effective at enhancing phagocytosis and binding and activating complement. One successful example is a human McAb directed against Rh(D), which can prevent haemolytic disease of the newborn.

In our view, it is naive to assume that human McAb will overcome all the limitations of their murine counterparts. Several problems will remain, some of which are unavoidable.

Irrespective of their origin, McAb tend to have a lower affinity than their polyclonal equivalents. There are several sound reasons for this and ". . . monoclonal antibodies will never be able to replace conventional antisera as the essential high affinity of an antiserum lies in the cooperative effects between multiple types of antibody." (Campbell 1985). Furthermore, many of the procedures used to produce a McAb might have been designed to ensure a low-affinity product. Such procedures should be modified to allow full maturation of the immune response. Using the lock and key analogy, insufficient time is usually given to enable the lock (on the B lymphocytes and memory cells) to adjust its shape by repeated single point mutations to that of the key (the relevant epitope). Another disadvantage of some McAb is poor stability.

As discussed earlier, the very specificity of a McAb may ensure its lack of efficacy in a clinical situation. "It is almost impossible to emphasize too often that the final use of an antibody should whenever possible determine the type of assay employed [to assess it]." (Campbell 1985). However, biological assays are seldom used, because of their complexity and lack of sensitivity. Nonetheless, nothing is more certain than that scientific ingenuity will overcome the limitations imposed by the affinity and specificity of McAb, once it is accepted that they exist. Thus it is reasonable to expect that by the end of this century methods will exist for the production and purification of large amounts of high-affinity human McAb. It may also become common to overcome the problem of "excessive" specificity by pooling different human McAb which bind to different and carefully selected epitopes. This will be especially important for the treatment of tumours and microorganisms.

There are two additional and intransigent problems that seem unavoidable, namely the need for stringent quality control and the high costs involved in producing and assessing a McAb-based therapeutic product. All products intended for systemic administration must meet strict regulatory requirements. It is not by chance that in a recent book relating to the therapeutic uses of McAb (Borrebaeck and Larrick 1990) by far the longest chapter relates to regulatory affairs. Its author (Brown 1990) notes that "We now know that a large proportion of cell lines used for the manufacture of biological medicines do in fact release oncogenes and viral agents that are pathogenic to man." There will always be some concern when virus transformed and/or neoplastic cells are involved in the manufacture of a product and virtually no limit to the range of testing that our regulatory authorities may demand.

". . . Specific Mabs can be generated more rapidly and with far less effort than that required for synthesis of conventional low molecular weight organic molecules." (Larrick et al. 1990). Nonetheless, the need for stringent quality control adds to the high cost of McAb. Even those of murine origin cost at least ten times more to produce, purify and assess than their polyclonal equivalents. This is not a problem when murine McAb are used in vitro or in vivo for diagnostic purposes since even RIS requires only 500 μg of antibody. However, a course of murine OKT3 (5 mg daily for 10–14 days) costs about $5000. Such costs will inhibit the use of cocktails of murine McAb or the gram amounts required, for example, to treat a patient with tricyclic antidepressant overdose. Human McAb will be still more expensive, as summarized by the statement in *Scientific American*: "Indeed all those new technologies are considerably more expensive than churning out old-fashioned murine MAbs." Cost is certain to prove a major hurdle in the developed world (and an insurmountable problem in the developing world) to the use of human McAb.

The therapeutic use of McAb has the makings of a Greek tragedy. Thus on the one hand it faces the Scylla of requiring cocktails to better imitate a polyclonal product and on the other the Charybdis of the immense cost of producing even a single McAb.

PcAb receive scant attention in the scientific and commercial press and many have questioned their continuing therapeutic role. But in contrast to McAb, "Conventional antiserum [polyclonal] will not only have antibodies to several determinants but also a family of antibodies of different structure which compete for each individual determinant." (Campbell 1985). This broad specificity together with their high affinity and stability ensures that polyclonal products are effective; the regulatory requirements for their manufacture are reasonable; and no culture medium has been devised that remotely approaches the efficiency and safety of the intact living animal. It will be difficult to reduce the cost of preparing highly purified McAb to less than £1000 per gram, but specific ovine Fab and avian IgY can be produced for about 10% and 2% of this sum respectively.

There is no doubt of the efficacy of human PcAb for replacement in immunodeficient subjects and for the treatment of disorders such as idiopathic thrombocytopenic purpura. Several companies have established the necessary plasmapheresis centres and production facilities, most in the USA. Factors curtailing their use will remain the risk of transferring viral diseases and causing allergic manifestations, for example in IgA-deficient individuals. What of non-human PcAb? Equine products will eventually be discarded because of the side-effects associated with their systemic administration and the decreasing availability of horses. Sheep provide the most obvious alternative because of their ease of handling, low cost and the enormous numbers available worldwide. Other alternatives, albeit only for oral use, include avian IgY obtained from hens' eggs and IgA from the milk of immunized cows.

Safety is paramount, especially for products designed to reduce morbidity rather than save lives. It is much less of a problem with orally than systemically administered antibodies and we see an important role for intact IgY and IgA in the prevention and/or treatment of gastroenteritis (e.g. due to rotavirus or *E. coli*). Furthermore, this role is equally applicable to veterinary and human healthcare. PcAb of animal origin require substantial modification prior to systemic administration if side-effects are to be avoided. Ovine (or caprine) IgG is to be preferred. The PcAb should be specific for their intended use and free of contaminating proteins, microorganisms and endotoxins. Specificity is achieved by means of an affinity chromatography step with the ligand coupled to an insoluble matrix. Removal of the Fc part of the IgG molecule prevents binding and activation of complement and phagocytes; Fab is preferred to $F(ab')_2$ because its single binding site avoids formation of immune complexes. We believe that ovine-specific Fab-based therapeutic products have much to offer, especially in view of their large volume of distribution; the rapid rate at which they diffuse from the plasma into the interstitial fluid; and their rapid rate of clearance. Being foreign, such products seem certain to induce a humoral immune response in the recipient, albeit to a lesser extent than intact murine McAb and not for 10 days or more. Consequently it would seem wise to limit the systemic administration of such products to a single course lasting a week or less.

In our view, therapeutic indications for ovine specific Fab may include intravenous infusion:

1. For snake, spider and scorpion envenomation. It will take at least a decade for human McAb to be available against each of the 20 or more toxic constituents that comprise a typical snake venom. It is most unlikely that such McAb can be provided at a cost acceptable to developing countries.
2. As a cocktail of Fabs of different specificities directed against the initiators, mediators and effectors of septic shock.
3. To correct the clinical manifestations of drug overdose or the ingestion of other toxic molecules.
4. For some viral and other infections.

References

Abramowicz D, Schandene L, Goldman M et al. (1989) Release of tumour necrosis factor, interleukin-2 and gamma-interferon in serum after injection of OKT3 monoclonal antibody in kidney transplant recipients. Transplantation 47: 606–608

Borrebaeck CAK, Larrick JW (eds) (1990) Therapeutic monoclonal antibodies. Stockton Press, New York

Britton KE, Mather SJ, Granowska M (1991) Radiolabelled monoclonal antibodies in oncology. III: Radioimmunotherapy. Nucl Med Commun 12: 333–347

Brock-Utne JG, Gaffin SL (1989) Endotoxins and anti-endotoxins (their relevance to the anaesthetist and the intensive care specialist). Anaesth Intensive Care 17: 49–55

Brown J (1990) Therapeutic monoclonal antibodies: European regulatory issues. In: Borrebaeck CAK, Larrick JW (eds) Therapeutic monoclonal antibodies. Stockton Press, New York, pp 321–363

Campbell AM (1985) Monoclonal antibody technology: The production and characterization of rodent and human hybridomas. Elsevier Science Publishers

Debets JMH, Leunissen KML, van Hooff HJ, van der Linden CJ, Buurman WA (1989) Evidence of involvement of tumour necrosis factor in adverse reactions during treatment of kidney allograft rejection with antithymocyte globulin. Transplantation 47: 487–492

Dillman RO (1989) Monoclonal antibodies for treating cancer. Ann Intern Med 111: 592–603

DiPiro JT, Hamilton RG, Wei JP (1992) Novel antibody drug products. Am J Surg 164: 77–84

Granowska M, Britton KE, Mather SJ et al. (1993) Radioimmunoscintigraphy with technetium-99m-labelled monoclonal antibody, SM3, in gynaecological cancer. Eur J Nucl Med 20: 483–489

Greene GL (1988) Monoclonal antibodies to human estrogen and progesterone receptors. In: Hubbard R, Marks V (eds) Clinical applications of monoclonal antibodies. Plenum Press, New York, pp 81–85

Groves DJ, Morris BA (1988) Production and use of bovine and ovine monoclonal antibodies. In: Hubbard R, Marks V (eds) Clinical applications of monoclonal antibodies. Plenum Press, New York, pp 187–197

Haber E, Runge MS, Bode C et al. (1988) Antibody-targeted plasminogen activators. In: Hubbard R, Marks V (eds) Clinical applications of monoclonal antibodies. Plenum Press, New York, pp 207–213

Hellström K-E, Hellström I (1990) Mouse antibodies to carcinomas. In: Borrebaeck CAK, Larrick JW (eds) Therapeutic monoclonal antibodies. Stockton Press, New York, pp 95–108

Hochman J, Inbar D, Givol D (1973) An active antibody fragment (Fv) composed of the variable portions of heavy and light chains. Biochemistry 12: 1130–1135

Hooks MA, Wade CS, Millikan WJ (1991) Muromonab CD-3: A review of its pharmacology, pharmacokinetics and clinical use in transplantation. Pharmacotherapy 11: 26–37

Jones PT, Dear PH, Foote J, Neuberger MS, Winter G (1986) Replacing the complementarity-determining regions in a human antibody with those from a mouse. Nature 321: 522–525

Keyler DE, Salerno DM, Murakami MM, Ruth G, Pentel PR (1991) Rapid administration of high dose antibody Fab fragments to dogs: Pharmacokinetics and toxicity. Fund Applic Toxicol 17: 83–91

Larrick JW, Gavilondo JV, Coloma MJ, Fry KE (1990) Construction of recombinant therapeutic monoclonal antibodies. In: Borrebaeck CAK, Larrick JW (eds) Therapeutic monoclonal antibodies. Stockton Press, New York, pp 17–34

Miles LEM, Hales CN (1968) Labelled antibodies and immunological assay systems. Nature 219: 186–195

Mudgett-Hunter M, Anderson W, Haber E, Margolies MN (1985) Binding and structural diversity among high affinity monoclonal anti-digoxin antibodies. Mol Immunol 22: 477–488

Padlan EA, Cohen GH, Davies DR (1986) Antibody Fab assembly: The interface residues between CH1 and CL. Mol Immunol 23: 951–960

Piqueras J (1989) Hepatotoxic mushroom poisoning: Diagnosis and management. Mycopathologia 105: 99–110

Reisfeld RA, Schrappe M (1990) Current status and future perspectives of chemoimmunoconjugates for the treatment of cancer. In: Borrebaeck CAK, Larrick JW (eds) Therapeutic monoclonal antibodies. Stockton Press, New York, pp 57–73

Schifferli JA (1992) Adverse effects of intravenous immunoglobulins. Transfusion Sci 13: 331–338

Steiner LA (1985) Immunoglobulin disulfide bridges: Theme and variations. Biosci Rep 5: 973–989

Steinitz M, Tamir S, Frodin J-E, Mellstedt H (1990) Human monoclonal anti-idiotypic antibodies against a murine monoclonal antibody (Mab 17–1A) as an anti-tumor vaccine. In: Borrebaeck CAK, Larrick JW (eds) Therapeutic monoclonal antibodies. Stockton Press, New York, pp 159–171

Swinnen LJ, Costanzo-Nordin MR, Fisher SG et al. (1990) Increased incidence of lymphoproliferative disorder after immunosuppression with the monoclonal antibody OKT3 in cardiac transplant recipients. N Engl J Med 323: 1723–1728

Timsina MP, Hewick DS (1992) Digoxin-specific Fab fragments impair renal function in the rabbit. J Pharm Pharmacol 44: 867–869

Wunner WH, Dietzschold B, Rupprecht CE, Koprowski H (1988) Monoclonal antibodies against rabies virus. In: Hubbard R, Marks V (eds) Clinical applications of monoclonal antibodies. Plenum Press, New York, pp 115–137

Yalow RS, Berson SA (1960) Immunoassay of endogenous plasma insulin in man. J Clin Invest 39: 1157–1162

2 Biology of the Immune Response

T. Poulton and F. Hay

Introduction

The last few years have seen dramatic changes in our understanding of the way that the cells of the immune system recognize antigen and communicate with each other. This increase in knowledge has simplified the concepts of immunology rather than increasing their complexity, and biochemists have succeeded in explaining and simplifying the phenomena observed by the immunologist.

This chapter will describe the elements of the immune response using bacteria entering through a skin lesion as a model example.

The immune system exists to recognize and dispose of foreign material, notably parasitic ("infectious") microorganisms. The immune mechanisms can be divided into two parts, innate and adaptive. The innate mechanisms, which are not enhanced by repeated infection with a given microorganism, are mediated by complement and phagocytic cells. This contrasts with adaptive mechanisms, which improve with reinfection; hence secondary infections are more effectively dealt with than primary ones. These mechanisms are mediated mainly by lymphocytes: B lymphocytes, which produce antibody, and T lymphocytes, which produce the so-called "cell-mediated" responses. Both systems act together, with antibody as perhaps the most significant link between the two.

Innate Immune System

The first line of defence of the innate immune system is to prevent entry of organisms into the body. The major defence against microbial attack is the skin and mucous surfaces. In the event of a break in the skin, bacteria encounter two major defence systems: complement (a humoral defence) and phagocytosis (a cellular defence).

Complement

Complement consists of a large number of serum components that, when activated sequentially, lead to inflammation, phagocytosis and direct microbial destruction.

Complement is activated by either of two pathways, the classical and the alternative. The latter, despite its name, is the most primitive pathway, and is directly activated by bacterial factors such as complex carbohydrates. Fixation of complement to the surface of an organism has three effects: (i) lysis, (ii) "opsonization" or absorption and phagocytosis by phagocytic cells, and (iii) cleavage of small soluble factors, which diffuse into the tissues and induce inflammation and chemotactic movement of phagocytes.

The key element in both complement pathways is fixation of C3 to the cell surface. C3 may bind directly to particle surfaces (and this can be inhibited by molecules on the surface of the host cells). C3 is converted to C3b through a C3 convertase. Direct adsorption of C3 to the cell surface is a relatively inefficient process compared with antibody-directed fixation. This is initiated by binding of the globular protein C1q, a subunit of the complex C1, to certain immunoglobulins. Conformational changes in C1 lead to the cleavage of C4a from C4, which reacts with C2 and leads to the formation of the C3 convertase C4b2b. C3b is both an opsonin and the basis for complement lysis of pathogens.

The final phase of both pathways is the formation of the membrane attack complex C5b6789n (MAC), which creates the hydrophobic lytic "plug" that is inserted into membrane bilayers. C3b produces its own amplification loop and induces the binding of many more molecules of C3b to the surface.

The release of the soluble factors C3a and C5a, the anaphylatoxins, stimulates chemotaxis of neutrophils and the degranulation of mast cells, releasing the mediators of inflammation.

Phagocytosis

Phagocytosis is the most primitive form of immunity. In higher animals this is restricted to specialized cells, the macrophages and polymorphs, and can be evaded by many organisms that are adapted to the host. Phagocytic ability is enhanced if pathogens are coated with complement and antibodies, the latter an example of the interaction of adaptive mechanisms with the innate response. Cells in every tissue can carry out these functions.

Macrophages

The major cell is the macrophage, a tissue descendent of the blood monocyte characterized by a horseshoe-shaped nucleus. The cytoplasm contains numerous lysosomes, which include acid hydrolases and peroxidase, agents important in the killing of ingested organisms. Phagocytosis of pathogens occurs naturally, but is greatly assisted by specialized receptors for immunoglobulin, the Fc receptors: FcγRI,-II,-III for IgG; FcαR for IgA; and receptors for the C3b and C3d complement components.

Monocytes migrating into the tissues take up a new role as fixed macrophages; these form a network known as the reticuloendothelial system. Most of these cells are organized to present antigen to promote lymphocyte function.

Some macrophages are specialized to present antigen to lymphocytes, and these cells are frequently found in lymphoid tissues. The classical antigen-presenting cell (APC) is the Langerhans cell in the skin. These cells take up antigen, migrate in the afferent lymphatics to the lymph nodes and present antigen to the T cells. Different APCs will present to B cells and T cells for reasons discussed later. An example is the follicular dendritic cell, which is found in the secondary follicles of the B cell areas of the spleen and lymph nodes.

Polymorphs

These cells can be divided into several groups: neutrophils, mast cells, basophils and eosinophils. All are phagocytic to some degree, but the most important cells for bacterial clearance are the neutrophils. Unlike macrophages they are short-lived and represent 60%–70% of total blood leucocytes. They have multilobed nuclei and many granules, lysosomes containing acid hydrolases, peroxidase and lysozyme and secondary granules containing lactoferrin and lysozyme. They can adhere to and penetrate endothelial cells lining blood vessels. Like macrophages they respond chemotactically to the complement cleavage products C3a and C5a.

Mast cells are tissue-based cells with similar functions to the circulating basophil. They release the inflammatory mediator histamine and slow reactive substance of anaphylaxis (SRSA), which is chemotactic for eosinophils. These factors are released during degranulation in response to allergen or antigen recognized by the IgE receptor on the surface of the cell. The effects of this are well known for their involvement in syndromes such as hay-fever. Mast cells are also important in response to immunity to parasites.

Eosinophils are predominantly involved in the responses to larger parasites such as worms and protozoa. In migrating into an inflammatory area they release histaminase, which dampens the inflammatory response.

Adaptive Immunity

In a primary response where innate mechanisms are not sufficiently effective, there is activation of adaptive immune mechanisms. If these adaptive mechanisms successfully produce recovery from the disease, the associated development of immunological memory will prevent further disease from reinfection.

The key cells of adaptive immunity are the T and B lymphocytes. They are produced in the bone marrow and thymus at a rate of 10^9 per day and represent 20% of total white blood cells. Whilst the sole function of the B cell is the production of antibody, the T cell is the cornerstone of acquired immunity. There are several subgroups, with a variety of functions including control of other cells such as B cells, lymphokine production and specific T cell cytotoxicity.

T and B lymphocytes in blood are heterogeneous in size and morphology but share many properties. Both are individually specific towards particular antigens, owing to the possession of surface receptors by which each lymphocyte can "recognize" its "own" antigen. Both can respond to antigens by proliferating to form a clone, some carrying out lymphocyte functions and others developing into memory cells.

The differences between T and B lymphocytes relate to their function in the adaptive immune response and to the way in which they recognize antigen. The most exciting recent development in immunology has been the elucidation of the way in which antigen is processed for recognition by T cells. This explains the highly specific roles of APCs and has finally explained the importance and relevance of the major histocompatibility complex (MHC). The MHC is a group of antigens on the surface of most cells which were known to be the antigens involved in graft rejection, and to "restrict" in some way the cellular immune response.

Immune Recognition

For B cells, the antigen receptor is the antibody molecule itself; each cell carries antibody of one specificity only. The T cell antigen receptor, termed Ti, is more complex. It consists of two different chains, alpha and beta, a heterodimer that, like the immunoglobulin molecule, contains variable and constant regions. Like the B cell, each T cell carries specificity for one antigen. Ti is complexed with a molecule called CD3, which is functionally linked to the Ti antigen receptor. CD3 has a larger cytosolic region than Ti and CD3 may be part of the complex that transmits the signal caused by antigen binding to the inside of the cell.

T and B cells respond both to soluble antigen and to antigen presented on the surface of APCs. In lymph nodes APCs include the interdigitating cells of the T cell areas and the follicular dendritic cells of B cell areas. Stimulation leads to activation, the growth of cells into blast cells and subsequent function. From this point the resemblance between T and B cells ends.

The B cell can respond to antigen presented on the surface of macrophages as "native" antigen. Unlike the B cell the T cell needs the antigen to be presented in the form of small peptides in association with the MHC. This is the group of antigens involved in transplant rejection. Class I is on all nucleated cells whilst class II is expressed on APCs and some lymphocytes. Different T cell subsets (helper and cytotoxic/suppressor) recognize antigen in association with different classes of the MHC. The complex on the helper T cells recognizes antigen associated with class II MHC; the cytotoxic cell recognizes antigen associated with class I. The molecule associated with helper T cells, CD4, and the molecule associated with cytotoxic cells, CD8, take part in the recognition of the MHC in each case. Hence helper T cells see antigen presented on APCs and the cytotoxic T cells see antigen in association with class I present on any nucleated cell (e.g. a virally infected epithelial cell). The way in which antigen can only be presented in association with the MHC is called HLA restriction. It is a further layer in determining the specificity of the adaptive immune response. The antigen is found in a groove in the MHC molecule and binds to both the MHC and the antigen receptor. The question that remained baffling was how did it get there?

Antigen is adsorbed to clathrin on the APC surface and endocytosed into intracellular compartments (endosomes). In certain cells, such as B lymphocytes, this fluid-phase uptake can be replaced by more efficient systems: binding to specific receptors on the cell surface such as specific surface immunoglobulin, or binding in the form of immune complexes to Fc receptors. Inside the endosome, limited proteolysis takes place and the antigen is broken into smaller fragments. Newly synthesized class II MHC interacts with this endosomal pathway. Class II MHC can recognize short sequence patterns in fragments of the antigen, patterns that will occur quite frequently and which have hydrophobic or polar amino acids. The fragments recognized differ from one MHC haplotype to another. The MHC becomes associated with the antigen, prevents it from further degradation, and returns it to the surface of the cell. Here the processed antigen is recognized by the antigen receptor on the CD4-carrying helper cell.

In summary, antigen for recognition by the T helper cell is taken up by APCs and processed into fragments. Some of these fragments will bind to the class II molecules. They are then presented on the surface of the APC and are recognized by the T helper cell–antigen complex.

The B cell has a different system of recognition. It does not need to recognize processed antigen because its receptor is antibody. It is clear that the B cell antigen receptor responds to unprocessed antigen and that this antigen is presented on APCs that present specifically to B cells rather than T cells. However, the B cell depends on the T cell in order to divide, and the T cell only recognizes antigen in association with the MHC. So the B cell also processes antigen and presents this to the T cell in order to activate.

Cytotoxic T cells recognize antigen in a similar way, but typically the peptides are produced from within the cell, as for example with viral peptides.

Both T and B cells require antigen to be presented, even though B cells do not require antigen to be processed. Typically the APCs for B cells, such as the marginal zone macrophages of the spleen and the follicular dendritic cells of the lymph node, are phagocytic whereas the APCs for the T cell are not.

Lymphocyte Function

Activation of the T and B cells involves recognition of antigen and MHC and, in addition, signals in the form of soluble factors which pass between the APC and the lymphocytes. These soluble factors are collectively called cytokines: monokines, if produced by monocytes; lymphokines if produced by lymphocytes; and interleukins if operating between cells of the immune system. The T cell recognizes the MHC–antigen complex and passes a signal to the macrophage which may be γ-interferon. Interleukin-1 (IL-1) released by the macrophage in response will, in the presence of antigen, stimulate the T cell, which enters the T cell cycle. Part of this cycle is the production of IL-2 in one set of T cells and the IL-2 receptor in another. IL-2 is specific for the T cell and induces T cell proliferation. This promotes clonal expansion of the

T cells and the development of cells secreting a wide variety of lymphokines, including those that promote proliferation of B cells, IL-4 and IL-5.

The Lymphoid Organs

Lymphoid stem cells originate in the bone marrow, differentiate in primary lymphoid organs and generate an immune response in secondary lymphoid organs. These include the spleen, which "filters" the blood, chains of lymph nodes, which drain lymph from the tissues, and mucosal-associated lymphoid tissue. There is a recirculation of lymphocytes, particularly of T cells, between tissues, blood and lymphoid organs.

The two lobes of the thymus are organized into lobules or follicles separated by connective tissue. Each lobe is organized into outer cortex and inner medulla. The cortex contains immature proliferating cells while the medulla contains more mature cells. Bone-marrow-derived cells become antigen-sensitive immunocompetent T lymphocytes in the thymus under the influence of a network of epithelial cells. These cells are rich in "self" antigens and probably control or prevent the appearance of lymphocytes that react with host antigens. Lymphocytes are densely packed in the cortex and are sparser in the medulla, which contains Hassall's corpuscles of unknown function. The B cell areas are not well defined in mammals, but in birds are produced in the bursa of Fabricius, a modified segment of the intestine. In mammals the B cells are produced in fetal liver and in the fetal and adult bone marrow. The bone marrow also serves as an important secondary lymphoid organ.

The generation of lymphocytes in primary lymphoid organs is followed by migration into secondary organs. In these sites the lymphocytes interact and are stimulated by antigen. They consist of the lymph nodes, spleen and various mucosal-associated lymphoid tissues (MALT).

The lymph nodes are found at junctions of lymphatic vessels and form a network that filters lymph from the tissue spaces and drains into the thoracic duct and then into the left subclavian vein. B cells are organized into primary and secondary follicles in the cortex of each node. Secondary follicles have a mantle of lymphocytes surrounding a pale germinal centre and are associated with memory. The adjacent "paracortical region" is populated by T cells with interdigitating APCs. The cortex also contains specialized antigen-presenting dendritic "macrophages". Lymphocytes enter through specialized blood vessels, the high endothelial venules (HEV), and leave through the efferent lymphatics.

The spleen contains red pulp and white pulp. The red pulp consists of an intricate sinusoidal complex in which blood is filtered by lining phagocytes. The white pulp comprises lymphoid tissue associated with arterioles. There are B and T cell areas, with plasma cells in the marginal zone.

A Typical Immune Response

Bacteria entering through a skin lesion will first encounter the innate immune response. Complement should be active within minutes, attempting to lyse the bacteria and simultaneously releasing the agents of inflammation, C3a and C5a. These and other factors both increase vascular permeability and attract phagocytic cells, which will engulf bacteria. Both mechanisms are enhanced by the presence of pre-existing antibodies.

During this time adaptive immune processes begin to mature. Most involve the passage of antigen or antigen-bearing cells to lymphoid tissue. Cells already resident in the skin will also be phagocytic, but some will be specialized APCs, such as Langerhans cells. Antigen is taken up by these cells, processed and presented at the surface in association with MHC. These cells can pass to the T cell areas of lymph nodes in the lymphatics and settle there as interdigitating cells, presenting antigen to the T cells. Free antigen will also pass through the lymphatics to the lymph nodes to be taken up by APCs in the follicles of B cell areas.

T and B cells form foci of activated and proliferating cells in the lymph nodes within a few days. The B cells form plasma cells, many of which remain in the lymph node and produce antibody which drains through the efferent lymphatics to the circulation. A greater proportion of T cells leave the lymph nodes, return to the circulation and migrate into the tissues where they carry out T cell functions: cytotoxicity of infected (particularly virally infected) cells; "help" for antibody production and phagocytosis; and the production of cytokines which activate a variety of immune and non-immune cells.

Immunoglobulin Structure and Function

Five different classes of immunoglobulin are found in serum. Each of the five classes serves a different function within the immune system. Binding of antigen triggers various effector functions and leads to removal of antigen. All classes can recognize a wide range of antigens, and all are based on the same basic structure of two "light" and two "heavy" chains.

General Structure

The basic immunoglobulin structure consists of two light (25 000 kDa) and two heavy chains (50–80 000 kDa) giving a total size of approximately 150 000 kDa. The light chains are of two types, kappa and lambda, which are present in all immunoglobulin classes. In contrast the heavy chain is structurally unique for all classes and subclasses. IgG, IgD and IgE exist as monomers of this unit; IgM is polymeric and IgA can also exist as a dimer. The heavy and light chains are organized into regions of more than 100 amino acids, called domains, which are held together by disulphide bonds. Some residues are the same in all immunoglobulin molecules, while others are highly variable – the so-called hypervariable region. The variable regions (V) and constant regions (C) are shown in Fig. 2.1.

The typical molecule (Fig. 2.1) contains V_L and C_L domains in the light chain and V_H, C_H1, C_H2 and C_H3 in the heavy chain, but immunoglobulins of a particular type have specific labels for their heavy chain domains, based on the heavy chain nomenclature used for each immunoglobulin (e.g. $C\alpha 3$

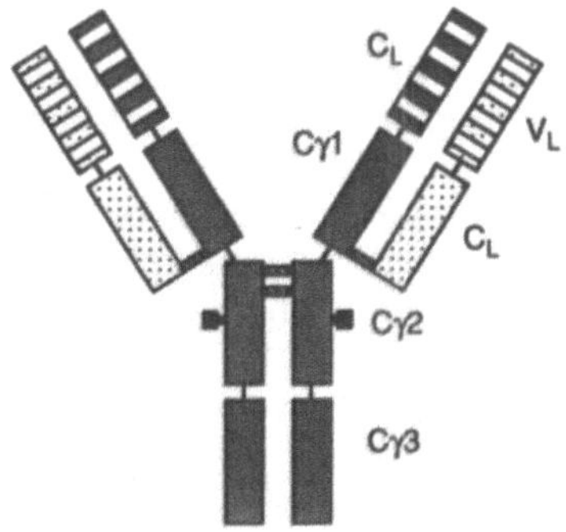

Fig. 2.1. The basic polypeptide structure of IgG. For all immunoglobulins, sequence variability is shown in that part of both the heavy and light chains referred to as the variable heavy (V_H) and variable light (V_L) chain domains. Other constant domains of the heavy chain are referred to as three discrete regions: C_H1, C_H2 and C_H3. The single constant light chain domain is termed C_L. This nomenclature applies to all classes of immunoglobulin. Additional terms are applied to the specific immunoglobulin classes, dependent on the heavy chain they possess. Consequently, C_H1, C_H2 and C_H3 for IgG, become Cγ1, Cγ2 and Cγ3. Carbohydrate units are shown diagrammatically (■). Sometimes these are present on the inside of the molecule, but for clarity are shown on the outside. The number of carbohydrate units varies between all the subclasses.

for IgA). The variable regions of these chains are the antigen-binding site. Disulphide bonds hold together the heavy and light chains and the two heavy chains. The number of intrachain bonds varies from one class or subclass to another. The molecule is flexible at the hinge region and this is the site at which proteolytic enzymes act. The cross-linking of domains makes the molecule rigid and ensures that the hypervariable regions from H and L function together.

The domains are typically folded into two layers. In the case of the variable regions this leads to three loops which fit closely. These loops are particularly variable and are the region of binding to antigen. The variable domains of the heavy and light chains form a surface with six of these loops, sufficient to contact large antigens over an area of up to 75 nm^2. The number of points of contact will influence the affinity of interaction.

The immunoglobulins are all members of the Ig supergene family, and related molecules are present on the surface of cells of the immune system, principally those involved in immune recognition.

Antibody Effector Function

Each Ig molecule is bifunctional, with one part binding to the target antigen and the other mediating the effector functions. These include: (i) elimination or neutralization of antigen (as for example with toxins); (ii) binding of antigen to tissues by interaction with Fc to assist phagocytosis, antigen processing or the release of antimicrobial factors; and (iii) fixation of complement. The enzyme papain splits IgG into two Fab fractions, which represent single arms of the antibody-binding region, and Fc, the region involved in effector functions.

IgG

IgG is the main immunoglobulin in serum (7–19 g/1, three-quarters of the serum Ig). The heavy chains are gamma chains. There are four subclasses: IgG_1, IgG_2, IgG_3 and IgG_4. These are similar in structure apart from a heavier γ3 chain in IgG_3. The number of interchain disulphide bonds is variable, with a larger number (15) between the heavy chains of IgG_3. The carbohydrate units lie between the the Cγ2 domains of all subclasses. Subclasses of IgG have different properties and different distributions in response to given antigens, e.g. anti-Rhesus antibodies are usually IgG_1 or IgG_3 while most antibodies to carbohydrates are IgG_2. Antibodies to factor VIII, which can arise after repeated injection of this protein in haemophiliacs, are often IgG_4, as are many autoantibodies.

The major functions of IgG are fixation of complement and binding to IgG receptors on phagocytic and antigen-processing cells. They increase phagocytic ability and the efficiency of antigen processing for presentation to T cells. Two subclasses, IgG_1 and IgG_3, are particularly involved in fixation of complement. Two molecules of the correct subclass are required to fix complement. IgG_2 is less effective and IgG_4 has no complement-fixing ability. Both IgG_1 and IgG_3 are cytophilic, i.e. they bind to cells with Fc receptors, particularly monocytes and granulocytes. This is important in phagocytosis and for efficient processing of antigen by APCs. The three common receptors for IgG are FcγRI, FcγRII and FcγRIII. The characteristics of these range from high-affinity interactions, which can bind single molecules of IgG (FcγRI), to low-affinity interactions (FcγRIII), which can only bind with high avidity when there is multiple interaction, i.e. two or more antibodies binding to an antigen and interacting with two or more receptors. The latter is particularly important in phagocytosis.

IgG is the only class of immunoglobulin to cross the placenta; maternally derived antibody is responsible for the immune protection of the newborn child.

IgM

IgM represents approximately 10% of the total serum immunoglobulin (0.5–2.0 g/l). The molecule is a pentamer of identical units, similar to the basic model, except that the heavy chain possesses an extra domain. The whole molecule is held together by disulphide bonds between the Cμ3 domains and is clearly seen in electron micrographs as a structure with radiating arms. It is stabilized by a further chain called the J or "joining" chain, which contains 137 amino acids. The structure of the J chain has not been analysed completely and so the illustration in Fig. 2.2 is only diagrammatic. The J chain assists polymerization by cross-linking cysteine residues in the Cμ3 region with disulphide bonds, and may increase resistance to proteolytic digestion.

The major function of IgM is fixation of complement. This is effected by binding of the first component of the classical pathway, C1q, to the C_H2 region of the molecule. C1q itself consists of six subunits, each of which has a helical collagen-like region that will react with the C_H2 regions of IgG and IgM. The

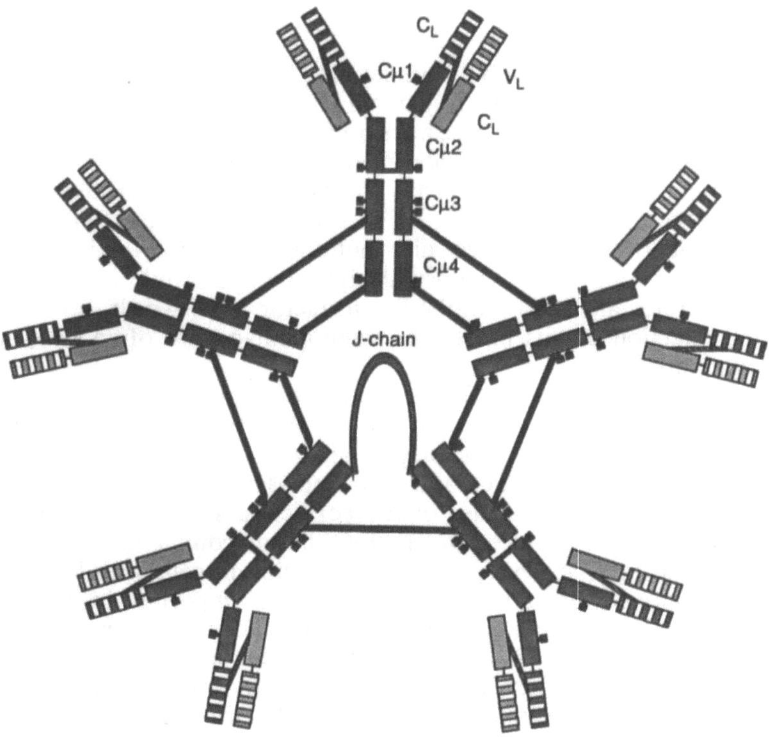

Fig. 2.2. The structure of IgM. The IgM molecule consists of five domains cross-linked by disulphide bonds. The IgM heavy chains contain a fourth constant domain, $C\mu4$.

affinity of this reaction is weak and the overall avidity is increased by the binding of several subunits to clusters of C_H2 regions. One IgM pentamer bound to antigen can activate complement, whereas it takes two adjacent IgG molecules to do the same. Consequently IgM may be several orders of magnitude more effective at fixing complement on a cell surface and as much as 1000 times more efficient at lysing a cell through complement fixation.

The function of complement is lysis and destruction of pathogens through the formation of a cascade of pore-forming complexes on the surface of the organism. An additional purpose is the enzymatic release of small soluble factors from the complement cascade, the anaphylatoxins, which induce inflammation and the chemotactic attraction of phagocytes to the area of invasion. Electron microscopy has revealed that IgM, on binding to antigen, alters from a star to a staple shape. This conformational change is probably involved in the ability of IgM to bind complement only when it is itself bound to antigen.

The primary response to antigenic challenge in infection is always IgM. Although the individual binding sites of IgM are usually of lower affinity than those of IgG, the ability of IgM to bind antigen with up to ten binding sites provides very high avidity to multivalent antigens. All B lymphocytes possess IgM on their cell surface, which is very similar to secreted IgM except for an absence of disulphide bonds between J chains and heavy chains. All B cells,

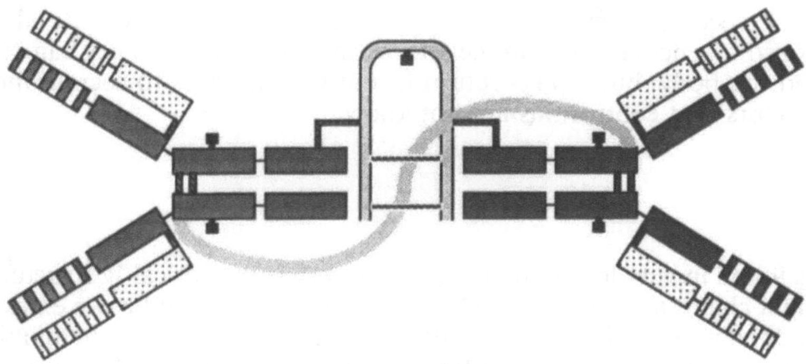

Fig. 2.3. Secretory IgA. Dimer IgA contains two moneric units of IgA (either IgA_1 or IgA $_2$) connected by a J chain. The secretory component is believed to be wrapped around the dimer and attached to Cα2 domains of each monomer.

when activated to produce antibody, begin by producing IgM, and then switch to producing a different antibody class. The secondary response is usually another class of antibody, determined by the antigen and its route of entry into the body.

IgA

IgA is the main type of immunoglobulin produced at mucous surfaces and epithelial interfaces, in secretions such as saliva, colostrum, milk, and all the secretions of the respiratory, alimentary and genitourinary systems. It is thought of as the most important antibody in mucosal immunity, but it also has the second highest immunoglobulin concentration in blood, after IgG. In man, serum IgA is almost entirely monomer and mucosal IgA is mainly dimer. In most other mammals serum IgA is also dimer. The functions of mucosal IgA are reasonably well known, but the precise function of serum IgA is unclear. It may react with an IgA receptor on phagocytes and induce phagocytosis.

IgA has two subclasses, IgA_1 and IgA_2. Both are present in serum and have a molecular size of approximately 385 000 kDa. In common with IgM, IgA possesses an additional C-terminal peptide which can bind covalently to the J chain in the dimer form of IgA (Fig. 2.3). This exists in an end-to-end formation linked by the Cα3 regions. IgA_1 is the most abundant form in serum but there is relatively more IgA_2 in secretions. Many organisms found in the urogenital, gastrointestinal and respiratory tracts produce enzymes that easily cleave IgA_1 but have less effect on IgA_2. In both subclasses carbohydrate is particularly abundant in the hinge region.

Secretory IgA (sIgA) is a dimer containing a J chain and an additional peptide, secretory piece (15 000 kDa). This is very resistant to denaturation and degradation, an important property in areas such as the gut. Most of the IgA at mucous surfaces exists in this form. The secretion of IgA is made possible by a five-domain member of the Ig supergene family, the poly-Ig receptor on epithelial cells in mucosae, which transports the dimeric IgA across the cell by a process of receptor-mediated endocytosis. The degraded receptor becomes secretory piece. The lymphocytes that secrete sIgA are sensitized by encountering antigen at the mucosal surface. They can "traffic" around the body, but always return to mucosal surfaces to secrete the IgA. The factors that control this are not known.

IgE

IgE is found in very low amounts in serum. It has the typical Ig structure with two light chains and two epsilon heavy chains. Like IgM it has an extra heavy chain domain, $C\epsilon 4$. It has a primary defence function against helminths and other large parasites, but in Northern Europe it is more often associated with allergens, which, for example, may cause hay-fever. Examples include pollen grains, with high sensitivity in Western Europe to the grasses (and in Britain, plane trees) and the house dust mite.

The basophil and its tissue equivalent, the mast cell, have surface IgE receptors. IgE binds very tightly to the receptor for IgE on mast cells without binding antigen. When antigen subsequently binds, this triggers the mast cell to "degranulate". Granules rapidly shed their contents outside the cell, releasing histamine and other substances, which promote inflammation.

IgD

IgD has a typical IgG-like structure, with the same number of domains. IgD is probably not important in serum and appears mainly as a cell surface receptor. It is found on B cells when they switch from virgin lymphocytes, with IgM on the cell surface, to memory cells with other classes on the cell surface.

General

The different functions of immunoglobulin types are reflected in the distribution of their receptors on cells. Even lymphocytes have Fc receptors, which may be involved in antigen presentation. IgA or IgE receptor-positive T cells help B cells to switch from IgM to IgA secretion. The mechanism of this is unknown.

The Immunoglobulin Genes

We inherit the genetic information to make many thousands of different antibodies. In the bone marrow this genetic information is rearranged such that each B lymphocyte receives the information to make only one antibody specificity. The genes for the two types of light chain are on different chromosomes with the genes for the heavy chains on a third chromosome.

The light chain is assembled from a *V* gene, which combines with a *J* (joining) gene. Human germline DNA has genes for about 2300 V regions (each with its own leader sequence gene), around five J regions and one constant region. In all cells in the body except B cells the DNA is retained, but as B cells are produced in the bone marrow much of this DNA is lost so that only one V and one J is left. This is a random process so that thousands of combinations of V and J regions are possible. Each combination will allow the lymphocyte to make a different antibody. The lymphocyte transcribes DNA into RNA, which is then processed by splicing of the VJ region to the C region prior to translation. When the light chain is secreted, the leader or signal sequence is removed.

The heavy chain V domain is assembled from a *V* gene, *D* (diversity) gene and a *J* (joining) gene. The joining of VDJ again occurs as the lymphocytes are produced. For 300*V*, 12 *D* and 4*J* genes the total number of combinations is $300 \times 12 \times 4 = 14\,400$. The joining of V to J or V to D or D to J is not always the same, giving rise to even more diversity; if the joining of a *V* gene to a *J* gene is moved along one codon, a new amino acid and therefore a new hypervariable region is produced. For the heavy chain, the extent of recombination produces even greater diversity since two joining events take place. The joining regions all contribute to the third hypervariable region, with the first two hypervariable regions coded for by *V* genes.

Triggering of B cells occurs when antigen binds to the antigen receptor on its surface. This is an IgM on a virgin B cell and immunoglobulin of another class on a memory cell. The B cell will secrete an antibody identical to that on its surface. L chains and H chains are made separately and come together in the lumen of the endoplasmic reticulum, always with an excess of L chains.

In a virgin B cell the VDJ genes are next to the μ chain gene; therefore this cell will make IgM and all the antibody in the primary response is IgM. If the lymphocyte meets antigen it will be activated and some will become memory cells. These memory cells undergo a "class-switch" because DNA is lost and the VDJ genes become aligned to another heavy chain gene. Somatic mutation only occurs in memory cells that have already switched class.

The ability to make different H and L chains is inherited. In addition, during a lifetime many new antibodies are produced because of (somatic) mutations in B cell DNA. Mutation is relatively common in Ig genes and increases during the lifetime of an individual as memory cells become more abundant.

References

Chapel H, Heaney M (1993) Essentials of clinical immunology, 3rd edn. Blackwell Scientific, Oxford.

Klaus GGB (1990) B lymphocytes. IRL Press, Oxford.

Male D, Champion B, Cooke A (1992) Advanced immunology, 2nd edn. Gower Medical, London.

Roitt I (1993) Essential immunology, 7th edn. Blackwell Scientific, Oxford.

Roitt I, Brostoff J, Male D (1992) Immunology, 3rd edn. Gower Medical, London.

3 Antibody Production in the Hen

J. Landon, J.A. Woolley and C. McLean

Summary

> It has, I believe, been often remarked, that a hen is only an egg's way of making another egg. (Samuel Butler, 1835–1902)

Antibodies of the IgG class are selectively transported across the oviduct from the hen's circulation to the egg yolk. From there they are transferred to the embryo and help to provide systemic immunity essential for survival during the first few weeks of a chicken's existence in a microbially hostile environment. Antibodies of the immunoglobulin (Ig) M and A classes are largely confined to the egg white and are ingested by the embryo to help to ensure local gastrointestinal immunity in early life. There is a substantial and rapidly increasing literature concerning the potential application of yolk-derived antibodies for both diagnostic and therapeutic purposes.

Yolk antibody levels are similar to, or slightly exceed, those in hen's blood. They comprise at least two subclasses of IgG, which differ in several significant ways from their mammalian counterparts and are often referred to as IgY. Thus, although comprising two light and two heavy chains, they are of larger molecular weight; their isoelectric point (pI) is about one pH unit lower; and the Fc portion of the molecule does not bind with protein A, protein G, complement, rheumatoid factor or macrophages. These differences offer advantages in the use of yolk-derived antibodies for some immunoassay procedures. Of especial importance, because of phylogenetic dichotomy, it has often proved possible to raise antibodies in hens directed against highly conserved mammalian macromolecules when this has not been accomplished in rabbits or other mammalian species.

On theoretical grounds, there are potential risks in administering avian antibodies systemically to man or animals. However, it seems likely that yolk-derived antibodies will prove to be safe when given by the oral route and will prove of value in the prevention and/or treatment of an extensive range of gastrointestinal infections in both clinical and veterinary medicine. Thus it has proved to be relatively simple to produce high titres of high-affinity IgY against numerous viruses, bacteria and parasites. Such antibodies may be more resistant to heat, acid and enzymatic cleavage than mammalian IgM and

IgA; the egg represents considerable "downstream" processing as compared with blood; and there may be advantages in the oral administration of yolk or whole egg suspensions, rather than purified IgY. This approach has already proved successful in the prevention of rotaviral diarrhoea in mice and cats and in the treatment of piglets infected with pathogenic *Escherichia coli*. Of particular importance in this regard is the simplicity and low cost of producing kilogram amounts of specific antibodies in egg yolk and the ease of oral therapy.

Background

History

Since the third century AD it has been common practice for farmers to feed raw eggs to calves with diarrhoea (scours). Klemperer, in 1893, appears to have been the first to show that antibodies synthesized by the hen in response to an immunogenic contact are transferred to the egg yolk. A few years later, Dzierjgowski (1901) conducted a series of studies in which hens were immunized with increasing amounts of diphtheria toxin. He showed that those hens which survived had developed active immunity and their antitoxins were transferred without modification to the egg yolk (but not the egg white) and thence to the embryo and chicken's blood. These studies were confirmed later in ducks (Fraser et al. 1934) and extended to the transfer of antibodies against a microbe, using egg yolk from hens that had been immunized with, or recently recovered from, Newcastle virus (Brandley et al. 1946).

By 1970 much was known about how antibodies are transferred to egg yolk (Patterson et al. 1962) and about the structure and function of avian immunoglobulins (Leslie and Clem 1969). It was also recognized that egg yolk antibodies could be substituted for serum IgY for immunoassay purposes (Aulisio and Shelokov 1967). However, most of the information relating to the production of egg antibodies and all information relating to their therapeutic potential has arisen during recent years.

Circulating Immunoglobulins in the Hen

Based on earlier work (Benedict et al. 1963; Orlans 1967) and on the antigenicity of the heavy (H) chains, Leslie and Clem (1969) concluded that the domestic hen has at least two immunoglobulin classes. One, with a molecular weight of about 900 000 Da, is very similar to mammalian IgM although having a significantly lower hexose content. The other has a similar structure to mammalian IgG with two H and two light (L) chains, but differs in a sufficient number of important respects (summarized in Table 3.1) to warrant the authors' suggesting a different name, immunoglobulin Y (IgY). Furthermore, based on its enzymatic cleavage with pepsin, they concluded that at least two subclasses of IgY exist, a view substantiated later by others. In the same year, Gallagher and Voss (1969) studied yolk-derived

Table 3.1. Comparison of mammalian IgG and avian IgY

	Mammalian IgG	Hen IgY
Structure	All comprise 2 H and 2 L chains	
Molecular weight (MW)	About 160 000	About 180 000
Heavy chain MW	—	About 67 000
%		75%
Light chain MW	—	About 22 000
%		25%
	Light chains shared with IgM and IgA	
Hexose chain %	1%	2.22%
Mean pI	7.8	6.8
Pepsin digestion	To $F(ab')_2$ + Fc	To ×2 Fab + Fc
Papain digestion	All to ×2 Fab + Fc	Only about 70% to ×2 Fab + Fc
In 1.15 M saline	No aggregation	Considerable aggregation
Extinction coefficient	—	15.1
Binding to:		
complement	Yes	No
macrophages	Yes	No
protein A	Yes	No
protein G	Yes	No
rheumatoid factor	Yes	No

specific anti-DNP IgY, which they had purified by affinity chromatography, and confirmed that its molecular weight was about 180 000 Da and that it had an extinction coefficient of 15.1.

Hen IgY has a higher content of Gly, Ala and Leu but a lower content of Asp, Thr, Ser and Lys than bovine IgG (Shimizu et al. 1988) and the difference in composition with regard to appropriate amino acids explains why avian IgY has a lower isoelectric point (pI) than mammalian IgG. Other relevant differences include the inability of the Fc part of IgY to bind to mammalian complement, rheumatoid factor and macrophages or to *Staphylococcus aureus* protein A or streptococcal protein G. It is also stated that on enzymatic cleavage with pepsin, IgY forms two molecules of Fab (as opposed to one molecule of $F(ab')_2$ with mammalian IgG). From the standpoint of oral therapy, it is relevant that IgY appears to be more heat-stable and more acid-resistant than mammalian IgG (Losch et al. 1986), so that pasteurization is possible without loss of binding (Yolken et al. 1988). It is also more resistant to enzymatic cleavage by chymotrypsin but more susceptible to trypsin and possibly pepsin (Shimizu et al. 1988).

Serum from hens contains IgA, as well as IgM and IgY, but no secretory component is detectable. Rose et al. (1974) recorded serum IgY levels of about 6 g/l, IgM of some 1.3 g/l, and a mean IgA level of 0.6 g/l. More detailed studies are indicated using improved analytical techniques, especially since there is evidence that circulating immunoglobulin levels vary with age (being higher in laying hens compared with chickens) and sex (being higher in laying hens than roosters) (Polson et al. 1980a). Furthermore, circulating immunoglobulins increase markedly in response to immunization and intramuscular injections of Freund's complete adjuvant (FCA) alone in one study caused an increase in serum IgY levels from about 13 g/l (viz. more than twice the value recorded above) to over 30 g/l (Tam and Benedict 1975).

However, there is little doubt that albumin is the dominant serum protein (at over 50% of the total protein concentration), with immunoglobulins normally comprising less than 30% of the total.

Response of Hens to Active Immunization

Following the intravenous injection of a large amount of bovine serum albumin (BSA), Patterson et al. (1962) detected the presence of specific antibodies in the circulation after 4 days, which, as discussed later, then appeared at the periphery of the yolk sac after a further similar interval. Yolk IgY levels directed against BSA peaked some 6 days after the serum peak while specific antibody levels in serum and yolk, after an intramuscular injection of influenza virus, appeared slightly earlier. It was subsequently found (French et al. 1970) that the humoral response in hens to an intramuscular injection of 40 μg of human serum albumin (HSA) was greatly enhanced in the presence of FCA. It was further shown that most of the specific IgY was being synthesized by macrophages and plasma cells present in the granuloma found at the site of injection; even after a single immunization in FCA, maximum antibody levels persisted throughout the 59-day study period; and 16-week hens had a greater immune response than 10-week-old chickens. The importance of including *Mycobacterium tuberculosis* in the adjuvant (or suitable alternatives such as *Bordetella pertussis* or *Nocardia rubra*) to ensure granuloma formation was demonstrated by Tam and Benedict (1975). The injection of FCA alone caused a marked increase in circulating IgY from about 13 to more than 30.0 g/l due to the presence of non-specific antibodies, and this was associated with an increase in serum levels of the acute-phase proteins and a decrease in albumin.

Most groups now use adjuvant, especially Freund's complete and incomplete adjuvants, and other adjuvants have been used, including a lipid emulsion system with a *Salmonella typhimurium* mitogen (McCune et al. 1992). Hens of about 20 weeks of age are preferred when raising antibodies to hapten–carrier conjugates and other macromolecules. A variety of immunization routes have been used, but most favour a single (or multiple) intramuscular injection into the pectoral muscle, which, even in the presence of adjuvants, does not appear to cause the hen discomfort or result in abscess formation. There seems no doubt that hens require less frequent immunizations than the commonly used mammalian species to maintain a maximally elevated antibody response (Polson et al. 1980a). Evidence is accumulating that smaller amounts of immunogen are required than for rabbits or sheep (Gassmann et al. 1990), but, as in mammals, the antibody response is partially related to the molecular weight of the immunogen. Thus it is excellent, for example, to haemocyanin (molecular weight 8×10^6 Da) but poor to the many low-molecular-weight components of Cape cobra venom (Polson et al. 1980b).

Information with regard to the affinity of IgY is limited. On the basis of the "sharpness" of the precipitation lines obtained by a tube and the Ouchterlony technique, Polson et al. (1980a) concluded that hen IgY had a higher affinity than rabbit antiserum. Bauwens et al. (1987, 1988) recorded an affinity constant (K) of 1.5×10^{10} l/mol for one of their avian antibodies raised against a vitamin D conjugate, which made possible the establishment of a sensitive radioimmunoassay and suggests that the values obtained for avian and mammalian antibodies are similar.

The humoral immune response to microbes has also been studied in detail and it may be possible to immunize hens with such organisms by ocular drops or by the intranasal or oral route (Dawson et al. 1980). Losch et al. (1986) obtained an antibody response persisting for over 200 days following intramuscular injection of *Brucella abortus* in FCA and concluded that hens, unlike mammals, do not have an anamnestic (greatly enhanced) response to a second or subsequent immunization, suggesting that memory cells play no part. Conversely, Schiemann and Montgomery (1991) found that hens initially immunized by the subcutaneous route with *S. typhimurium* had a considerably greater IgY response to the later oral administration of this microorganism, thereby favouring the existence of memory cells. The question of whether or not hens have an anamnestic response requires answer. The absence of such a response might explain the need for a prolonged immune response to a single contact with an immunogen. Because in mammals it is accepted wisdom that the primary immune response involves predominantly IgM, it is difficult to explain the rapid increase in yolk antibodies, which as discussed later are of the IgY type, within a few days' exposure to influenza virus (Patterson et al. 1962). However, others did not find an increase in specific IgY until some 28 days following immunization with canine distemper virus (Schmidt et al. 1989a), which would be in accord with current teaching, provided there had been a much earlier IgM response.

As discussed later, these and other questions of a fundamental nature require further detailed study using improved analytical techniques.

Composition and Formation of Hens' Eggs

An average hen's egg in the UK weighs about 60 g and comprises the central yolk (of some 15 ml volume) and surrounding egg white. These two components have a very different composition and function. For example, 100 g of yolk provides nearly ten-fold more energy than the same amount of egg white due largely to its high lipid content (Table 3.2).

Egg Yolk

Egg yolk contains the yellow-coloured vitellines, which comprise various lipoproteins, including LDL and HDL, as the dominant component and the major source of energy for the embryo and newly hatched chicken. The protein components are referred to as the levitins and comprise alpha levitin

Table 3.2. Composition of hens' eggs

Per 100 g	kJ	Protein	Fat (cholesterol)	Carbohydrate
Egg yolk	1402	16.1	30.3 (1.25)	Trace
Egg white	153	9.0	Trace	Trace

(mainly ovalbumin), beta levitin (mainly alpha-2 glycoprotein) and gamma levitin which is the IgY fraction (Hatta et al. 1990). There is a significantly higher ratio of IgY to albumin in yolk than in serum.

In contrast to egg white, the yolk contains no detectable, or only very small, amounts of IgM, IgA or secretory product but large amounts of at least two subclasses of IgY. On the basis of their Fc bands, pI, sialic acid content (1–2 moles per mol of IgY), papain digestion products, isoelectric focusing (Loeken and Roth 1983) and amino acid composition (Shimizu et al. 1988), the two or more subclasses of IgY in egg yolk are identical to those in the hen's circulation. The amount of IgY present has been found to increase from about 25 mg/yolk in non-immunized hens to about 75 mg/yolk after immunization (Carroll and Stollar 1983). However, others report still higher values of up to 250 mg/egg (Losch et al. 1986) and more accurate figures will require the availability of improved analytical procedures and extraction techniques. At present all that can be concluded is that yolk IgY concentrations approximate to those in serum.

Egg White

Egg white contains only traces of lipids and carbohydrates but substantial amounts of protein. At least 40 different proteins are present (Langeland 1983), of which more than 90% comprises relatively small molecules and especially ovalbumin, transferrin, ovamucoid and lysozyme. Much of the remainder is made up of IgM, at about 150 mg/l, IgA at about 700 mg/l and free secretory component with no detectable IgY (Rose et al. 1974) or from 0.3% to 1% of that present in serum or yolk (Dawson et al. 1980). Actual values depend on many factors, including the analytical techniques used and, as discussed later, most of the molecules present in the white play important roles after their ingestion into the gastrointestinal tract of the embryo and newborn chick. Of particular potential significance, egg white also contains significant amounts of protease inhibitors (Schmidt et al. 1989b).

Egg Formation

Hens have a single ovary containing myriad small ova located in the lumbar area of the abdomen. At sexual maturity the largest ova are about 0.1 cm in diameter and yolk material is deposited on the surface of selected ova during a phase of rapid growth and the largest is deposited in the infundibulum and surrounded by the vitelline membrane. Each egg is fully formed in the 24 h after ovulation as it travels down the infundibulum by the deposition of egg white followed by the shell membrane and finally the shell. In studies using ^{131}I-IgY, Patterson et al. (1962) found that there was a 24–48 h interval between its intravenous injection and appearance initially on the periphery of the yolk. Thus this is the time required for the selective transport of IgY from the hen's circulation to the yolk.

Active transport of IgY involves its binding by the Fc part of the molecule to specific receptors facing the maternal circulation. These then migrate to a pit region on the membrane and aggregate to form a coated vesicle, which in turn transports intact IgY across the cell for release into the yolk sac (Loeken and Roth 1983). This is a similar mechanism to that operating to transfer IgG across the human placenta or the intestinal tract of the newborn piglet.

Immunological Protection of the Newly Hatched Chicken

The newly hatched chick enters an extremely hazardous environment where a wide range of pathogenic organisms await the immunologically compromised. In the weeks before it is protected by its own endogenous antibodies, the chicken must depend for its survival on the passive immunity provided by its mother via the egg. Its continued existence depends on adequate defences both in the gastrointestinal tract against orally ingested pathogens and in its blood against systemic infections. In general terms, the egg white provides the former and the yolk the latter in a manner analogous, respectively, to milk and colostrum in most mammalian species.

Gastrointestinal Protection

The chicken, unlike the newborn mammal, depends immediately on pecking its feed, often from an extremely unhygienic surface. Thus it is fortunate that the egg white, which has passed into the amniotic cavity and then been ingested into the gastrointestinal tract of the embryo, contains a variety of protective components. As discussed earlier, these include IgM, IgA and its secretory component. Fortunately, these will be directed against those microorganisms that the mother hen had encountered and that therefore will be present in the immediate surroundings of the newborn chick. There is also evidence that during the days immediately before hatching, the embryo ingests some IgY that passes from the yolk sac to the egg white because these are no longer separated by an intact vitelline membrane (Kramer and Cho 1970).

In addition to immunoglobulins, egg white provides several other protective macromolecules. These include substantial amounts of transferrin, which bind irreversibly any iron present in the gut and thereby deprive *E. coli* and other iron-requiring microbes of an essential growth and multiplication factor. Another component of egg white, lysozyme, has a powerful destructive effect on many microorganisms.

Systemic Protection

This is provided by IgY, which is actively transported from the hen's circulation to the yolk sac and thence to the chicken's circulation via the yolk sac's endothelium, which is equivalent to the transplacental transfer of this immunoglobulin in humans. Again these will be directed specifically against the microorganisms to which the mother was, and probably continues to be, exposed. These antibodies will bind to any appropriate invading organisms and, via its Fc, serve to bring complement and macrophages into intimate contact to initiate their destructive effects. Hens kept in crowded surroundings are prone to develop systemic infections, therefore it is common practice to maintain a vigorous programme of protective vaccination, which, in turn, will ensure that the egg yolk contains relatively high titres of the appropriate specific IgY.

Extraction of Antibodies from Egg Yolk

There are significant advantages in giving a whole egg suspension orally for the prevention or treatment of gastrointestinal infections. Costs are reduced; losses are avoided; pasteurized raw eggs have a constipative effect; such preparations are a valuable source of energy; and IgM, IgA and other protective molecules (such as transferrin) are provided in addition to IgY. Given that egg white provides the natural protection to gastrointestinal pathogens in chickens, it would seem unwise to prefer an egg yolk to a whole egg suspension and there is evidence that the more proteins that are present the better protected are the egg immunoglobulins against an acid environment and proteolytic degradation.

There are circumstances, for example in the supply of antibodies for some diagnostic purposes, when it is appropriate to purify partially or completely the IgY from other yolk constituents. Several techniques have been introduced for this purpose, all of which involve the initial separation of the egg white (with its IgM and IgA) from the yolk and often washing of the latter. The next step is to separate the hydrophobic lipids from the hydrophilic protein fraction since ". . . almost 50% of the yolk is non-aqueous material . . ." (Jensenius et al. 1981) and it is helpful if at this step some of the small molecular weight, non-IgY proteins are removed together with the lipids. Some loss of IgY is inevitable during this step because of entrapment within the lipid fraction, but the slight improvement in yield obtained by including one or more wash steps must be weighed against the time and labour involved.

Methods to separate the lipid and protein components include ultra-centrifugation and use of organic solvents such as chloroform (Aulisio and Shelokov 1967; Ntakarutimana et al. 1992) and pre-cooled (at −20°C) propane-2-ol (Bade and Stegemann 1984). However, the most popular methods involve lipid precipitation with 3.5% (Polson et al. 1985) or 4.4% (Hassl and Aspock 1988) polyethylene glycol 6000, dextran sulphate and calcium chloride (Jensenius et al. 1981), or with magnesium chloride and phosphotungstic acid (Vieira et al. 1984). A recent innovation has been to use various gums, which are common food additives, for this purpose (Hatta et al. 1990). Thus gums such as carrageenan have a slight negative charge and bind with, and aggregate, lipoproteins, which are positively charged. The resultant aqueous phase, which contains the IgY, is gin-clear and suitable for most purposes. Further purification from low molecular weight proteins is simple and involves the precipitation of the IgY by a high (12%) concentration of polyethylene glycol or by ammonium or sodium sulphate.

Total IgY can be purified on a DEAE column (Bade and Stegemann 1984); using pre-cooled (−20°C) ethanol (Polson et al. 1985); by hydrophobic interaction chromatography (Hassl and Aspock 1988); or by FPLC on a Mono Q column (Gassmann et al. 1990). Finally, specific IgY can be prepared by means of affinity chromatography (Gallagher and Voss 1969; Carroll and Stollar 1983; Gottstein and Hemmeler 1985; Kuhlmann et al 1988; Thalley and Carroll 1990; Ntakarutimana et al. 1992). The product will be more than 99% pure and suitable for structural and related studies. However, such complete purification is only likely to be required on a large scale if avian IgY or its $F(ab')_2$ or Fab fragments prove to be safe and practical for systemic administration to patients.

Comparison of Avian and Mammalian Antibody Production

Currently, polyclonal antibodies for diagnostic or therapeutic use are raised in guinea-pigs (seldom), rabbits, goats, sheep, donkeys (seldom) and horses. During the course of many years, immunization protocols and processing procedures have been improved and are well defined. Thus it must be asked why groups should dilute their efforts and devote scarce resources to a study of antibody production in hens. This question is of especial relevance at a time when there is a general move to the use of murine, humanized or human monoclonal antibodies. Consideration of the latter is beyond the scope of this review, which will limit itself to a comparison of the advantages and disadvantages that may be gained by the use of avian, as compared with mammalian, polyclonal antibodies. These are summarized in Table 3.3.

General Considerations

Many of the potential advantages of using hens and egg yolk-derived IgY are minor, such as their stability in intact eggs for at least 6 months (Ricke et al. 1988). Thus, in a major review of polyclonal antibody production, Hurn and Chantler (1980) concluded that hens are "... best avoided if possible". Nor would it seem likely that avian IgY (or its fragments) can replace ovine Fab for systemic administration in, for example, the treatment of envenoming, septic shock or drug overdose. Thus, they are likely to be more immunogenic than their mammalian counterparts because of differences in structure as the result of evolutionary dichotomy, larger molecular weight and greater degree of glycosylation. Nonetheless, this remains to be proved and an American group (Carroll et al. 1992) is producing yolk-derived IgY for use in the treatment of rattlesnake envenomation. This group points out that such antibodies are less likely to cause side-effects than intact equine antibodies because the Fc part of IgY does not activate complement or bind macrophages.

There is some evidence, although again this requires further study, that hens mount a humoral response to smaller amounts of immunogen given

Table 3.3. Comparison of avian and mammalian antibody production

Related to the use of hens
1. Home Office regulations relating to the housing of hens are not unduly onerous and their use does not generate an emotional response from animal rights and similar groups
2. Once housing is available, hens are inexpensive to purchase and maintain (approximately £15 per hen per year)
3. They are easy to handle and tolerate all adjuvants without systemic or local complications
4. Blood samples are easy to obtain for initial assessment
5. Only microgram amounts of immunogen need to be given at infrequent intervals to obtain an excellent prolonged humoral immune response
6. Evolutionary dichotomy from mammalian species helps to ensure an excellent antibody response to highly conserved mammalian macromolecules.

Related to the use of eggs
1. Antibody levels in egg yolk approximate to those in serum
2. Eggs represent considerable downstream processing as compared with blood and it is both simple and inexpensive to purify IgY from the yolk
3. Egg white and especially yolk are a rich source of calories, which may be of value during oral therapy
4. Egg white contains many non-immunoglobulin antimicrobial factors, including transferrin and lysozyme, which may be of value when fed orally
5. Egg white contains proteolytic enzyme inhibitors which protect antibodies during their passage to the small intestine
6. Each hen lays over 260 eggs per year and each egg contains over 15 ml of yolk. This is equivalent to 4000 ml of antiserum per year, the productive capacity of one sheep
7. Antibodies retain their activity for at least 6 months when stored in an inactive egg

Related to yolk IgY
1. IgY is likely to be more immunogenic than mammalian IgG or its fragments when administered systemically to humans (or animals) because of:
   (i) the evolutionary dichotomy of avian and mammalian immunoglobulins
   (ii) its larger molecular weight (180 000 as compared with 160 000 Da)
   (iii) its greater hexose content
2. It may be difficult to cleave a subclass of IgY to Fab with papain and to produce $F(ab')_2$ with pepsin
3. Information regarding the K value of yolk IgY is limited
4. IgY does not bind rheumatoid factor or activate complement, which is an advantage for some diagnostic and possibly therapeutic purposes
5. The low pI of yolk IgY facilitates its use in rocket immunodiffusion assays for mammalian immunoglobulins
6. IgY is more heat, acid and enzyme resistant than mammalian IgG and therefore may be more suitable for pasteurization and oral therapy

at less frequent intervals than mammals. If correct, this is of obvious importance with regard to scarce and expensive macromolecules, such as human parathyroid hormone. However, the main diagnostic importance of avian IgY lies in the possibility of raising high-affinity antibodies against highly conserved mammalian molecules that are not immunogenic in mammalian species, such as rabbits and sheep. In 1983 Carroll and Stollar successfully produced IgY in hens to calf thymus RNA polymerase, which, despite its large molecular weight of about 140 000 Da, had not proved to be immunogenic in rabbits or guinea-pigs and concluded ". . . the use of laying hens as hosts for immunization may be generally applicable to other highly conserved mammalian antigens". This prediction has been amply justified with examples including the serine protease kallikrein (Burger et al. 1985), the alpha subunit of insulin receptors from rat hepatocytes (Song et al. 1985), proliferating cell nucleur antigen (PCNA) from calf thymus tissue (Gassmann et al. 1990) and the highly conserved enzyme, rat liver cytosolic casein kinase II (Goueli et al. 1990).

As well as binding to the macromolecules in question, these avian IgY have been shown to block the catalytic activity of the enzymes studied. In the case of PCNA, a total of 30 μg per hen, in three divided amounts, produced a good response (with 3.2% of the total IgY being specific for this protein, as shown by affinity chromatography), whereas no rabbits produced suitable antisera.

Economic Considerations

Cost is not a major problem with regard to the provision of antibodies for diagnostic products, although it is important to produce sufficiently large amounts to allow distribution to many laboratories (Gardner and Kaye 1982). As discussed later, the main role for avian IgY may be for oral administration in the prevention and treatment of gastrointestinal infections in both human and animal healthcare. Here cost is a major consideration, especially if such antibodies are to be used as a food supplement given to all subjects at risk during an epidemic or on exposure to a risk situation, such as hospital admission. Clearly, the use of yolk-derived IgY rather than mammalian-derived antibodies will depend in part on their resistance to heat, acid and an extensive range of proteolytic enzymes. However, acceptability of such an approach will be determined largely by cost.

It should be possible to provide IgY for oral administration at less than 10% of the cost of specific ovine serum IgG. A battery hen produces 268 eggs per year, with each egg containing over 15 ml of yolk with an IgY content similar to, or slightly higher than that of, serum. Thus each hen provides the equivalent of more than 4000 ml of antiserum per year, which is the maximum productive capacity of a large sheep. In a recent study, Ntakarutimana et al (1992) found IgY amounts of about 180 mg per egg, of which over 10% was specific for the immunogen used (human transferrin). Against this must be set the fixed and variable costs totalling about £12 per year (*The Agricultural Budgeting and Costing Book*, November 1991), which are less than 10% of those involved with sheep. A further gain accrues from the fact that an egg represents considerable "downstream" processing as compared with blood because it is unnecessary to centrifuge off red cells. Furthermore, a suspension of whole raw egg is extremely nutritious and palatable, whereas unprocessed serum causes diarrhoea and is unpalatable.

Uses of Avian Antibodies

Antibodies are required for both the human and animal healthcare professions for their diagnostic and therapeutic applications (Table 3.4). This will be considered in the following sections.

Table 3.4. Clinical applications of antibodies

Diagnostic
In vivo (imaging)
In vitro (as a primary or secondary reactant in immunoassay)
Therapeutic
Extracorporeal
Gastrointestinal
Systemic:
to deliver therapy ("magic bullet")
for therapy

For Diagnostic Purposes

Antibodies are used in vivo in a number of imaging techniques, such as to detect areas of myocardial ischaemia. Monoclonal antibodies are preferred for this purpose because of their homogeneity and defined specificity. Their high cost (about $1500 per gram) is irrelevant because only small amounts are injected. It is extremely unlikely that yolk-derived IgY is sufficiently specific or safe for intravenous use and there are no papers in the literature on the subject. In contrast, there are many publications relating to the in vitro use of avian antibodies, both as a primary and a secondary reagent in immunoassay. The first dates from 1967 when Aulisio and Shelokov showed that yolk-derived IgY from hens immunized with Rous sarcomavirus could replace serum antibodies for the detection of this virus by an indirect fluorescence procedure. Indeed, they commented that yolk antibodies were much easier to assess and caused less non-specific fluorescence.

Immunoassays can be divided into three general catagories, namely those that use no labelled reagent (non-labelled immunoassays), those based on the use of labelled analyte (such as radioimmunoassay) and others that use labelled specific antibodies (including immunometric assays). Yolk-derived IgY has proved to be suitable for all three categories and is available against an extensive range of haptens, macromolecules and microorganisms (Table 3.5).

Haptens

Antibodies to four different prostaglandins have been raised in hens by immunization with appropriate keyhole limpet haemocyanin conjugates; extracted from the egg yolk; and used to develop specific, sensitive radioimmunoassays (Fertel et al. 1981). The antibodies could be used at a 1:30 000 dilution and gave results comparable to those using rabbit antibodies. Bauwens et al. (1987, 1988) extracted specific IgY from the yolks of eggs collected from hens immunized with a 1,25-dihydroxyvitamin D-3-hemisuccinate–BSA conjugate. The mean affinity constant from one hen was 1.25×10^{10} l/mol and it was used at a dilution of 1:1500 with a tritiated label in a radioimmunoassay with a sensitivity of 5 pg/tube. They concluded that the avian IgY provided a more sensitive and specific assay (as demonstrated by extensive cross-reactivity studies) than that obtained with a rabbit antiserum.

Macromolecules

Non-labelled immunoassays depend on the formation of large antigen–antibody complexes, which scatter light in solution or form a precipitation line in a gel, as in radial immunodiffusion and rocket immunoelectrophoresis. For example, Kint et al. (1987) developed a nephelometric assay for the measurement of transferrin in human serum using IgY and noted that the signal was enhanced ten-fold in the presence of 8% sodium chloride. More recently, Ntakarutimana et al. (1992) described a similar assay using affinity-purified IgY and obtained results that correlated closely with those found using a rabbit antiserum.

Altschuh et al. (1984) wrote "In view of the relatively large quantities of reagents required in a technique such as rocket immunoelectrophoresis, the ease and low cost of producing antibody in chicken egg is of particular relevance." This technique depends on differences in the charge of the analyte to be measured and the antibodies used and it is not possible therefore to measure mammalian IgG or IgM levels using a mammalian IgG (without prior treatment of one to alter its pI). The authors point out that avian IgY can be used without pre-treatment because of its significantly lower pI and they used such antibodies to measure human IgG and IgM and rabbit IgG. Vieira and his group (1984) raised antibodies in hens against both the 1–34 and 53–84 amino acid sequence of human parathyroid hormone. Each hen was immunized by the intradermal route with 50 μg of one of the peptides in Freund's complete adjuvant at monthly intervals and after 4 months it was possible to extract IgY from the yolk for use in a radioimmunoassay for this hormone.

Larsson and Sjoquist (1988) have pointed out the advantages of using chicken antibodies in immunoassays on samples containing rheumatoid factor, an IgM anti-IgG autoantibody that binds to the Fc part of the molecule and is present in patients with a variety of disorders, including rheumatoid arthritis and systemic lupus erythematosus. Thus in a latex particle agglutination assay, false positives were obtained with such samples when the particles were coated with any of a range of mammalian IgG but not with chicken IgY. They further pointed out that this advantage would extend to other types of immunoassay, including nephelometry, and also avoid problems due to protein A, protein G or anti-human IgG, which are often used as labelled second antibodies.

Viruses, Bacteria and Parasites

Yolk antibodies have proved to be suitable for the detection of an extensive range of pathogenic microorganisms and their products (Table 3.5). For example, they have been used for the detection of plant viruses, in enzyme-linked immunosorbent assays (ELISA), and made possible some 3000 assays per day for citrus tristeza virus in an orange grove eradication programme (Bar-Joseph and Malkinson 1980).

Avian antibodies extracted from egg yolk are used extensively in clinical practice for rapid viral diagnosis. The large amounts available allow for detailed quality control and distribution to many laboratories for a prolonged

Table 3.5. Avian antibodies produced to date

	Reference
To haptens	
Dinitrophenyl (DNP)	Gallagher & Voss (1969)
PGE_2, PGF_2, 6-keto-$PGF_1\alpha$ and thromboxane B_2	Fertel et al. (1981)
1,25-dihydroxyvitamin D	Bauwens et al. (1987)
To macromolecules	
Diphtheria toxin	Dzierjgowski (1901), Fraser et al. (1933)
Bovine serum albumin (BSA)	Patterson et al. (1962)
Human serum albumin (HSA)	French et al. (1970), Polson et al. (1980b), Losch et al. (1986)
Haemocyanin	Polson et al. (1980b)
Amandin	Polson et al. (1980b)
Tetanus toxoid	Polson et al. (1980b)
Venoms from *Bitis arietans* and *Naja nivea*	Polson et al. (1980b)
Calf thymus RNA polymerase	Carroll & Stollar (1983)
Human IgG and IgM	Altschuh et al. (1984)
Rabbit IgG	Altschuh et al. (1984)
Human parathyroid hormone fragments 1–34 and 53–84	Vieira et al. (1984)
Kallikrein	Burger et al. (1985)
Alpha subunit of insulin receptor	Song et al. (1985)
Human transferrin	Kint et al. (1987), Ntakarutimana et al. (1992)
Venoms from *Crotalus atrox* and scorpion	Thalley & Carroll (1990)
Mixture of venoms from *C. atrox, C. adamanteus* and *Agkistrodon contortrix*	Thalley & Carroll (1990)
Venoms from *C. durissus terrificus, Trimeresurus flavoviridis* and *A. halys*	Carroll et al. (1992)
Proliferating cell nuclear antigen	Gassmann et al. (1990)
Cell-associated glucosyltransferase	Hamada et al. (1991)
Rat liver cytosolic casein kinase II	Goueli et al. (1990)
C-terminal peptide of alpha tubulin from *Arabidopsis thaliana*	McCune et al. (1992)
To viruses	
Newcastle virus	Brandley et al. (1946)
Influenza virus type A	Patterson et al. (1962), Gardner & Kaye (1982)
Rous sarcomavirus	Aulisio & Shelokov (1967)
Citrus tristeza virus and tobacco mosaic virus	Bar-Joseph & Malkinson (1980)
Eight different plant viruses	Polson et al. (1980a)
Rotavirus	Bartz et al. (1980), Yolken et al. (1988), Hiraga et al. (1990)

Table 3.5. (*cont.*)

	Reference
To viruses cont.	
Influenza virus type B, parainfluenza virus 1 and 3	Gardner & Kaye (1982)
Adenovirus group antigen	Gardner & Kaye (1982)
Respiratory syncytial virus	Zrein et al. (1986)
Canine distemper virus	Schmidt et al. (1989a)
To bacteria and parasites	
Amoebiasis antigen	Polson et al. (1980b)
Mycoplasma gallisepticum	Glisson & Kleven (1984)
Echinococcus granulosus	Gottstein & Hemmeler (1985)
Brucella abortus	Losch et al. (1986)
E. coli	Shimizu et al. (1988), Kuhlmann et al. (1988)
Four different ruminal bacteria	Ricke et al. (1988)
Toxoplasma gondii protein	Hassl & Aspock (1988)
Salmonella typhimurium	Schiemann & Montgomery (1991)
Chlamydiae	Kunz et al. (1991)

period (Gardner and Kaye 1982). Another advantage is that viruses are often cultured in eggs prior to their use for immunization, so that the presence of any contaminating macromolecules will not elicit an immune response in hens, whereas they would in mammals. Such antibodies have been used with a fluorophore label (Gardner and Kaye 1982), while Zrein et al. (1986) used IgY directed against the nucleocapsid of respiratory syncytial virus to develop a very sensitive indirect immunoenzymometric assay to detect the virus in nasal secretions from children. The latter authors also noted that the IgY obtained from just ten eggs was sufficient for more than one million assays. Egg-derived antibodies have been used for immunohistochemistry to detect canine distemper virus in brain (Schmidt et al. 1989a) and chlamydia in formalin-fixed paraffin sections (Kunz et al. 1991).

Based on studies with *Echinococcus granulosus*, Gottstein and Hemmeler (1985) concluded that chicken egg IgY was excellent for diagnostic parasitology and their use has been extended to bacteriology. For example, Shimizu et al. (1988) raised such antibodies against a virulent strain of *E. coli*, which had been pre-treated with formalin, for use in a simple ELISA based on microtitre plates coated with lipopolysaccharide and rabbit anti-chicken IgY labelled with alkaline phosphatase.

For Therapeutic Purposes

There is considerable interest worldwide in the therapeutic potential of exogenous antibodies (Table 3.4). They are being used to bring radionuclides and toxic molecules, such as ricin, into the immediate environment of tumour cells, but probably only monoclonal antibodies are of a specificity adequate to bind onto the surface antigens of particular cell types and thereby deliver "magic bullets". Any type of antibody can be employed for extracorporeal use, provided it is available in adequate amounts, can be covalently coupled to an insoluble support without loss of activity and binds to the circulating analyte of concern with adequate specificity and affinity. There is no mention in the literature of the use of yolk-derived IgY for this purpose, but it should be noted that they avoid the theoretical risk of slow virus transfer.

The use of egg-derived antibodies for systemic and especially oral use will be considered separately.

Systemic Use

Antibodies can bind to and neutralize the toxic effects of molecules such as botulinus toxin or drugs. They can bind to microorganisms to prevent their attachment to gastrointestinal cells or to cause their aggregation or destruction by macrophages and complement within the body. Exogenous antibodies for therapeutic purposes were first introduced in 1891 by Von Behring and Kasato. Serum derived from horses previously immunized with diphtheria or tetanus toxoid was shown to provide passive immunity and significantly improve the prognosis of patients with diphtheria and tetanus respectively. This approach was soon extended to the treatment of snake envenomation by Calmette (1894) and there are now more than 70 centres worldwide that provide equine antibodies or antibody fragments directed against the toxic components of most snake, spider and scorpion venoms.

Studies conducted by Polson et al. (1980b) showed that yolk-derived IgY from hens immunized with tetanus toxoid protected mice against the lethal effects of tetanus toxin. However, they were unable to produce neutralizing avian antibodies against venoms from the puff-adder (*Bitis arietans*) or Cape cobra (*Naja nivea*) in contrast to rabbits, which produced highly effective antivenoms. Recently, Thalley and Carroll (1990) have successfully raised IgY against the venom of *Crotalus atrox* (rattlesnake) and a scorpion, which protected mice against multiple lethal amounts of both venoms. They recorded that their product had a specific activity some 20-fold that of an equine counterpart, which, unlike IgG(T) derived from horses, will not cause complement-mediated side-effects because complement does not bind to the Fc part of IgY. They are also immunizing hens with a mixture of venoms with the aim of providing a polyspecific avian antivenom for use in the USA (Carroll et al. 1992).

As discussed earlier, it is possible to produce kilogram quantities of yolk-derived antibodies at low cost. This raises the important question of whether such IgY may become the preferred treatment for envenomation, drug overdose, septic shock and similar clinical states. Such antibodies do not appear to have been given systemically to man and there are several reasons for advising caution. Thus, many subjects are allergic to egg proteins (Langeland 1983) and, as discussed earlier, IgY will probably prove to be more immunogenic than mammalian IgG and, especially, ovine Fab. Nonetheless, studies are required to compare the immunogenicity of IgY with that of ovine Fab and to determine the incidence of egg protein allergies in the general population.

Gastrointestinal Use

There is an extensive and rapidly increasing literature indicating that yolk-derived antibodies have enormous potential for the prevention and/or treatment of a wide range of gastrointestinal infections. Its oral administration will not be associated with any side-effects, in contrast to the use of many antibiotics. Furthermore, its low cost opens up the veterinary as well as the medical market and the developing as well as the developed world. Whole egg suspensions from appropriately immunized hens may prove to be suitable to curtail epidemics and protect those at risk (such as the immunocompromised and very young) from gastrointestinal infections when entering a new environment, such as a hospital or play school. As discussed in the introduction, this appears to have been appreciated for many centuries because it is the custom of many farmers to feed raw eggs, often in milk, to animals with scours.

Rotavirus infection is one of the most common causes of morbidity throughout the world and is responsible for over one million deaths per year in infants and young children. In 1980 Bartz et al. immunized hens with a simian strain of rotavirus and showed that IgY extracted from their egg yolks prevented epidemic diarrhoea in 3-day-old mice given 5000 infective doses of murine rotavirus. Yolk extracts from non-immunized hens were ineffective. It was subsequently reported that over 95% of individual eggs in the USA and all pasteurized egg pools contain low but significant levels of IgY directed against rotavirus, which infects virtually all hens. Furthermore, even after pasteurization these antibodies bound to and inhibited viral growth in culture and cross-reacted with human strains (Yolken et al. 1988). The Mount Sinai group further found that immunizing the hens with rotavirus produced a considerable increase in antibody levels, which, as above, could protect young mice against rotavirus gastroenteritis. Such antibodies can also protect specific pathogen-free cats against a human strain (strain 3) of rotavirus (Hiraga et al. 1990), leading to the statement that ". . . continuous administration of chicken egg yolk immunoglobulins would provide a rational means of protection . . .".

All reports to date suggest that avian antibodies, like their equivalent IgG in colostrum or serum-derived products, are effective in preventing rotaviral enteritis but not in its treatment.

Some of the most important recent work on the use of IgY relates to the production of such antibodies against virulent strains of *E. coli* and indicates that they are effective for both prevention and treatment. Hens immunized with formalin-treated virulent *E. coli* have been shown to transfer specific IgY into the yolk, which binds to these bacteria and causes their aggregation and inhibits multiplication (Shimizu et al. 1988). In a series of studies in Munich, hens were immunized with four different strains of inactivated *E. coli*, with the production of specific IgY directed against pili antigens. These were extracted from egg yolk, purified by affinity chromatography and used to develop a simple, sensitive ELISA. It was noted that specific antibody levels increased rapidly to very high values, which were maintained for a prolonged period (Kuhlmann et al. 1988). It was stressed that there was no need to isolate IgY for oral consumption and that a "cocktail" of eggs could be formulated, collected from hens immunized with different pathogens. For example, diarrhoea in piglets is usually due to *E. coli*, rotavirus or coronavirus but may on occasion follow infection with transmissible gastroenteritis, enteric viral diarrhoea or *Salmonella*. The authors commented that hens produced about 20 times more antibody per kilogram of body weight than a cow and that eggs were an inexpensive alternative to providing passive immunity with colostrum or a serum-based product, and concluded "In human medicine it could be imaginable to use egg antibodies . . . in the event of epidemics (typhoid, cholera) after natural catastrophies. Further clinical applications for egg yolk antibodies could be the protection of low birth weight or immunodeficient infants . . .".

In the second of their series of papers, the Munich group showed that suspensions of whole eggs were more resistant to heat, acid and enzymatic degradation than yolk suspensions, which they attributed in part to the fact that egg white contains protease inhibitors (Schmidt et al. 1989b). They noted that, even in 1893, Klemperer was adding sodium bicarbonate to neutralize gastric acid when giving antibodies in goats' milk and that, more recently, magnesium and aluminium hydroxide were being used for this purpose (Tacket et al. 1988). Finally, they pointed out that enzymatic cleavage of IgY to $F(ab')_2$ or Fab would not be detrimental and concluded that ". . . the application of egg suspension is to be preferred to that of globulin fractions or antibody isolates. This will also have financial and technical advantages." This was proved in the next paper, based on the use of piglets with artificial jejunal fistulae, which allowed direct sampling from the gut (Wiedemann et al. 1990). Thus no IgY could be detected following oral administration of purified IgY or a yolk suspension, but large amounts were present if egg white was added or whole egg suspensions used, which they attributed to the fact that egg white contains powerful enzyme inhibitors. Addition of sodium bicarbonate to whole egg suspension resulted in a 40% increase in jejunal IgY levels. Lysozyme, avidin and ovatransferrin present in egg white all have antibacterial properties, while ovamucoid inhibits porcine (but not human) trypsin and other ovinhibitors offer IgY protection against both trypsin and chymotrypsin.

Subsequently the Munich group (Jungling et al. 1991) showed that specific IgY markedly inhibited the adhesion of enterotoxigenic *E. coli* to isolated porcine enterocytes and, in the final paper (Wiedemann et al. 1991), demonstrated the beneficial effects of whole egg lyophilisates from hens immunized with *E. coli* in a successful series of trials. Giving the equivalent of one egg twice daily for 3–9 days protected piglets against multiple oral doses of pathogenic *E. coli* and was as effective as giving a mixture of wide-spectrum antibiotics. In the first of two field trials, 92% of 299 piglets, aged 2–14 days and with *E. coli*-induced diarrhoea, were rapidly cured by administration of 4 g daily of whole egg lyophilisate. In a second trial, all 37 piglets given the lyophilisate were rapidly cured, whereas 21 piglets given egg yolks from non-immunized hens were no better until given antibiotics (necessitated by the death of one piglet).

Perhaps the most surprising study in this context related to the prevention of dental caries by yolk-derived IgY from suitable immunized hens. In a project involving over 1100 hens, Hamada et al. (1991) showed that chicken antibodies produced against cell-associated glucosyltransferase from *Streptococcus mutans* effectively blocked the catalytic activity of this enzyme, prevented adherence of the bacteria to smooth surfaces, and significantly reduced plaque formation and dental caries in rats fed a high sucrose diet.

Alternatives to Avian Antibodies for Therapy

Various important questions arise with regard to the oral use of IgY. Do yolk antibodies and especially egg white proteins cross the gastrointestinal tract in the first few days of life or during gastrointestinal infections and thereby induce allergic effects in some subjects? It has been recommended that ". . . further studies are required before IgY becomes a common additive for human products . . ." (Shimizu et al. 1988). Yolken et al. (1988) have echoed this concern for the newborn but concluded that, for example, passive immunity directed against rotaviral infection is required by older subjects and noted that the ability to pasteurize egg products without impairing IgY activity is an obvious advantage. It is also important to consider the various alternatives to IgY that are available for the prevention and/or treatment of gastroenteritis.

Antibiotics are used frequently, but are ineffective against viruses, may lead to the development of resistant strains of bacteria, and often cause side-effects, including diarrhoea. Murine monoclonal antibodies have been shown to be effective in protecting against pathogenic strains of *E. coli* (Sherman et al. 1983). However, their specificity may be a disadvantage and their cost prohibitive for oral use. Others have successfully used serum-derived antibodies from appropriately immunized animals for this purpose and as the basis for various colostrum supplements. Very high circulating antibody levels can be achieved at reasonable cost, but unprocessed serum is not suitable for oral use. It is unpalatable and often induces diarrhoea, probably due to the presence of small molecular weight peptides. The need to take blood, separate off the red cells and then partially purify the immunoglobulin fraction adds considerably to costs, which is important especially with regard to veterinary products.

Mammals obtain gastrointestinal passive immunity during the first few hours of life by orally ingesting colostrum and thereafter milk. Characteristically, colostrum contains large amounts of IgG and has been used successfully to protect infants against viral infection. However, supplies of colostrum are limited and calves are usually born outside normal working hours and are remarkably adept at obtaining all available supplies. The high lipid content of colostrum is also apt to cause diarrhoea. Conversely, milk is available in virtually limitless amounts at relatively low cost and is a potential competitor to IgY. The dominant immunoglobulin found in milk (as opposed to colostrum) is IgA, which, with its secretory unit, is more resistant to acid denaturation and enzymatic cleavage than IgG (Lindh 1975). Milk is also easy to pasteurize and spray-dry, but on the debit side, its immunoglobulin concentration is much lower than an egg's and production and distribution costs may be greater. Many groups have used milk to treat gastrointestinal infections. For example, Tacket et al. (1988) protected all volunteers against oral doses of pathogenic *E. coli* by means of a milk immunoglobulin concentrate from cows immunized with this bacteria. Subsequently this group (Tacket et al. 1992) was successful in a similar approach to the prevention of dysentery due to *Shigella flexneri*.

A careful comparison of milk- and egg-derived antibodies is required as to their efficacy in treating and/or preventing gastrointestinal infections, their relative cost, and their safety. Thus it remains to be determined if it is the raw eggs, the milk or both that has led for many centuries to farmers adopting such treatment for animals with scours.

References

Altschuh D, Hannache G, van Regenmortel MHV (1984) Determination of IgG and IgM levels in serum by rocket immunoelectrophoresis using yolk antibodies from immunized chickens. J Immunol Meth 69: 1–7

Aulisio CG, Shelokov A (1967) Substitution of egg yolk for serum in indirect fluorescence assay for Rous sarcoma virus antibody. Proc Soc Exp Biol Med 126: 312–315

Bade H, Stegemann H (1984) Rapid method of extraction of antibodies from hen egg yolk. J Immunol Meth 72: 421–426

Bar-Joseph M, Malkinson M (1980) Hen egg yolk as a source of antiviral antibodies in the enzyme-linked immunoassay (ELISA): A comparison of two plant viruses. J Virol Meth 1: 179–183

Bartz CR, Conklin RH, Tunstall CB et al. (1980) Prevention of murine rotavirus infection with chicken egg yolk immunoglobulins. J Infect Dis 142: 439–441

Bauwens RM, Devos MP, Kinit JA et al. (1988) Chicken egg yolk and rabbit serum compared as sources of antibody for radioimmunoassay of 1,25-dihydroxyvitamin D in serum or plasma. Clin Chem 34: 2153–2154

Bauwens RM, Kint JA, Devos MP et al. (1987) Production, purification and characterization of antibodies to 1,25-dihydroxyvitamin D raised in chicken egg yolk. Clinica Chimica Acta 170: 37–44

Benedict A, Hersh RT, Larson C (1963) The temporal synthesis of chicken antibodies. J Immunol 91: 795–802

Brandley CA, Moses HE, Jungherr EL (1946) Transmission of antiviral activity via the egg and the role of congenital passive immunity to Newcastle disease in chickens. Poultry Sci 25: 397–398

Burger D, Ramus MA, Schapira M (1985) Antibodies to human plasma kallikrein from egg yolks of an immunized hen: Preparation and characterization. Thromb Res 40: 283–288

Calmette A (1894) Proprietes du serum des animaux immunises contre le venin des serpents, et therapeutique de l'envenimation. CR Acad 68: 720–725

Carroll SB, Stollar BD (1983) Antibodies to calf thymus RNA polymerase II from egg yolks of immunized hens. J Biol Chem 258: 24–26

Carroll SB, Thalley BS, Theakston RDG, Laing G (1992) A comparison of the purity and efficacy of affinity purified avian antivenoms with commercial equine crotalid antivenoms. Toxicon 30: 1017–1025

Dawson GJ, Chang PW, Yates VJ et al. (1980) Neutralizing antibodies to CELO and avian adenovirus-associated viruses in the albumen of chicken eggs. Avian Dis 24: 890–895

Dzierjgowski MSK (1901) Contribution a l'etude de l'heredite dans l'immunite artificielle vis-a-vis de la diptherie. Arch Sci Biol 8: 429–440

Fertel R, Yetiv JZ, Coleman MA et al. (1981) Formation of antibodies to prostaglandins in the yolk of chicken eggs. Biochem Biophys Res Comm 102:1028–1033

Fraser DT, Jukes TH, Branion HD et al. (1934) The inheritance of diptheria immunity in ducks. J Immunol 26: 437–446

French VI, Stark JM, White RG (1970) The influence of adjuvants on the immunological response of the chicken. Immunology 18: 645–655

Gallagher JS, Voss EW (1969) Molecular weight of a purified chicken antibody. Immunochemistry 6: 199–206

Gardner PS, Kaye S (1982) Egg globulins in rapid virus diagnosis. J Virol Meth 4: 257–262

Gassmann M, Thommes P, Weiser T et al. (1990) Efficient production of chicken egg yolk antibodies against a conserved mammalian protein. FASEB J 4: 2528–2532

Glisson JR, Kleven SH (1984) *Mycoplasma gallisepticum* vaccination: Effects on egg transmission and egg production. Avian Dis 28: 406–415
Gottstein B, Hemmeler E (1985) Egg yolk immunoglobulin Y as an alternative antibody in the serology of echinococcosis. Z Parasitenkd 71: 273–276
Goueli SA, Hanten J, Davis A et al. (1990) Polyclonal antibodies against rat liver cytosolic casein kinase II (CK-2) cross-react with CK-2 from tissues and nuclear form (PK-NZ) of the enzyme. Biochem Int 21: 685–694
Hamada S, Horikoshi T, Minami T et al. (1991) Oral passive immunization against dental caries in rats by use of hen egg yolk antibodies specific for cell-associated glucosyltransferase of *Streptococcus mutans*. Infect Immun 59: 4161–4167
Hassl A, Aspock H (1988) Purification of egg yolk immunoglobulins. J Immunol Meth 110: 225–228
Hatta H, Kim M, Yamamoto T (1990) A novel isolation method for hen egg yolk antibody, "IgY". Agric Biol Chem 54: 2531–2535
Hiraga C, Kodama Y, Sugiyama T et al. (1990) Prevention of human rotavirus infection with chicken egg yolk immunoglobulins containing rotavirus antibody in cat. Kansenshogaku-Zasshi 64: 118–123
Hurn BA, Chantler SM (1980) Production of reagent antibodies. Methods Enzymol 70: 104–142
Jensenius JC, Andersen I, Hau J et al. (1981) Eggs: Conveniently packaged antibodies. Methods for purification of yolk IgG. J Immunol Meth 46: 63–68
Jungling A, Wiedemann V, Kuhlmann R et al. (1991) Chicken egg antibodies for prophylaxis and therapy of infectious intestinal diseases. IV. In vitro studies on protective effects against adhesion of enterotoxigenic *Escherichia coli* to isolated enterocytes. J Vet Med B 38: 373–381
Kint JA, Huys A, Leroy JG (1987) Egg yolk antibody for nephelometric immunoassay of transferrin in human serum. Arch Int Phys Biochem 95: B215
Klemperer F (1893) Über natürliche Immunität und ihre Verwertung für die Immunisierungstherapie. Arch Expl Pathol Pharmakol 31: 356–382
Kramer TT, Cho HC (1970) Transfer of immunoglobulins and antibodies in the hen's egg. Immunology 19: 157–167
Kuhlmann R, Wiedemann V, Schmidt P et al. (1988) Chicken egg antibodies for prophylaxis and therapy of infectious intestinal diseases. I. Immunization and antibody determination. J Vet Med B 35: 610–616
Kunz US, Pospischil A, Paccaud MF (1991) Immunohistochemical detection of chlamydiae in formalin-fixed tissue sections: Comparison of a monoclonal antibody with yolk derived antibodies. Zent Vet B 38: 292–298
Langeland T (1983) A clinical and immunological study of allergy to hens' egg white. Allergy 38: 399–412
Larsson A, Sjoquist J (1988) Chicken antibodies: A tool to avoid false positive results by rheumatoid factor in latex fixation tests. J Immunol Meth 108: 205–208
Leslie GA, Clem LW (1969) Phylogeny of immunoglobulin structure and function. J Exp Med 130: 1337–1352
Lindh E (1975) Increased resistance of immunoglobulin A dimers to proteolytic degradation after binding of secretory component. J Immunol 114: 284–286
Loeken MR, Roth TF (1983) Analysis of maternal IgG subpopulations which are transported into the chicken oocyte. Immunology 49: 21–28
Losch U, Schranner I, Wanke R et al. (1986) The chicken egg, an antibody source. J Vet Med B 33: 609–619
McCune C, Goddard RH, Cho SO, Wick SM (1992) Use of the lipid emulsion system and *Salmonella typhimurium* mitogen adjuvant to stimulate IgG production in chickens. J Immunol Meth 155: 267–270
Ntakarutimana V, Demedts P, von Sande M, Scharpe S (1992) A simple and economical strategy for downstream processing of specific antibodies to human transferrin from egg yolk. J Immunol Meth 153: 133–140
Orlans E (1967) Fowl antibody. VIII. A comparison of natural, primary and secondary antibodies to erythrocytes in hen sera, their transmission to yolk and chick. Immunology 12: 27–37
Patterson R, Younger JS, Weigle WO et al. (1962) Antibody production and transfer to egg yolk in chickens. J Immunol 89: 272–278

Polson A, Coetzer T, Kruger J et al. (1985) Improvements in the isolation of IgY from the yolks of eggs laid by immunized hens. Immunol Invest 14: 323–327

Polson A, von Wechmar MB, Fazakerley G (1980b) Antibodies to proteins from yolk of immunized hens. Immunol Comm 9: 495–514

Polson A, von Wechmar MB, van Regenmortel MHV (1980a) Isolation of viral IgY antibodies from yolks of immunized hens. Immunol Comm 9: 475–493

Ricke SC, Schaefer DM, Cook ME, Kang KH (1988) Differentiation of ruminal bacterial species by enzyme-linked immunosorbent assay using egg yolk antibodies from immunized chicken hens. Appl Environ Microbiol 54: 596–599

Rose ME, Orlans E, Buttress N (1974) Immunoglobulin classes in the hen's egg: Their segregation in yolk and white. Eur J Immunol 4: 521–523

Schiemann DA, Montgomery AL (1991) Immune responses in chickens against *Salmonella typhimurium* monitored with egg antibodies. Vet Microbiol 27: 295–308

Schmidt P, Hafner A, Reubel GH et al. (1989a) Production of antibodies to canine distemper virus in chicken eggs for immunohistochemistry. J Vet Med B 36: 661–668

Schmidt P, Wiedemann V, Kuhlmann R et al. (1989b) Chicken egg antibodies for prophylaxis and therapy of infectious intestinal diseases. II. In vitro studies on gastric and enteric digestion of egg yolk antibodies specific against pathogenic *Escherichia coli* strains. J Vet Med B 36: 619–628

Sherman DM, Acres SD, Sadowski PL et al. (1983) Protection of calves against fatal enteric colibacillosis by orally administered *Escherichia coli* K99-specific monoclonal antibody. Infect Immun 42: 653–658

Shimizu M, Fitzsimmons RC, Nakai S (1988) Anti-*E. coli* immunoglobulin Y isolated from egg yolk of immunized chickens as a potential food ingredient. J Food Sci 53: 1360–1366

Song CS, Yu JH, Bai DH et al. (1985) Antibodies to the alpha-subunit of insulin receptor from eggs of immunized hens. J Immunol 135: 3354–3359

Tacket CO, Binion SB, Bostwick E et al. (1992) Efficacy of bovine milk immunoglobulin concentrate in preventing illness after *Shigella flexneri* challenge. Am J Trop Med Hyg 47: 276–283

Tacket CO, Losonsky G, Link H et al. (1988) Protection by milk immunoglobulin concentrate against oral challenge with enterotoxigenic *Escherichia coli*. N Engl J Med 318: 1240–1243

Tam LQ, Benedict AA (1975) Elevated 7S immunoglobulin and acute phase proteins in adjuvant-injected chickens. Proc Soc Exp Biol Med 150: 340–346

Thalley BS, Carroll SB (1990) Rattlesnake and scorpion antivenoms from the egg yolks of immunized hens. Biotechnology 8: 934–938

Vieira JGH, Oliveira MAD, Russo EMK, Maciel RMB, Pereira AB (1984) Egg yolk as a source of antibodies for human parathyroid hormone (hPTH) radioimmunoassay. J Immunoassay 5: 121–129

Wiedemann V, Kuhlmann R, Schmidt P et al. (1990) Chicken egg antibodies for prophylaxis and therapy of infectious intestinal diseases. III. In vivo tenacity test in piglets with artificial jejunal fistula. J Vet Med B 37: 163–172

Wiedemann V, Linckh E, Kuhlmann R et al. (1991) Chicken egg antibodies for prophylaxis and therapy of infectious intestinal diseases. V. In vivo studies on protective effects against *Escherichia coli* diarrhoea in pigs. J Vet Med B 38: 283–291

Yolken RH, Leister F, Wee SB et al. (1988) Antibodies to rotaviruses in chickens' eggs: A potential source of antiviral immunoglobulins suitable for human consumption. Pediatrics 81: 291–295

Zrein M, Obert G, van Regenmortel MHV (1986) Use of egg-yolk antibody for detection of respiratory syncytial virus in nasal secretions by ELISA. Arch Virol 90: 197–206

4 Catalytic Antibodies

G. Gallacher

Introduction

In 1986 two groups, working independently, showed that antibody combining sites could do more than simply bind determinants – they could catalyse chemical reactions. These results, together with more recent developments, are reviewed here with particular reference to their implications for the therapeutic potential of catalytic antibodies.

Catalysis via Transition-State Complementarity

The above groups were guided by current understanding of the way enzymes bring about catalysis. Central to this understanding is the theory of transition state stabilization first outlined by Linus Pauling in 1946 and gradually elaborated by other investigators to become the predominant theory of the mechanism of enzyme action (Schowen 1978; Kraut 1988). The enzyme active site is believed to be specifically complementary to the high-energy transition state of a reaction rather than to reactants in the ground state. Preferential binding of the transition state stabilizes this high-energy species and lowers the activation energy of the reaction. Pauling also anticipated the discovery of enzyme inhibitors that structurally resemble transition states such that the enzyme has higher affinity for inhibitor than for substrates. We now refer to these compounds as transition state analogues and their discovery and exploitation to produce therapeutic agents has contributed to the general acceptance of the transition state theory of enzyme catalysis. It is interesting to note that although Pauling referred to antibody binding in his discussion of enzyme inhibition, he did not anticipate the reverse situation – namely, that antibodies with combining sites complementary to analogues of reaction transition states should possess catalytic properties. This hypothesis was put forward by William Jencks in 1969 and it was this principle that guided the two groups in their discovery of catalytic antibodies.

The successful groups were headed by Richard Lerner, at the Research Institute of Scripps Clinic, and by Peter Schultz, at the University of California (Berkeley). Their initial investigations addressed antibody-catalysed hydrolysis of esters and carbonates. The mechanisms of ester hydrolysis, either free in solution or catalysed by enzymes, are among the most intensively studied of all reactions. In solution, base-promoted ester hydrolysis proceeds via a charged tetrahedral transition state (Fig. 4.1) and certain hydrolytic enzymes are believed to preferentially stabilize just such a transition state. These enzymes are inhibited by tetracoordinated organophosphorus compounds bearing a negative charge (Fig. 4.1) (Thorset et al. 1982). Thus organophosphorus compounds are recognized analogues of the transition state involved in ester hydrolysis and, in their quest for catalytic antibodies, the above groups investigated antibodies that bound phosphonate or phosphate esters.

Antibody-Catalysed Hydrolysis of Labile Esters

The Scripps group (Tramontano et al. 1986) synthesized the rather complex phosphonate [1]* and found that monoclonal antibodies raised against this transition state analogue catalysed hydrolysis of the structurally related, though somewhat simpler, ester [2] (Fig. 4.2). The catalysed reaction was monitored by HPLC and shown to follow Michaelis–Menten kinetics, with a Michaelis constant (K_m) of 1.9 μM and a first-order rate constant (k_{cat}, or turnover number) of 0.027 s^{-1}. The rate acceleration provided by the catalyst was almost 1000 times greater than background, as judged by the ratio of the apparent first-order rate constants for catalysed and non-catalysed reactions, $k_{cat}/k_{non\text{-}cat}$. Consistent with preferential binding by the antibodies of the hapten to which they were elicited, the catalysed reaction was inhibited by the phosphonate [3] (Fig. 4.2) with an inhibition constant approximately ten times lower than the Michaelis constant for the substrate [2]. In contrast to enzymes, which are usually tolerant of small changes in substrate structure, antibody-catalysed hydrolysis was shown to be very specific. A range of esters similar to [2] but differing in the aromatic ring substituents was not accepted as substrate by the catalytic antibody; this reflects the highly specific nature of antibody binding. The participation of a histidine imidazole in the catalysis was considered and the possibility of using cofactors, particularly metal ions, to increase the potency of catalytic antibodies was discussed.

The Berkeley group adopted a slightly different approach (Pollack et al. 1986). They investigated the myeloma protein MOPC167, an immunoglobulin A (IgA) molecule that was known to bind nitrophenylphosphorylcholine [4]; this catalysed hydrolysis of the corresponding carbonate [5] (Fig. 4.3). Release of nitrophenolate on hydrolysis greatly facilitates monitoring of this reaction, by following the increase in absorbance at 400 nm. The catalysed reaction showed saturation kinetics and the following parameters were reported:

* The numbers in brackets refer to the numbered structures shown in Figs 4.2–4.5 and Structures 4.1–4.7.

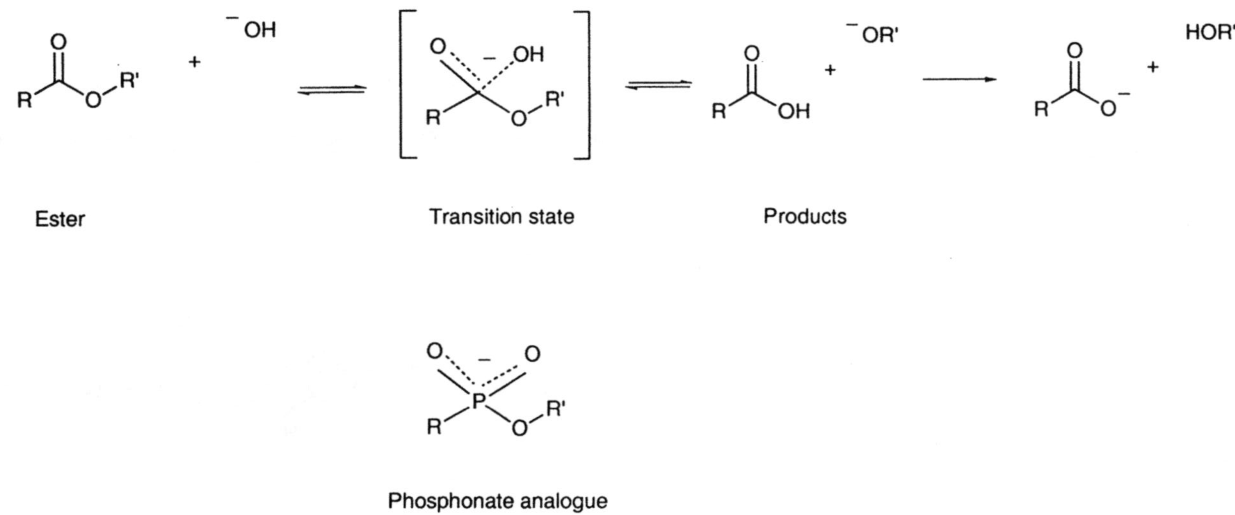

Fig. 4.1. Base-promoted ester hydrolysis proceeds via an unstable tetrahedral transition state carrying a negative charge and tetracoordinated phosphorus compounds bearing a negative charge, such as phosphonate monoesters, provide stable analogues of this high-energy species.

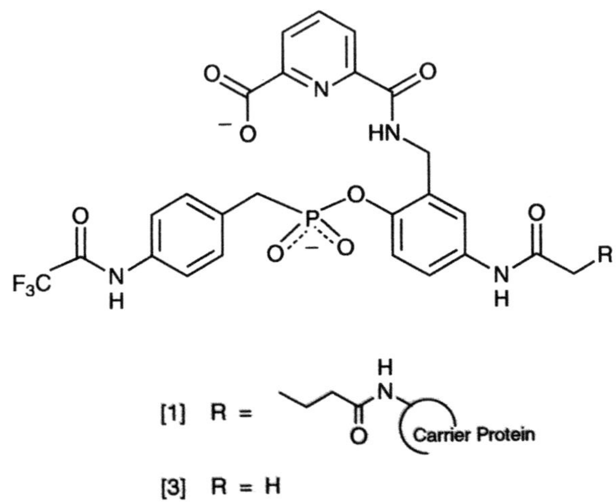

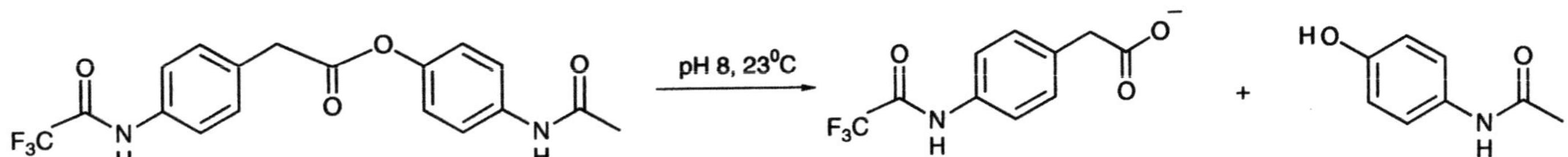

[2]

Fig. 4.2. Monoclonal antibodies elicited by the phosphonate immunogen [1] catalyse hydrolysis of the structurally related, though somewhat simpler, ester [2] and the catalysis is inhibited by the phosphonate [3] (Tramontano et al. 1986).

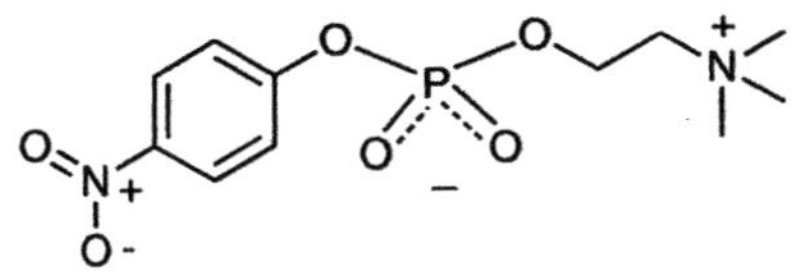

[4]

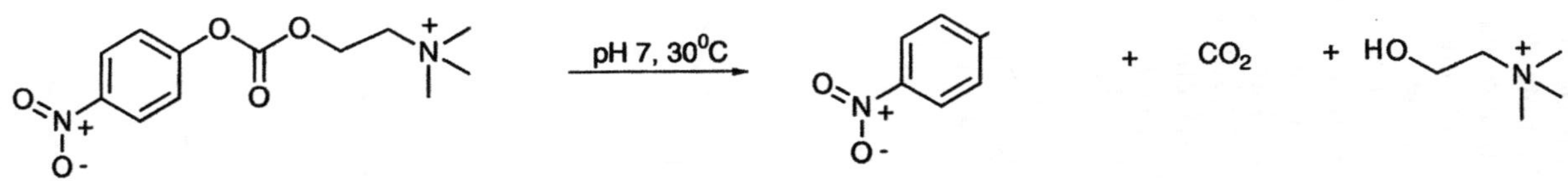

[5]

Fig. 4.3. The myeloma protein MOPC167 binds the choline phosphate [4] and catalyses ıydrolysis of the corresponding choline carbonate [5].

k_{cat}= 0.0067 s^{-1}, K_m = 208 μM, and $k_{cat}/k_{non\text{-}cat}$ = 770. Catalysis was pH dependent with hydroxide ion as a reactant. Evidence was presented implicating a tyrosine residue in the catalysis. The phosphate [4] inhibited the catalysed hydrolysis with an inhibition constant (K_i) of 5 μM.

Having demonstrated catalytic antibodies, both groups recognized that this new development offered the potential of designing and producing novel specific catalysts for use in fundamental research, biotechnology, medicine and industry. Therapeutic applications were suggested almost immediately; for example, Massey (1987) speculated on the development of antibodies to hydrolyse virus coat proteins. Once discovered, developments in this new area have been rapid.

Less than 2 years after their first report the Scripps group (Tramontano et al. 1988) described the production of a monoclonal antibody that catalysed ester hydrolysis with kinetic characteristics similar to those of some enzymes. The antibody (designated 50D8) was raised against the phosphonate [6] (Structure 4.1), which is effectively their original immunogen minus the dipicolinic acid moiety. At pH 8 it was found to catalyse hydrolysis of the ester [7] with a k_{cat} of 20 s^{-1}, a K_m of 1.5 mM, and a $k_{cat}/k_{non\text{-}cat}$ of 6

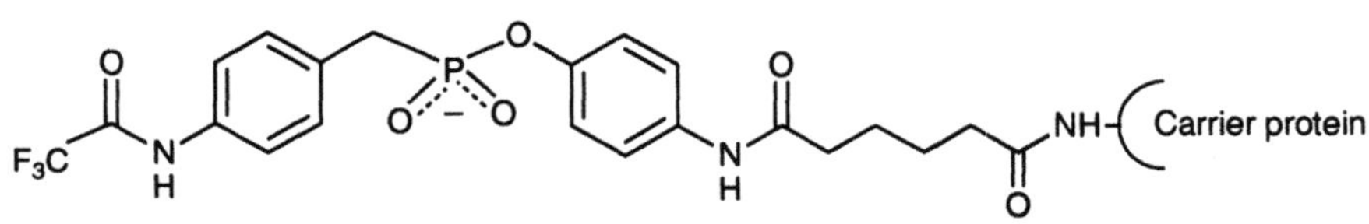

[6]

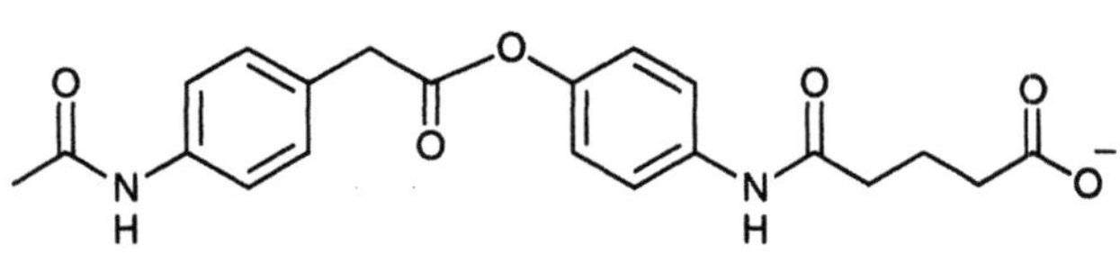

[7]

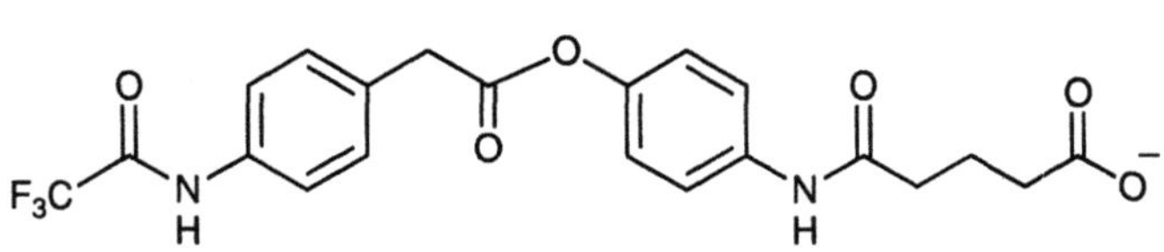

[8]

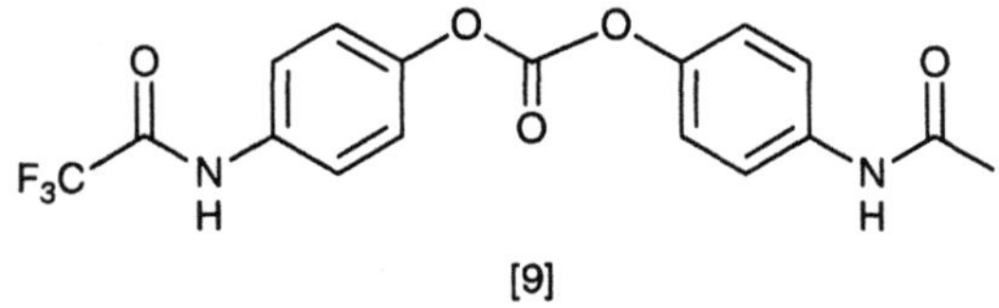

[9]

Structure 4.1

$\times 10^6$. Various experiments implicated tyrosine residues in the mechanism of catalysis. Surprisingly, the ester [8], which more closely resembles the haptenic determinant, exhibited slower turnover ($k_{cat} = 2\ s^{-1}$) and reduced acceleration over background ($k_{cat}/k_{non\text{-}cat} = 1 \times 10^5$). This finding is of considerable importance for the design of catalytic antibodies for specific substrates. Where high rates of turnover are required it may be desirable to optimize binding energy close to the region of the molecule where the reaction occurs and to reduce interactions at distant sites. This may be a difficult balance to achieve in situations in which the substrate is invariant (the situation likely to be encountered in proposed therapeutic applications); investigation of minor variations in immunogen structure is essential. Also noteworthy was the failure of antibody 50D8 to catalyse hydrolysis of the related carbonate [9], which would be expected to be more labile than the esters [7] and [8] (Structure 4.1).

The revelations, firstly of modest catalytic activity in antibodies and subsequently of a catalytic antibody with a turnover number similar to some enzymes, were of immense importance. Investigation of these systems should provide much insight into the mechanisms underlying protein-mediated catalysis. However, though the potential of specific catalytic antibodies for therapeutic and other applications was immediately apparent, the above hydrolyses are of labile aryl esters. Antibodies intended for biotechnological applications will be required to catalyse hydrolysis of more stable compounds such as alkyl esters and amides. It would also be desirable to develop antibodies to catalyse a range of different reactions. Indeed, considerable effort has been concentrated on extending both the power and scope of catalytic antibodies.

Hydrolysis of More-Stable Compounds

Shortly after reporting their results with aryl esters the Scripps group (Janda et al. 1988), in collaboration with Stephen Benkovic at Pennsylvania State University, published details of a monoclonal antibody that catalysed hydrolysis of an aryl amide. The antibody (NPN43C9) was raised against the phosphonamidate immunogen [10] and catalysed hydrolysis, at pH 9, of the nitroanilide [11] (Structure 4.2) with a k_{cat} of 0.001 s^{-1}, a K_m of 562 μM, and a $k_{cat}/k_{non\text{-}cat}$ of 2.5×10^5. This was the first indication that antibodies are able to catalyse hydrolysis of amides and, because many applications can be envisaged for amide hydrolysis (peptide hydrolysis is an example), this result was of great significance. Lerner's group (Janda et al. 1989) and the group headed by Schultz (Pollack et al. 1989) have now raised monoclonal antibodies that catalyse hydrolysis of stable alkyl esters. In each case the catalysed hydrolysis was stereospecific with, in one case, discrimination between R and S enantiomeric substrates and, in the other, between substrates epimeric at one chiral centre. Both groups indicated that such catalysts would be particularly valuable for organic synthesis (e.g. synthesis of chiral drugs). However, it seems equally likely that the ability to hydrolyse unactivated esters with exquisite specificity will be exploited to

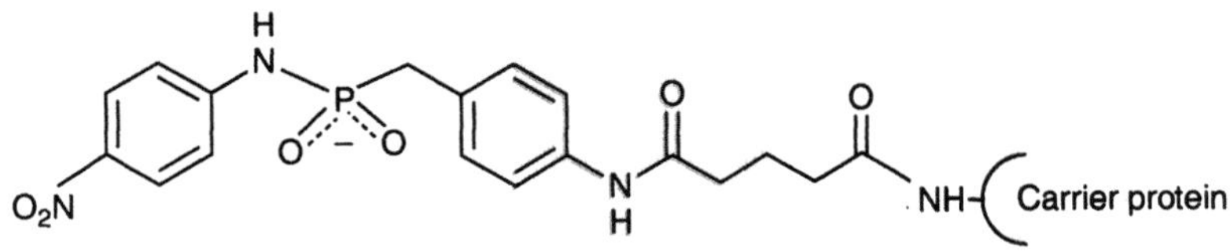

[10]

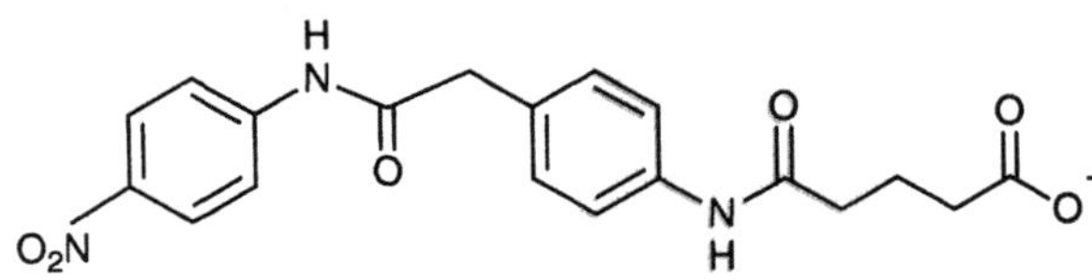

[11]

Structure 4.2

produce novel therapeutic agents (for instance, the activation of prodrugs in vivo).

Catalysis via Other Strategies

Further strategies have been explored in the search for antibodies with catalytic properties. Schultz's group has taken the myeloma antibody MOPC315, which binds 1-substituted 2,4-dinitrophenyl compounds, and introduced imidazole at the binding site. The original antibody recognizes and very slowly hydrolyses reactive esters of 2,4-dinitrophenyl substituted alkylcarboxylic acids. In one approach imidazole was chemically linked to the antibody to give a semisynthetic product (Pollack and Schultz 1989) and, in a second approach, imidazole was introduced via a histidine substitution in a recombinant fragment of the antibody (Baldwin and Schultz 1989). In each case the introduced imidazole produced an increase in the rate of catalysed hydrolysis. The increase was by a factor of approximately 10 for the semisynthetic antibody, and approximately 50 for the recombinant antibody fragment. Lerner's group has pursued the association of metal ion cofactors to increase the power of hydrolytic catalytic antibodies. In one strategy (Iverson and Lerner 1989) a transition metal complex was employed as cofactor. Monoclonal antibodies were raised against the cobalt (III) complex [12] (Fig. 4.4) in which two of the ligand sites are provided by a peptide haptenic determinant. Hydrolytic activity was reported in several antibodies and the activity of one antibody, designated 28F11, was described in detail. This antibody catalysed hydrolysis of the peptide substrates [14]

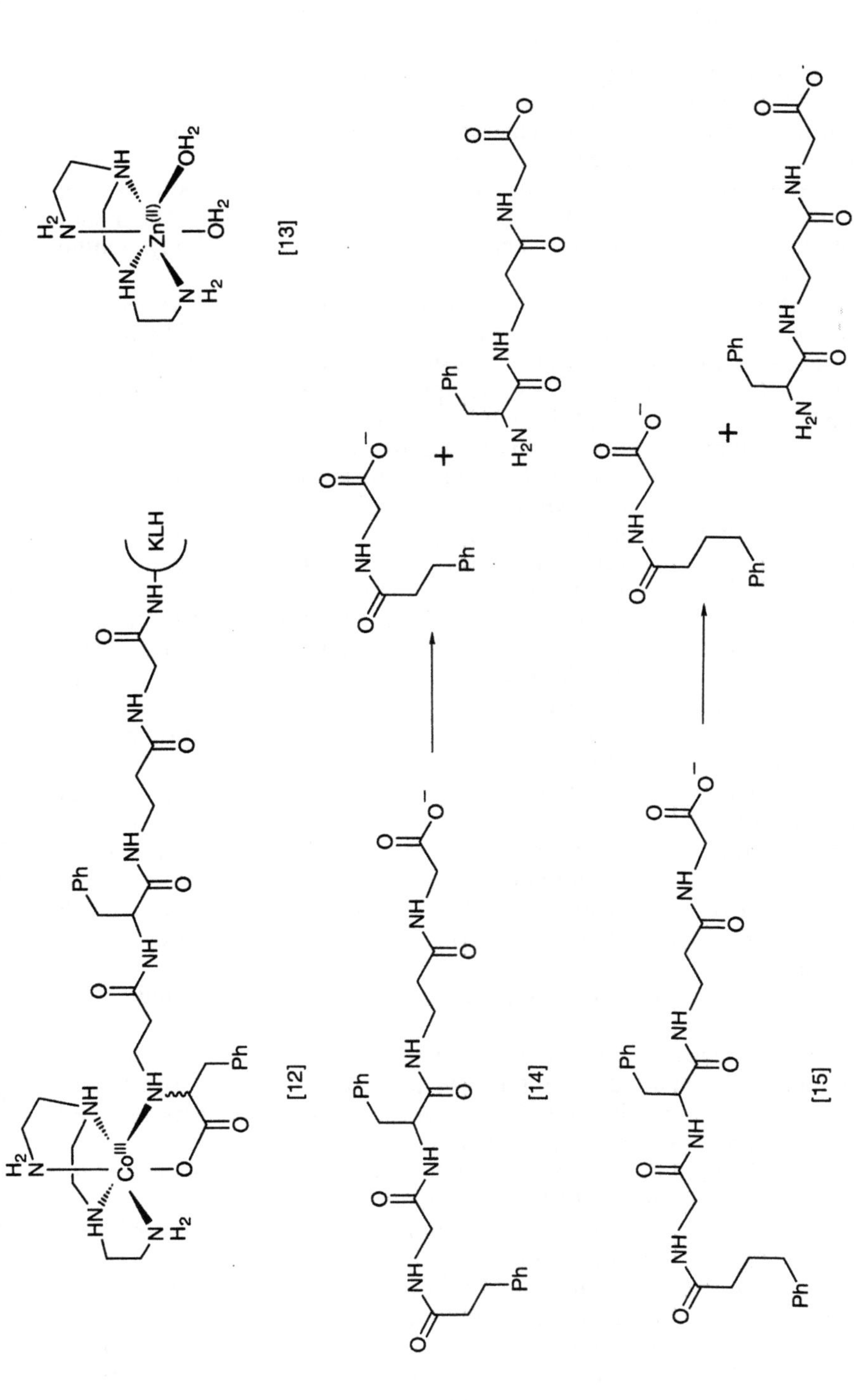

Fig. 4.4. Monoclonal antibodies elicited by the cobalt (III) complex [12], catalyse hydrolysis of the peptide substrates [14] and [15] by using the zinc (II) complex [13] as a cofactor.

and [15] and was dependent on participation of transition metal complexes such as the zinc (II) complex [13] (Fig. 4.4). The reaction was monitored by thin-layer chromatography and the k_{cat} was estimated to be 6×10^{-4} s^{-1} at pH 6.5. The hydrolysis was sequence specific though the particular amide bond hydrolysed was unexpected. Thus the metal complex in the immunogen is replaced by an acyl amino terminus in peptides [14] and [15] and this amide bond was expected to be the site of hydrolysis, whereas the actual site was the next amide in the sequence, between glycine and phenylalanine. This result was attributed to a conformational change bringing the glycine–phenylalanine amide bond near the metal ion.

The importance of the demonstration of alkyl amide hydrolysis transcends the rather slow rate of reaction and lack of control over the site of hydrolysis and is, perhaps, the most important result to date with respect to the potential of catalytic antibodies for therapy. It establishes that antibodies can catalyse hydrolysis of peptide bonds in a sequence-specific manner. A series of small improvements on this theme of metal-ion-assisted antibody catalysis might lead to catalysts with specific proteolytic activity sufficient to fulfil Massey's vision of an antiviral catalytic antibody. One such improvement might be to use a metal complex–peptide determinant involving a transition state analogue rather than the substrate template used in the above example. Lerner's group has, in fact, explored a more audacious approach (Iverson et al. 1990). They have engineered, via site-directed mutagenesis, a metal ion binding site into an antibody combining site. Taking an antibody (4-4-20) known to bind fluorescein as the starting point, three histidine residues were substituted into the light chain to give a metal binding site modelled on carbonic anhydrase B. Expression of the mutant light chain together with the native heavy chain in *Escherichia coli* gave a mutant antibody that simultaneously bound transition metal ions, such as copper (II) and zinc (II), and fluorescein. Evidence for the simultaneous nature of the binding was provided by metal-ion-mediated quenching of fluorescence of antibody-bound fluorescein. Though not catalytic, this system provides a model for future antibody constructs that will bind metal cofactor and substrate and efficiently catalyse hydrolysis and/or redox reactions.

Additional strategies that have provided catalytic antibodies include:

1. The use of charged groups in the haptenic determinant to induce complementary charged groups in the antibody combining site where they can react with substrate (Shokat et al. 1989), sometimes referred to as a "bait and switch" strategy (Janda et al. 1990).
2. The use of alternative transition state analogues such as secondary alcohols (Shokat et al. 1990) that do not carry a charge.
3. The generation of DNA libraries for immunoglobulin V regions of both heavy and light chains and the development of vectors for coexpression of these regions to yield functional Fab fragments from which catalytic Fab can be selected (Huse et al. 1989). Such combinatorial libraries allow screening of the immunological repertoire without prior immunization of an animal. Major advances are anticipated from the merging of these methods with systems that screen directly for catalytic activity rather than binding.

Catalysis of Other Types of Reaction

The scope of reactions catalysed by antibodies has also been greatly increased (cf. Lerner et al. 1991). Two examples are a Claisen rearrangement and a photolytic reaction. The particular Claisen reaction is the rearrangement of chorismate [16] to prephenate [17]. This 3,3-sigmatropic rearrangement is central to the formation of aromatic amino acids in bacteria and other organisms and is catalysed by the enzyme chorismate mutase. There is considerable evidence to suggest that the electrocyclic transition state for this reaction, either free in solution or in the active site of the enzyme, involves a conformation approaching the chairlike bicyclo (3.3.1) structure depicted in Fig. 4.5. Furthermore, the most powerful known inhibitor of chorismate mutase is the bicyclic compound [18]. In March 1988 a group led by Donald Hilvert at Scripps (Hilvert et al. 1988), and Schultz's group (Jackson et al. 1988) both reported that monoclonal antibodies raised against [18] catalysed the rearrangement of chorismate to prephenate. Both groups coupled [18] through the secondary hydroxyl but used slightly different derivatives for conjugation to carrier protein. Hilvert described a rate enhancement above background of approximately 2×10^2, and Schultz of 1×10^4 (the enzyme

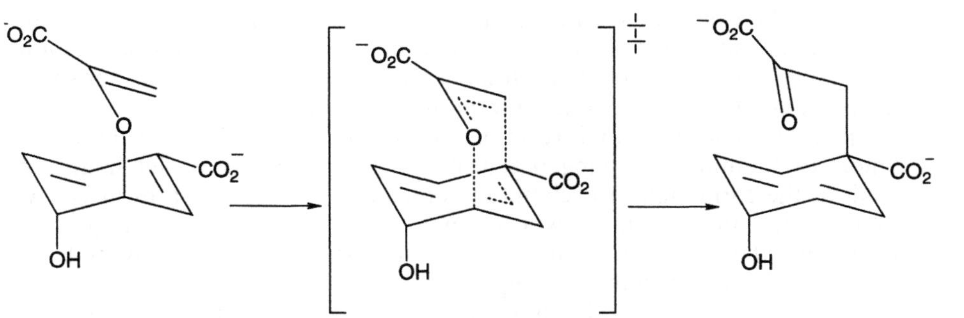

[16] Transition state [17]

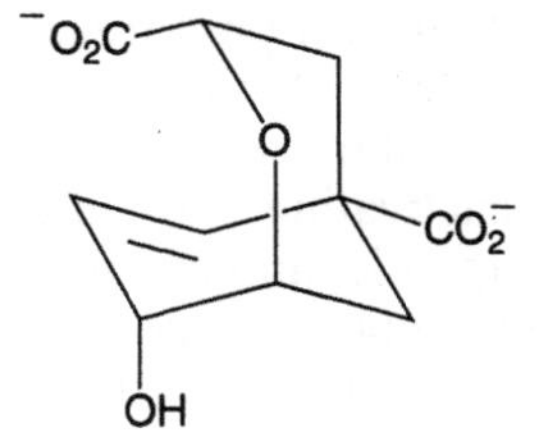

[18]

Fig. 4.5. The 3,3-sigmatropic rearrangement of chorismate [16] to prephenate [17] is believed to proceed via a chairlike bicyclo (3.3.1) transition state, a stable analogue of which is provided by the bicyclic compound [18].

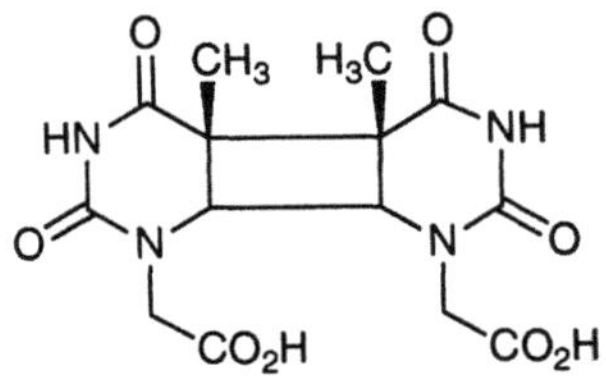

[19]

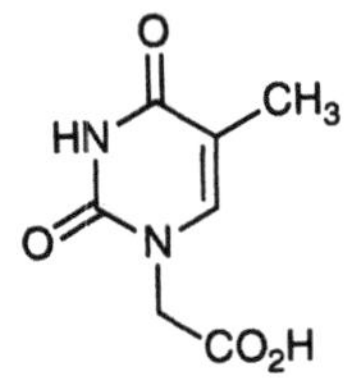

[20]

Structure 4.3

gives an increase of 3×10^6). The Scripps antibody (1F7) has been shown to be enantiospecific with only the natural enantiomer, (−)chorismate, being accepted as a substrate (Hilvert and Nared 1988). Furthermore, Hilvert has introduced the DNA encoding the Fab fragment of the antibody (1F7) into a chorismate mutase-deficient yeast (*Saccharomyces cerevisiae*). Antibody-rescue of the metabolism of the yeast, when grown in medium lacking phenylalanine, was then demonstrated (Tang et al. 1991). This work is clearly pertinent to the therapeutic applications of catalytic antibodies. Within 5 years of their discovery, catalytic antibodies have been shown to substitute for an important enzyme in a living organism. This encourages the suggestion that catalytic antibodies might eventually provide enzyme substitutes for some of the metabolic disorders encountered in medicine.

The catalysis of a photolytic reaction is illustrated by cleavage of cyclobutane dimers of thymine. In living organisms, exposure to ultraviolet light can result in the formation of cyclobutane dimers of pyrimidine bases in DNA. Photoreactivating enzymes, which employ light in the visible region to regenerate the monomers, are one of the instruments used by cells to repair this lesion. Schultz's group has obtained catalytic antibodies with photoreactivating activity (Cochran et al. 1988) raised against an immunogen consisting of the carboxymethylthymine dimer [19] (Structure 4.3) coupled to carrier protein. One of the antibodies was shown to catalyse photolysis of the carboxymethylthymine dimer to give two equivalents of the monomer [20]. Moreover the turnover number (k_{cat} of 1.2 min^{-1} for the antibody compares favourably with that of a photoreactivating enzyme from *E. coli*, DNA photolyase (k_{cat} = 3.4 min^{-1}). Certain rare human cancers are known to have their origins in defects of mechanisms for repair of pyrimidine dimers, and substitution of photoreactivating antibodies for the deficient enzymes is an intriguing possible therapeutic application for catalytic antibodies.

Recently, Schultz's group reported another example of antibody catalysis with possible future implications for the modification of nucleic acids, this time involving hydrolysis of phosphate esters (Scanlan et al. 1991). Antibodies raised against the α-hydroxyphosphonate [21] were reported to catalyse hydrolysis of the phosphate [22] (Structure 4.4). The rate of catalysed hydrolysis was moderate, but the result is significant in extending catalysed hydrolyses to include phosphates. Further progress can be

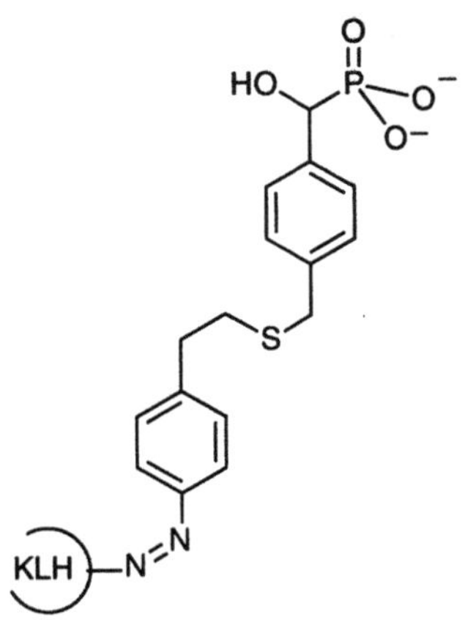

[21]

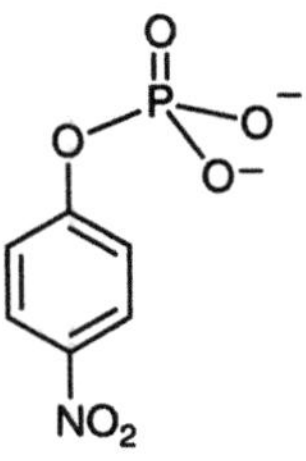

[22]

Structure 4.4

expected with the incorporation of concepts derived from ester and amide hydrolysis.

Polyclonal Catalytic Antibodies

All of the examples of catalytic antibodies discussed so far have been monoclonal. Early attempts (Raso and Stollar 1975) to generate polyclonal catalytic antibodies were discouraging. However, following the successful work of Lerner and Schultz, indications that polyclonal catalytic antibodies could be obtained began to emerge. Polyclonal antibodies were shown to form a template for a photochemical reaction (Balan et al. 1988) and IgG isolated from autoimmune serum from a human subject has been reported to catalyse hydrolysis of vasoactive intestinal peptide (Paul et al. 1989). It would be very surprising if monoclonal antibodies possessed properties not possessed by polyclonal antibodies: our group has shown that very effective polyclonal catalytic antibodies can indeed be generated (Gallacher et al. 1991). Antibodies were raised in sheep against the phosphate [23] and were found to catalyse hydrolysis of the corresponding carbonate [24] (Structure 4.5) with catalytic parameters similar to those reported previously for monoclonal catalytic antibodies. Remarkably, these polyclonal antibodies also catalyse hydrolysis of the corresponding nitroanilide [25] (Gallacher et al. 1992) with kinetic parameters that compare favourably with those of monoclonal antibody NPN43C9-catalysed hydrolysis of the structurally similar nitroanilide [11]. It is pointed out in other chapters that very large quantities of high-quality polyclonal antibodies are easily obtained for therapeutic applications. Our demonstration extends this valuable resource to supplies of catalytic

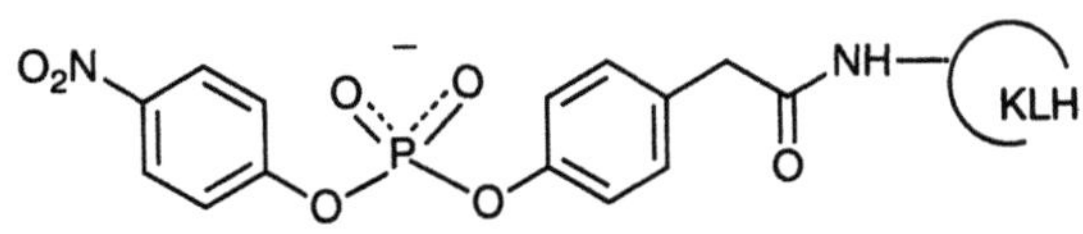

[23]

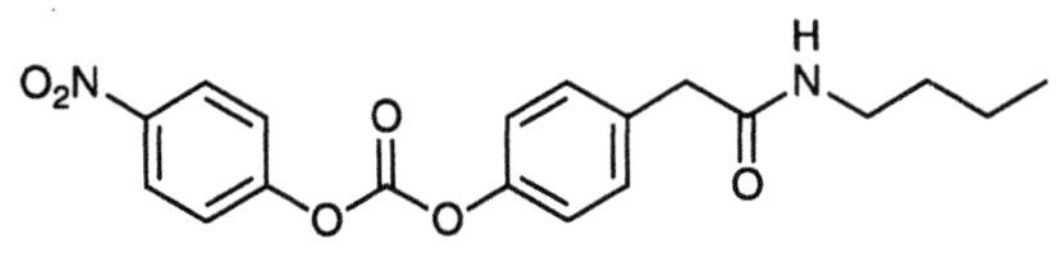

[24]

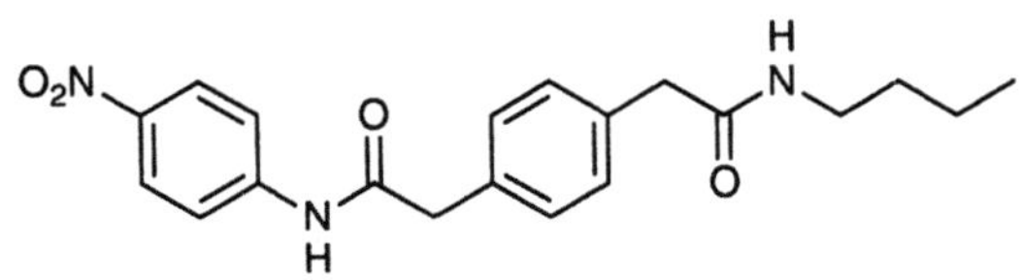

[25]

Structure 4.5

antibodies. Furthermore, in addition to considering passive immunization with catalytic antibodies, we can now consider eliciting the host's own catalytic antibodies via active immunization.

Developing Therapeutic Catalytic Antibodies

Progress in catalytic antibody research has now reached the stage at which several groups are actively pursuing therapeutic applications of these new agents. This is evident from both the patent and the academic literature. Thus, in a patent application published in 1989, Powell et al. described potential therapeutic applications of catalytic antibodies. A difluoroketone analogue of the transition state for peptide hydrolysis presumably hydrated was outlined for the generation of monoclonal antibodies designed to hydrolyse peptide bonds, and therapies based on peptide hydrolysis were indicated. Massey's earlier speculation on antibody-catalysed hydrolysis of viral coat proteins was elaborated with reference to human immunodeficiency virus (HIV). A method for preventing attachment of HIV coat protein gp120 to the T helper cell CD4 receptor and thereby precluding entry of the virus into the T cell was described via catalytic antibody-mediated hydrolysis of the gp120 glycoprotein.

The procedure conveyed inclusion of transition state analogues into short synthetic peptide sequences of HIV gp120 for the production of catalytic antibodies. Other examples concerning antibody catalysis of peptide hydrolysis for therapy were: reduction of hypertension via hydrolytic inhibition of renin; amelioration of toxic effects of tumour necrosis factor via hydrolysis of this cytokine; and prevention of allergic reactions via hydrolysis of IgE. The patent application also described antibodies raised against phosphonates for the hydrolysis of ester groups in bacterial lipopolysaccharide. Treatment of Gram-negative septicaemia and shock via antibody-mediated ester hydrolysis was suggested. Finally, the publication relates an example of activation of a prodrug by catalytic antibody. Cytarabine, an established antineoplastic agent with important side-effects, can be converted into its 5′-galactoside to give a prodrug of cytarabine. It is suggested that more effective targeting of the antimetabolite at a tumour may be achieved by linking an antibody that specifically binds tumour cells to a catalytic antibody that hydrolyses the galactosyl prodrug. The immunogen for these antibodies would be a transition state analogue in which the acetal moiety in 5′-galactosyl cytarabine is replaced by an amidine.

Therapies involving destruction of toxic molecules in vivo using specific catalytic antibodies are a particularly attractive goal. Organophosphorus nerve agents have received particular attention, not least because investigations into treatments based on binding antibodies have been disappointing. The generation of antibodies that could catalyse hydrolysis of the nerve agent soman [26] (Structure 4.6) was discussed by Green and Glikson (1991) at a recent biotechnology conference. Hydrolysis of phosphonate esters such as soman proceeds via a transition state in which phosphorus is pentacoordinate with a trigonyl bipyramidal structure. Green and Glikson reported investigation of vanadium compounds as transition state analogues, but had encountered problems as a result of their complex chemistry. More recently, Hillerns and Rehder (1991) published the successful synthesis of several oxovanadium alkoxides, including the pentacoordinate complex [27] (Structure 4.6), as potential haptens for the production of antibodies with phosphatase activity. A third group working towards the generation of antibodies with phosphoryl-transfer reactions has published synthesis of stable pentacoordinated phosphorus derivatives, including the compound [28], with functionality that will permit coupling to carrier protein (Moriarty et al. 1990). Schultz's successful demonstration of antibodies with phosphatase activity was discussed above and is also relevant here. With such intense activity in this area it seems likely that the production of antibodies capable of catalysing hydrolysis of the nerve agents will be achieved.

Catalysis of ester hydrolysis is by far the most firmly established ability of catalytic antibodies and efforts designed to obtain catalytic antibodies for therapeutic applications by exploiting this esterolytic ability are beginning to produce exciting results. Consideration of biologically active and medically important compounds that contain an ester functional group as part of their structure leads rapidly to recognition of cocaine [29] (Structure 4.7) as a potential target for catalytic antibodies. Cocaine is an addictive drug, abuse of which creates problems, both for individuals and for society as a whole. There are two ester moieties in cocaine [29], a benzoyl ester and a methyl ester. Several research groups are pursuing the development of catalytic

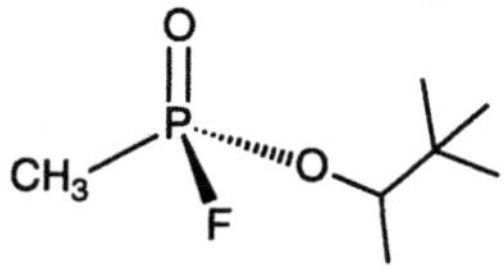

[26]

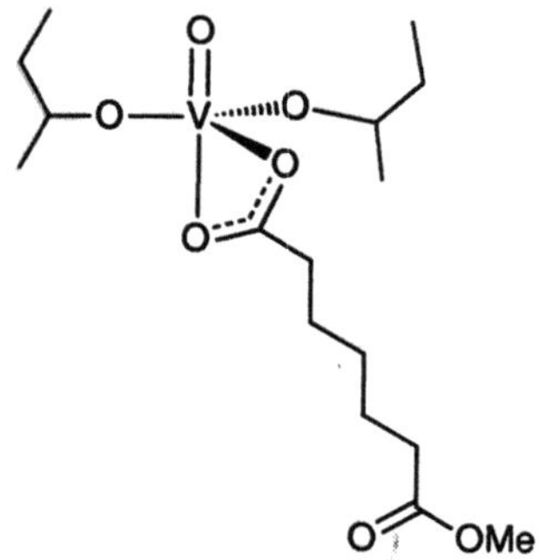

[27]

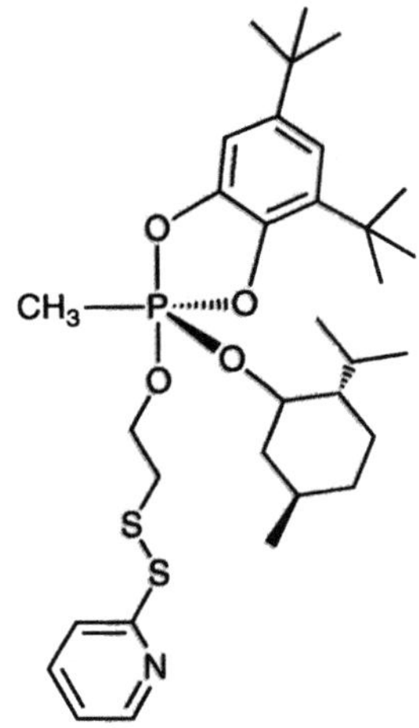

[28]

Structure 4.6

antibodies that will inactivate cocaine via hydrolysis of one or other of the ester moieties, and very recently two groups reported some impressive early results. Both groups targeted hydrolysis of the benzoyl ester of cocaine [29] to give methyl ecgonine [30] (Structure 4.7) and benzoic acid. Both groups hope to reduce the addictive properties of cocaine by using catalytic antibodies to rapidly inactivate the drug as it is administered. The first group – investigators at Monsanto and Searle – reported synthesis of the phenylphosphonate

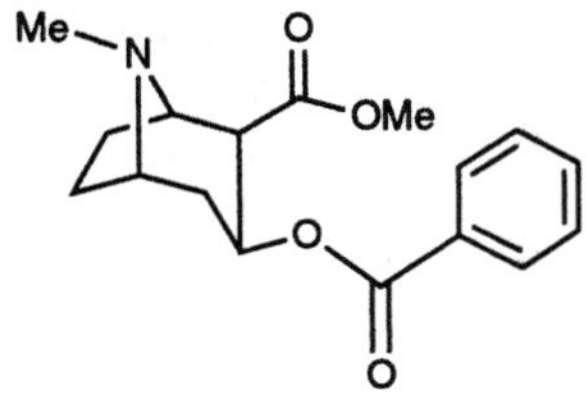

[29]

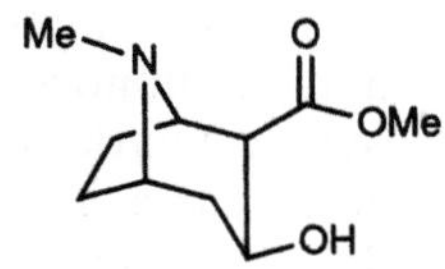

[30]

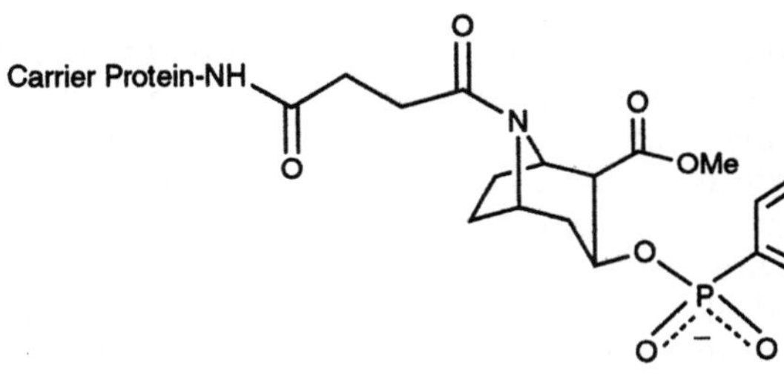

[31]

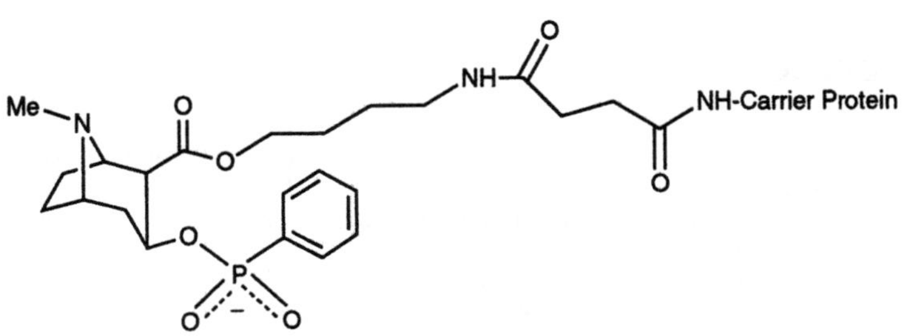

[32]

Structure 4.7

[31] (Structure 4.7), an analogue of the presumed transition state of the above hydrolysis (Chandrakumar et al. 1993). These workers reported the generation of monoclonal antibodies that bound the transition state analogue [31] and indicated that investigation of their catalytic activity was in progress. The second group, an academic group led by Donald W. Landry at Columbia University, reported synthesis of the phenylphosphonate [32] (Structure 4.7),

which is an alternative analogue of the above transition state (Landry et al. 1993). In addition to describing the generation of monoclonal antibodies, this group reported that 29 monoclonal antibodies were characterized and two were found to possess catalytic activity. The catalytic activity of the antibodies was not great and the investigators indicated that repetitive generation and screening would be expected to furnish more powerful catalytic antibodies. These results are, however, very exciting because they bring the prospect of therapeutic catalytic antibodies significantly closer.

Conclusion

In conclusion, it is clear that, since the discovery of catalytic antibodies in 1986, there has been rapid progress with considerable expansion of both the scope and the power of catalysis. Many groups are pursuing the development of catalytic antibodies that will be used therapeutically. Applications include: neutralization of toxic molecules; activation of prodrugs; enzyme replacement; inactivation of hormones, enzymes and antibodies; and the use of catalytic antibodies as antiviral, antibacterial and anticancer agents. Most of these proposals involve hydrolysis, which was the first reaction for which antibody catalysis was demonstrated and the reaction for which most progress has been achieved. Many of the proposals are extensions of applications in which binding antibodies have found success, in particular the treatment of poisoning and targeting of prodrugs, and it seems likely that catalytic antibodies will find their first therapeutic use in one of these areas.

References

Balan A, Doctor BP, Green BS, Torten M, Ziffer H (1988) Antibody combining sites as templates for selective organic chemical reactions. J Chem Soc Chem Commun 106–108

Baldwin E, Schultz PG (1989) Generation of a catalytic antibody by site directed mutagenesis. Science 245: 1104–1107

Chandrakumar NS, Carron CP, Meyer DM et al. (1993) Phenylphosphonate monoester analogues of cocaine, potential haptens for the generation of catalytic antibodies. Bioorgan Med Chem Lett 3: 309–312

Cochran AG, Sugasawara R, Schultz PG (1988) Photosensitised cleavage of a thymidine dimer by an antibody. J Am Chem Soc 110: 7888–7890

Gallacher G, Jackson CS, Searcey M et al. (1991) A polyclonal antibody preparation with Michaelian catalytic properties. Biochem J 279: 871–881

Gallacher G, Searcey M, Jackson CS, Brocklehurst K (1992) Polyclonal antibody-catalysed amide hydrolysis. Biochem J 284: 675–680

Green BS, Glikson M (1991) Towards catalytic antibodies for the degradation of toxic agents. In: Kamely D, Chakrabarty AM, Kornguth SE (eds) Biotechnology: Bridging research and applications. Kluwer Academic, Boston, USA, pp 249–264

Hillerns F, Rehder D (1991) Functionalised oxovanadium alkoxides – potential haptens. Chem Ber 124: 2249–2254

Hilvert D, Nared KD (1988) Stereospecific Claisen rearrangement catalysed by an antibody. J Am Chem Soc 110: 5593–5594

Hilvert D, Carpenter SH, Nared KD, Auditor MTM (1988) Catalysis of concerted reactions by antibodies: The Claisen rearrangement. Proc Natl Acad Sci USA 85: 4953–4955

Huse WD, Sastry L, Iverson SA et al. (1989) Generation of a large combinatorial library of the immunoglobulin repertoire in phage lambda. Science 246: 1275–1281
Iverson BL, Lerner RA (1989) Sequence-specific peptide cleavage catalysed by an antibody. Science 243: 1184–1188
Iverson BL, Iverson SA, Roberts VA et al. (1990) Metalloantibodies. Science 249: 659–662
Jackson DY, Jacobs JW, Sugasawara R, Reich SH, Bartlett PA, Schultz PG (1988) An antibody catalysed Claisen rearrangement. J Am Chem Soc 110: 4841–4842
Janda KD, Benkovic SJ, Lerner RA (1989) Catalytic antibodies with lipase activity and R or S substrate specificity. Science 244: 437–440
Janda KD, Schloeder DS, Benkovic SJ, Lerner RA (1988) Induction of an antibody that catalyses the hydrolysis of an amide bond. Science 241: 1188–1191
Janda KD, Weinhouse MI, Schloeder DM, Lerner RA (1990) Bait and switch strategy for obtaining catalytic antibodies. J Am Chem Soc 112: 1274–1275
Jencks WP (1969) Catalysis in chemistry and enzymology. McGraw-Hill, New York
Kraut J (1988) How do enzymes work. Science 242: 533–540
Landry DW, Zhao K, Yang GXQ, Glickman M, Georgiadis TM (1993) Antibody-catalysed degradation of cocaine. Science 259: 1899–1901
Lerner RA, Benkovic SJ, Schultz PG (1991) At the crossroads of chemistry and immunology: Catalytic antibodies. Science 252: 659–667
Massey RJ (1987) Catalytic antibodies catching on. Nature 328: 457–458
Moriarty RM, Hiratake J, Liu K (1990) New synthetic route to unsymmetrically substituted pentacoordinated phosphorus. Hydrolytically stable chiral monocyclic oxyphosphoranes. J Am Chem Soc 112: 8575–8577
Paul S, Volle DJ, Beach CM, Johnson DR, Powell MJ, Massey RJ (1989) Catalytic hydrolysis of vasoactive intestinal peptide by human autoantibody. Science 244: 1158–1162
Pauling L (1946) Molecular architecture and biological reactions. Chem Eng News 24: 1375–1377
Pollack SJ, Schultz PG (1989) A semisynthetic catalytic antibody. J Am Chem Soc 111: 1929–1931
Pollack SJ, Hsiun P, Schultz PG (1989) Stereospecific hydrolysis of alkyl esters by antibodies. J Am Chem Soc 111: 5961–5962
Pollack SJ, Jacobs JW, Schultz PG (1986) Selective chemical catalysis by an antibody. Science 234: 1570–1573
Powell MJ, Rees AR, Massey RJ (1989) PCT Patent Application, International publication number WO 89/10754
Raso V, Stollar BD (1975) The antibody-enzyme analogy. Comparison of enzymes and antibodies specific for phosphopyridoxyltyrosine. Biochemistry 14: 591–599
Scanlan TS, Prudent JR, Schultz PG (1991) Antibody-catalysed hydrolysis of phosphate monoesters. J Am Chem Soc 113: 9397–9398
Schowen RL (1978) In: Gandour RD, Schowen RL (eds) Transition states of biochemical processes. Plenum Press, New York, pp 77–114
Shokat KM, Ko MK, Scanlan TS et al. (1990) Catalytic antibodies: A new class of transition-state analogues used to elicit hydrolytic antibodies. Angew Chem Int Ed Engl 29: 1296–1303
Shokat KM, Leumann CJ, Sugasawara R, Schultz PG (1989) A new strategy for the generation of catalytic antibodies. Nature 338: 269–271
Tang Y, Hicks JB, Hilvert D (1991) In vivo catalysis of a metabolically essential reaction by an antibody. Proc Natl Acad Sci USA 88: 8784–8786
Thorset ED, Harris EE, Peterson ER et al. (1982) Phosphorus-containing inhibitors of angiotensin-converting enzyme. Proc Natl Acad Sci USA 79: 2176–2180
Tramontano A, Ammann AA, Lerner RA (1988) Antibody catalysis approaching the activity of enzymes. J Am Chem Soc 110: 2282–2286
Tramontano A, Janda KD, Lerner RA (1986) Catalytic antibodies. Science 234: 1566–1570

5 Immunotherapy for Drug Toxicity

A.J. Heath

Introduction

The potential use of immunotherapy in the treatment of drug-induced toxicity has been recognized for decades (Colburn 1980). Antibodies have been raised in horses, rats, rabbits, sheep and goats against a variety of drugs such as aspirin (Hooker and Boyd 1940), chloramphenicol (Hamburger and Douglass 1969), colchicine (Terrien et al. 1990), strychnine (Hooker and Boyd 1940), digoxin (Butler and Chen 1967), imipramine (O'Callaghan et al. 1987), desmethylimipramine (Pond et al. 1991), nortriptyline (Sabouraud et al. 1990), amitriptyline (Sidki 1991, personal communication) and phencyclidine (Owens and Mayersohn 1986). However, only one product – digoxin-specific ovine Fab fragments (Digibind, Digidote) – is marketed. This treatment has been available for almost 20 years yet remains the only commercially available immunotherapeutic antidote against drug-induced poisoning. Why is this so?

Treatments specifically produced as antidotes to drug-induced toxicity are very likely to have limited indications and be designated as orphan drugs. From a commercial perspective such antidotes are not likely to be profitable. However feasible the technology may be in a university laboratory, significant investment is necessary both to produce adequate clinical documentation and for large-scale production. Furthermore, monoclonals for use as therapeutic antibodies to drugs have several disadvantages compared with polyclonals (see Chapter 1). It has become increasingly clear that monoclonal technology, while unsurpassed in its diagnostic applications, has limitations when applied to therapeutics. In this setting, antibodies raised against several epitopes may be advantageous, resulting in greater efficacy. Nonetheless, monoclonal technology has received much focus in recent years, leaving an impression that a polyclonal product is old-fashioned and out of date. While this may be true with respect to unprocessed horse serum, significant advances have been made in polyclonal technology over the last decade. Experience with Digibind shows that the problems of hypersensitivity and serum sickness experienced with unprocessed horse serum can be avoided by using ovine Fab fragments. Improvements in immunization protocols and manufacturing techniques have been made, which should allow the production of specific, affinity purified, ovine Fab at an acceptable cost.

Table 5.1. Factors determining the proportion of drug ingested to be neutralized by Fab

Amount of drug ingested
Formulation (sustained release)
Amount vomited, lavaged or absorbed to charcoal
Bioavailability:
amount absorbed
first-pass effect (kinetics may differ at high concentrations)
Rate of equilibration between the central (toxic) compartment and other tissues
Rate and route of elimination of drug, antibody and drug–antibody complex

Feasibility

Which drugs are then amenable to neutralization by antibodies? One mole of Fab will combine with one mole of drug. Therefore, 10 mg of a toxin (such as a tricyclic) with a molecular weight of about 300 is stoichiometrically equivalent to 1.7 g of purified, specific Fab fragments. In such cases, an overdose may require treatment with several hundred grams of Fab if all the drug ingested is to be neutralized (Sullivan 1986). Tricyclic antidepressants (TCA) are the most common cause of death in the Western world in patients who arrive alive at hospital following a drug overdose. If, indeed, a smaller quantity of anti-TCA Fab fragments than that required for stoichiometric equivalence can affect outcome, then such therapy can become a clinical reality (see below). Several factors work together in determining how much of a drug or toxin must be neutralized with an antibody to positively affect morbidity and mortality (Table 5.1).

Why Fab Fragments?

Cleaving IgG into two separate antibody binding fragments (Fab) and at the same time removing the Fc fragment changes the pharmacokinetic profile without affecting the binding capacity of the molecule (Colburn 1980). The smaller molecular weight (about 50 000) results in a larger volume of distribution. This may explain the greater efficacy and quicker onset of action of digoxin-specific Fab fragments than intact digoxin-specific antibodies (Lloyd and Smith 1978). Because of their smaller size, Fab fragments are mostly eliminated through the kidneys. Elimination is more rapid than for whole immunoglobulin eliminated via the reticuloendothelial system. A further advantage of Fab fragments is that the total amount of foreign protein administered to neutralize a given quantity of drug is reduced.

Safety

Whole immunoglobulins, particularly of equine origin, are immunogenic. On repeat exposure there is a risk of an IgE-mediated anaphylactic reaction. This risk is markedly less with Fab fragments than with whole immunoglobulin

(Kirkpatrick 1991). Serum sickness is another major complication of treatment with whole immunoglobulin, with symptoms appearing from a week up to a month after exposure. Serum sickness occurs in up to 70% of patients treated for crotalid envenomation with whole equine immunoglobulin antidote. Serum sickness, like allergic sequelae, occurs in up to 10% of patients treated for viper bites with an $F(ab')_2$ antivenin (Persson 1992). Experience with Digibind (Kirkpatrick 1991) has shown an overall incidence of adverse reactions of 0.8%. No anaphylaxis has been reported. Clearly, the smaller Fab affinity-purified molecule is to be preferred both for its efficacy and its safety.

Digoxin

In 1967, Butler and Chen showed that antibodies raised in rabbits immunized with digoxin–bovine serum albumin conjugates specifically bound to digoxin, with cross-reactivity to digitoxin. Affinity-purified ovine Fab fragments were thereafter shown to reverse digoxin-induced ventricular tachycardia in dogs (Curd et al. 1971). Five years later, Smith et al. (1976) reported their successful use in an acute digoxin overdose in man; in 1982 a series of 26 patients was published (Smith et al. 1982). In Europe, Digidote has been used in both digitoxin and digoxin poisoning (Smolarz et al. 1984). Immune Fab (Digibind) was granted orphan drug status and a product licence by the FDA in 1986. Since then two major studies have been published confirming its efficacy and safety: a multicentre trial reporting 150 cases (Antman et al. 1990) and a post-marketing surveillance study including 717 adults (Hickey et al. 1991) and 29 children (Woolf et al. 1992). The use of Digibind in the USA has been estimated at about 2500 treatments/year (Hickey et al. 1991).

Digitalis Intoxication: Clinical Features

Digitalis intoxication may be acute or chronic. Chronic intoxication is probably the most prevalent drug reaction encountered in clinical practice (Mahdyoon et al. 1990). It is difficult to diagnose and often complicated by a myriad of possible drug interactions. The patient is typically elderly, on several medications for cardiovascular disease, and has elevated blood urea, nitrogen and creatinine levels. Unlike acute poisoning, most patients are normokalaemic. Serum digoxin levels in toxic and non-toxic patients overlap (Smith and Haber 1970) and are of little help in excluding a diagnosis of digoxin toxicity. Nevertheless, a better understanding of the pharmacokinetics of digoxin and increased awareness of the problem has resulted in a perceived reduction in the incidence of digitalis intoxication (Smith 1988). In-hospital mortality has been reported to be 4.6% in definitely intoxicated patients (Mahdyoon et al. 1990). Although unusual, chronic digitalis poisoning does occur in children. Typically, the patient is a neonate with underlying cardiac disease. In this group of patients mortality is much higher: in a series published by Woolf et al. (1992), four of 11 patients with chronic poisoning died.

Acute digitalis intoxication may result from accidental or deliberate ingestion of cardiac glycosides, including pharmaceuticals such as digoxin and digitoxin and plants such as the foxglove, lily of the valley and oleander species. In children, acute intoxication may result from accidental iatrogenic overdose in a hospital setting or, more commonly, in toddlers who all too easily find somebody else's medication within easy reach at home. Although serum digoxin levels are higher in acute than chronic poisoning, mortality may be lower: of 18 poisonings in Woolf et al.'s series, only three died. In adolescents and adults, acute digitalis poisoning is usually a result of intentional overdose.

Digoxin is rapidly absorbed and has a large apparent volume of distribution (V_d) (adults 7–8 l/kg; neonates 10 l/kg; infants 16 l/kg; Ellenhorn and Barceloux 1988). The initial V_d is small, and therefore high concentrations will be found if plasma samples are taken early on in the course of intoxication before the patient is in the elimination phase. About 60%–80% of digoxin is excreted through the kidneys unchanged. The terminal half-life is about 36 h. Digitoxin has a much smaller V_d (0.54 l/kg), is cleared mostly by hepatic metabolism, and has a longer half-life (about 100 h) (Table 5.2).

Acute digitalis poisoning is characterized by visual symptoms (colour aberrations or transient blindness), nausea and vomiting, mental status changes, hyperkalaemia (a level of 6 mEq/l indicates a plasma digoxin level of about 10 ng/ml (12.8 nM) and conduction disturbances. Cardiac symptoms may take up to 6 h to present. T wave inversion, S–T segment depression, a Q–T interval shortening, prolonged P–R interval and varying degrees of atrioventricular (AV) block are often seen on the electrocardiograph (ECG).

In adults, ventricular arrhythmias from increased automaticity are the immediate cause of death in 70% of patients, severe AV block in 20% and pump failure in 10% (Bismuth et al. 1977). Ventricular arrhythmias present often as a characteristic fascicular tachycardia (Wieland and Marchlinski 1986). Serious toxicity in children is more often heralded by sinus bradycardia and/or varying degrees of AV conduction block (Woolf et al. 1992). In acute poisoning, age, hyperkalaemia, a plasma digoxin concentration greater than 15 ng/ml, and conduction disturbances such as ventricular tachycardia or

Table 5.2. Digitalis pharmacokinetic parameters

	Digoxin	Digitoxin
Peak effect (h)	3–6	4–12
Peak $T_{1/2}$ (h)	30–45	Over 100
Duration of action	3–6 days	2–3 weeks
Gastrointestinal absorption (%)	50–80	90–100
Protein binding (%)	25	95
Excretion	Urinary (60%–80%)	Enterohepatic cycle; urinary (33% active)
Toxic blood level	Over 2 ng/ml	Over 40 ng/ml
Standard adult V_d (l/kg)	5–7	0.54

(Modified from Ellenhorn and Barceloux 1988.)

Table 5.3. Differences in acute and chronic digoxin poisoning

Acute intoxication	Chronic toxicity
All ages – often no history of cardiovascular disease	Older patient with underlying cardiovascular disease
Nausea, vomiting characteristic	Not always seen
Hyperkalaemia	Normo- or hypokalaemia common
Serum digoxin correlates with toxicity	Normal serum digoxin does not rule out toxicity

high-grade AV block are serious prognostic factors. The clinical picture in chronic poisoning is more diffuse and consequently more difficult to interpret (Table 5.3)

Mechanisms of Action and Pharmacokinetics of Digoxin Immune Fab

Cardiac glycosides bind reversibly to cardiac receptors. Digoxin-specific fragments reverse digitalis-induced dysrhythmias, conduction disturbances, myocardial depression and inhibition of the (sodium–potassium) ATPase pump by pulling digoxin off the receptor (Smith et al. 1982; Zucker et al. 1982). The affinity of digoxin immune Fab (Digibind) for digoxin is in the range of 10^9–10^{10} M^{-1}, which is greater than the affinity of digoxin for the (sodium–potassium) ATPase pump. The affinity of digoxin antibody fragments for digitoxin is about 10^8–10^9 M^{-1}. The effect of an infusion of digoxin immune Fab should be seen within 30 min of completion of a 30-min infusion. A rapid and large (10–20-fold) increase in total digoxin concentration in plasma occurs as the free digoxin concentration drops to zero and the potassium level falls (Fig. 5.1). In patients with normal renal function the half-life of the Fab–digoxin complex is 10–20 h.

Clinical Experience with Digoxin Immune Fab

In 1990 Antman and colleagues presented the results of a multicentre trial of digoxin immune Fab from 21 medical centres in 150 patients with life-threatening digitalis intoxication treated between 1974 and 1986. The youngest patient was a few hours old, the oldest 94 years old. Acute poisoning accounted for 49%: 39% had taken an overdose with suicidal intent and 10% were accidental. The remaining 51% of patients were on long-term digitalis therapy and presented with chronic intoxications. The median of serum concentrations was 8.0 ng/ml. Five patients with digitoxin intoxication had a median concentration of 156 ng/ml. The median dose of Fab fragments given was 200 mg; the maximum dose given was 1600 mg. Of 148 protocols that could be evaluated, 80% had resolution of all signs and symptoms, a further 10% improved and 10% showed no response. The median time to response was 19 min after terminating the Fab infusion. Seventy-five per cent of patients had some evidence of response by 60 min.

Only 14 adverse events were considered to be related to the administration of Fab – most common were the rapid development of hypokalaemia (16 patients) or an exacerbation of existing congestive heart failure (four patients). Reasons for partial or non-responses were underlying heart disease as the true cause of suspected digitalis toxicity, too low a dose of Fab and treatment of patients already moribund. Antman et al. (1990) concluded that a treatment response can be expected in at least 90% of patients with life-threatening toxicity.

In 1991 an observational, post-marketing surveillance study reported experience from the treatment of 717 adult patients from 487 hospitals (Hickey et al. 1991). In contrast to the clinical trial reported by Antman et al. (1990), these patients were older (mean age 75 years for women and 72 years for men). Most (94%) patients had an underlying cardiovascular disorder. About one-third had severe impairment of renal function and a further 43% mild to moderate impairment. Only 17% of patients were treated because of a single drug overdose; these patients had higher serum digoxin concentrations (Table 5.4). Only 7% of these patients had renal impairment. The severity of toxicity observed in this study was less than that in the Antman et al. (1990) study and the dose of Fab used was less. The median dose was 120 mg and the most frequently administered dose 80 mg. Fifty per cent of patients had complete reversal of signs of toxicity, 24% partial reversal and 12% no response to

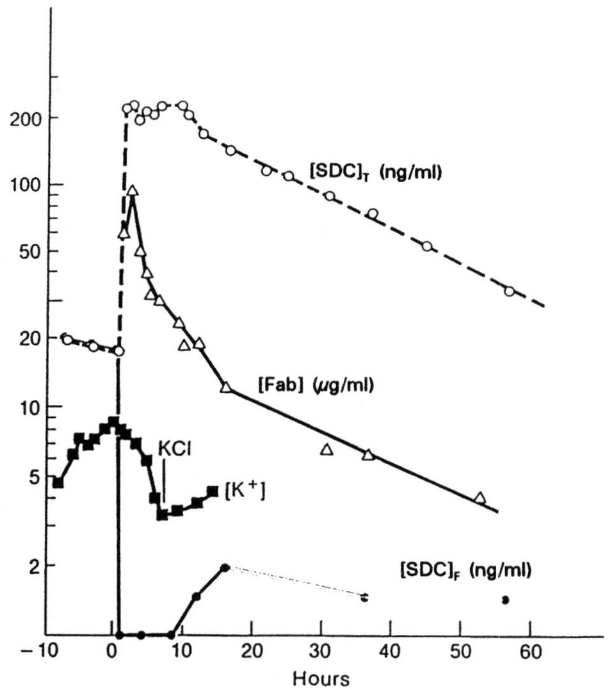

Fig. 5.1. Time course of serum potassium concentration in mEq/1 ([K^+], ■—■); total serum digoxin concentration ([SDC]$_T$, O·····O); free serum digoxin concentration ([SDC]$_F$, ●—●); and serum concentration of sheep digoxin-specific Fab fragments ([Fab], △—△). The scale on the vertical axis is logarithmic. On the horizontal axis, 0 denotes the time at which administration of digoxin-specific Fab fragments was started. (From Smith et al. 1976.)

Table 5.4. Amount of digoxin ingested and serum digoxin level by type of dosing in 717 patients[a]

Type of dosing	No.	%	Amount ingested (mg/day or mg): percentiles of the distribution				Serum concentration[b] (ng/ml): percentiles of the distribution			
			No. with amount specified	10%	Median	90%	No. with amount specified	10%	Median	90%
Maintenance	508	71	419	0.13	0.25	0.25	492	2.5[c]	4.2	8
Loading or in-hospital treatment	58	8	50	0.25	0.81	1.98	53	2.2[d]	4.6	9
Single ingestion (patients with heart disease)	85	12	55	1.0	5.0	17.7	83	4[e]	9	24
Single ingestion (patients without heart disease)	35	5	22	3.2	10.0	25.0	32	5	11	25
Unknown or unspecified	31	4	—	—	—	—	26	3.7	7	18

[a] Values for three patients with digitoxin intoxication are excluded; [b] values exceeding 5 ng/ml were rounded to the nearest integer; [c] 27 values <2.0 ng/ml; [d] one value <2.0 ng/ml; [e] two values <2.0 ng/ml.
(From Hickey et al. 1991.)

treatment. The response was not reported or uncertain in 14% of patients. However, only four patients were concluded by an independent cardiologist to be possible treatment failures. It is noteworthy that there was no clear relation between the initial response to treatment and the proportion of the estimated adequate dose actually administered. Only 52 patients (7%) had an adverse event possibly or probably related to Fab treatment (see below). None of the 171 (24%) deaths could be attributed to Fab.

Experience is now accumulating regarding the use of Fab fragments for severe digitalis intoxication in children. Woolf et al. (1992) reported 28 children with digoxin and one with digitoxin intoxication treated at 21 centres between 1974 and 1986. The serum digoxin concentrations ranged from 3.0 to 100 ng/ml (mean 13.8). Cardiac dysrhythmias and hyperkalaemia were seen in all patients. In 27 of the 29 patients, digitalis toxicity resolved after the administration of Fab. Three patients were retreated with Fab. Seven patients died of complications unrelated to the administration of Fab. No allergic reactions to Fab were observed. Digitalis intoxication in children differs from that in adults – children with healthy hearts tolerate higher digitalis concentrations and may possibly be revived later on in the course of intoxication than adults.

Adverse Events: Experience with Fab Fragments

Seven to nine per cent of patients treated with Fab experience an adverse event (Antman et al. 1990; Hickey et al. 1991). No deaths have been attributed to Fab.

Hypokalaemia. A decline in serum potassium is often seen within an hour of Fab administration and is completed within 4 h (Antman et al. 1990). With careful clinical management this complication can be avoided.

Recrudescent Digitalis Toxicity. Twenty of 717 patients (2.8%) (Hickey et al. 1991) were classed as recrudescent toxicity. Sixteen cases occurred within 3 days of Fab treatment; four patients had a recurrence of toxicity from 4 to 11 days after treatment. Recrudescent toxicity was more frequent among patients receiving less than the estimated adequate dose of Fab.

Allergic Responses. Six possible or probable allergic responses (0.8%) were reported in the post-marketing surveillance study (Hickey et al. 1991). Four of these responses occurred in patients with histories of allergies or asthma (0.5%); two were in patients with no such history (0.3%) (Table 5.5). Four reactions occurred during or shortly after an infusion of Fab. No anaphylactoid responses were observed, although one patient was treated twice with Fab.

Withdrawal of Inotropic and Chronotropic Effect of Digitalis. In Hickey et al.'s study (1991) five (0.7%) patients with congestive heart failure deteriorated because of withdrawal of the inotropic effect of digitalis. Withdrawal of the chronotropic effect of digitalis can result in a rapid ventricular response to an underlying atrial fibrillation.

Table 5.5. Allergic reactions to digitalis-specific Fab fragments

Case	Age and sex	Dose of Fab fragments	Onset of reaction	Nature of reaction	Allergies
1	28F	120 mg	During infusion	Skin rash, flushing, periorbital oedema	Penicillin, tetracycline, asthma
2	64F	40 mg	30 min	Rash	Cefaclor
3	61M	840 ng	Same day	Rash	Penicillin
4	63F	120 mg	90 min	Chills	None
5	73F	320 mg	11 days	Thrombocytopenia	None
6	54F	520 mg	16 days	Urticaria	Naproxen

(Modified from Kirkpatrick 1991.)

Digoxin Immune Fab Fragments in Patients with Renal Impairment

Fab, in contrast to IgG, is excreted mostly through the kidneys. Pharmacokinetic studies in patients with renal failure (Clifton et al. 1989; Colucci et al. 1989; Erdmann et al. 1989; Nuwayhid and Johnson 1989; Sinclair et al. 1989; Ujhelyi et al. 1991; Allen et al. 1991) show that the half-life of both free and bound Fab is prolonged in renal failure, with free serum digoxin rebounding after several days, rather than after 12 h as in patients with normal renal function. Recrudescent toxicity was not, however, observed in any of the six cases reported above. Wenger (1991) reviewed the use of Fab in patients with renal impairment in the original multicentre trial (Antman et al. 1990), the post-marketing surveillance study (Hickey et al. 1991) and data on file with the manufacturer. Patients with poor renal function showed no sign of a poorer response to Fab, either in terms of percentage of patients responding, onset of effect, or recrudescence. Twenty-eight patients were functionally anephric. One of these patients showed signs of recrudescense 10 days after Fab treatment. Although recrudescent toxicity in patients with renal failure seems rare, plasmapheresis has been recommended (Rabetoy et al. 1990) following Fab therapy to remove the Fab–digoxin complex. This procedure should obviate the risk of delayed toxicity. A large digitalis load together with an inadequate Fab dose and poor renal function may be the most likely setting for recrudescence. However, experience to date does not support the routine use of plasmapheresis in this group of patients.

Cross-Reactivity of Digoxin-Specific Fab Fragments

Digitoxin

Five patients (median serum digitoxin concentration 156 ng/ml) in the Antman et al. study (1990), one patient in the Woolf et al. study (1992) and three patients reported by Hickey et al. (1991) all responded to treatment with Digibind. Similar experience in digitoxin poisoning has been reported from France, where digitoxin is more commonly prescribed (Aeberhard et al. 1980; Bouffard et al. 1982). Although the affinity of digoxin–immune Fab may be one order of magnitude greater for digoxin than digitoxin, clinical evidence to date does not support the use of a different dosage regimen for digitoxin.

Cardiac Glycosides from Plant Poisoning

Nerium oleander (common oleander) poisoning is not uncommon in tropical and subtropical parts of the world, and deaths have occurred in both adults and children. Antibody used in the quantification of digoxin by radioimmunoassay cross-reacts with cardiac glycosides found in oleanders (Osterloh et al. 1982). Digoxin-specific Fab has been shown to reverse oleander-induced cardiac dysrhythmias in a canine model (Clark et al. 1991). However, because massive doses were used, it is difficult to conclude that smaller doses would be equally efficacious in man. It is equally difficult to draw any conclusions from two cases published in which Digibind was used in oleander poisoning. In one case a very low dose was given (Shumiak et al. 1988) and in the other case the patient died (Blum and Rieders 1987). Repeat administration or a larger dose of Fab may possibly be required. The role of digoxin-specific antibodies is even less clear as regards the foxglove, lily of the valley and yew. Digibind had no demonstrable effect in a serious case of yew berry poisoning (Cummins et al. 1990) in a 5-year-old autistic girl. However, yew contains the cardiac glycoside taxine, which is not similar to that found in the foxglove and lily of the valley. Until more experience is published, the physician should be prepared to treat severe poisoning with lily of the valley and foxglove with digoxin-specific Fab, aware that the dose required is yet to be determined.

Management of Digitalis Overdose with Digoxin-Specific Fab Fragments

Indications

Several factors should be considered before the administration of digoxin-specific Fab antibodies (Table 5.6). In less serious cases in patients who are haemodynamically stable, the severity of toxicity should be assessed by determining the amount of digoxin ingested and the serum digoxin concentration. In symptomatic patients with acute toxicity, it may be difficult to assess the amount absorbed: here the serum digoxin concentration is only useful in confirming the diagnosis and is of little help in determining the amount of Fab fragments indicated for neutralization (see below). In a symptomatic patient who has taken a large quantity of digitalis, Fab fragments are indicated irrespective of the plasma concentration, or if serum digoxin concentrations exceed 5 ng/ml (Marchlinski et al. 1991). Plasma concentrations are most helpful in assessing the severity of toxicity in chronic intoxications. At least 6 h should have passed after the last ingestion of digoxin for the serum digoxin concentration to be helpful in calculating the amount of Fab fragments necessary for stoichiometric equivalence.

Table 5.6. Questions raised before administering digoxin immune Fab (ovine) antibody

1. Is the rhythm/ECG abnormality due to digoxin toxicity?
2. Is haemodynamic compromise present?
3. Other considerations:
    - Is toxicity severe (amount ingested and serum concentration)?
    - What is the anticipated time course for reversal of toxicity (renal function)?
    - Is digoxin needed for ventricular rate control (atrial fibrillation) or inotropy?
    - Is there a history of severe allergies?
    - Are other factors present which predispose to severe toxicity, such as increased age, heart disease or abnormal thyroid function?

(Modified from Marchlinski et al. 1991.)

In patients with poor renal function, the elimination of digoxin is slowed. In this situation (mostly elderly patients), Fab fragments may be indicated to avoid a prolonged period of temporary pacemaking.

Skin Testing

Antman et al. (1990) reported the results of skin testing in 94 cases; only one patient had erythema. None of these patients had an allergic reaction following the intravenous infusion. Because allergy testing can delay therapy, it is not generally indicated before treatment with Fab. However, skin testing should be considered in patients known to be allergic to ovine proteins or who have previously received antibodies or Fab fragments raised in sheep. A 42-year-old woman (Hickey et al. 1991) was treated with Fab twice, approximately 2 months apart; no adverse event was reported. However, in this situation skin testing may be advisable, as in patients known to react to papaya (papaya extracts are used for discolysis as well as in the preparation of Fab fragments). A positive reaction may not constitute a contraindication for use of Fab fragments in a life-threatening situation, but should prepare the physician to take adequate precautions, such as treatment with antihistamines or other antiallergic drugs (Kirkpatrick 1991).

Dosage

The currently recommended dosage of Fab is an equimolar dose, administered by the intravenous route during 15–30 min, to achieve neutralization of the body load of digoxin or digitoxin. A dose of 80 mg of Fab fragments neutralizes approximately 1 mg of digoxin or digitoxin. The manufacturer's dosing recommendations are based on (a) the number of tablets ingested or (b) a serum digoxin concentration. If the dose of digoxin is unknown and assay unavailable, up to 800 mg antidote is recommended for an adult. Unfortunately, calculation of the amount of antidote required based on the number of tablets taken must account not only for bioavailability (80%) but "losses" through vomiting, gastric lavage, charcoal or metabolism. In most cases less than 60% of an acute, ingested dose will enter the systemic circulation.

Calculations based on the total body load of digitalis derived from serum digoxin or digitoxin concentrations assume that a steady state exists. A stat concentration in an acutely sick patient after a massive overdose does not reflect accurately a concentration taken after repeated dosing, because volumes of distribution in the distribution or elimination phases differ. Calculations based on V_d in steady state will overestimate the amount of antidote required. Volumes of distribution may vary in the very young or aged, and assays of digoxin are frequently erroneous at very high levels. Further, pharmacodynamics vary; children are more resistant to digoxin (Lewander et al. 1986), whereas patients with cardiovascular disease, electrolyte shifts (particularly potassium and magnesium) or hypothyroidism may show signs of toxicity at serum digoxin concentrations within the normal range. So far, the minimal optimal dose required to obtain a satisfactory cardiac response has not been determined. Recrudescent toxicity was observed in only 2.8% of patients (Hickey et al. 1991), although 42.8% received a dose below the estimated adequate dose. When the antibody is infused over a short period of time about half the dose of Fab fragments is cleared before enough digoxin has rediffused from the tissue for binding. Alternative dosing regimens have therefore been proposed (Jaeger et al. 1992). For adults, Schaumann et al. (1986) propose an initial infusion of 160 mg over 15 min and a further 160 mg over the next 7 h. Can then digoxin-specific Fab fragments be safely given simply on a body weight basis? In the multicentre clinical trial reported by Antman et al. (1990), the median peak serum digoxin concentration was 8.0 ng/ml with an upper quartile of 13.1 ng/ml. Even accepting the validity of dosing based on serum concentrations, ten vials (400 mg) will be adequate for 75% of patients. Recrudescence seems more likely to occur in patients with chronic poisoning. Because calculations based on "guesstimates" of the number of tablets taken or on stat serum concentrations overestimate the amount of antidote required, initial dosing in acute poisoning should be based on body weight: for most adults about 400 mg, for newborn, one vial (40 mg). Repeated doses should be given as and when indicated by the clinical response. Up to 1600 mg has been given with no signs of toxicity (Hickey et al. 1991).

In chronic poisoning serum digoxin concentrations are more likely to reflect a steady state and thus the calculation of the total load of digoxin from the serum digoxin concentration and V_d more accurately reflect the quantity of antidote necessary. Usually, four to six vials (160–240 mg) is adequate for chronic intoxication.

Once Fab fragments have been given, further monitoring of digitalis toxicity must be based on clinical signs and kalaemia, because total serum digoxin concentrations are markedly elevated. Fab fragment therapy is known to interfere with digoxin immunoassays causing spurious serum digoxin concentrations. In the presence of Fab, TDx FPIA with ultrafiltration is the assay of choice (Ujhelyi et al. 1992). Free digoxin concentrations may be useful in patients with renal impairment where there is concern for recrudescence (Allen et al. 1991); however, this laboratory capability is not always readily available.

Supportive Therapy

The introduction of digoxin-specific antibody fragments into clinical medicine has changed the management of digitalis intoxication. Nonetheless, supportive therapy forms the basis for the management of mild to moderate intoxication, and should be seen as a complement, rather than alternative, to the use of Fab fragments in severe toxicity. Most patients with an acute poisoning vomit profusely and further emesis is unnecessary. Gastric lavage may be indicated, although both emesis and lavage may increase vagal tone, precipitating or worsening an AV block or bradycardia. Therefore atropine should be given prior to emptying the stomach. This procedure should be terminated with the deposition of 50–100 g of activated charcoal (1 g/kg in children). Severe hyperkalaemia should be treated with glucose, insulin and bicarbonate. Careful monitoring of potassium is essential because potassium levels rapidly fall following the administration of Fab fragments. A temporary pacemaker should be placed early on in the course of severe poisoning. Phenytoin is the drug of choice for managing arrhythmias characterized by enhanced automaticity and for converting atrial tachycardia with block to sinus rhythm (Bayer 1991). Fab therapy together with careful monitoring and optimal intensive care can reduce morbidity and mortality associated with digitalis intoxication.

Other Indications

Whole IgG digoxin antibodies have been studied in deoxycorticosterone acetate-salt hypertensive rats, and in rats with aortic coarctation and elevations in digitalis-like factors (Huang and Smith 1984; Kunes et al. 1985). On the basis of these studies, and the possible role of endogenous digitalis-like factor (EDRF) in pregnant women with toxaemia, Goodlin (1988) treated a 31-year-old woman 25 weeks pregnant with severe toxaemia with two 10 mg doses of Digibind. A marked decline in blood pressure was seen after each dose. To date, the role of anti-digoxin antibodies in patients with elevated EDRF or toxaemia of pregnancy remains to be elucidated.

Colchicine

To date, colchicine is the only drug other than digoxin to which Fab antibodies have been raised and successfully given to treat a poisoned patient. Colchicine has been used in the therapy of acute gout for over 200 years. It is still widely prescribed in many countries, particularly France, where it is also used to treat primary biliary cirrhosis, Behçet's disease and familial Mediterranean fever. Colchicine is widely distributed in the body. Once in the cell, colchicine binds reversibly to microtubules (tubulin), impairing cellular function by inhibiting mitosis in metaphase. The half-life of the tubulin–colchicine complex is about 36 h (Jaeger et al. 1992). Colchicine is rapidly absorbed after oral administration, with peak concentrations seen in 0.5–2 h. Colchicine has a large V_d and low systemic clearance (Sabouraud et al. 1992a). Two major active metabolites are formed: 2-demethylcolchicine (10%) and 3-demethylcolchicine (33%). Most colchicine is excreted in the faeces; in subjects with normal renal function about 10%–20% is excreted in the urine. Colchicine accumulation leads to prolonged toxicity, particularly in elderly patients or those with cardiac, renal, hepatic or gastrointestinal disease. The severity of poisoning and mortality rate correlate well with the dose ingested. Ingestion of 0.5–0.8 mg leads to death in 10%–50% of cases; ingestion of more than 0.8 mg/kg is invariably fatal (Bismuth et al. 1986).

Signs and symptoms of toxicity appear after an initial delay of 2–12 h. The first 1–3 days are characterized by an intestinal and a circulatory phase with nausea, vomiting, diarrhoea and abdominal pain. This is followed by an aplasia phase and a recovery phase with alopecia. Shock, an adult respiratory distress syndrome (ARDS) and death usually occur within the first week. Haemodialysis and haemoperfusion cannot significantly increase the elimination of colchicine and do not affect the course of the poisoning. If an antibody is to be effective, it must reverse the intracellular binding of colchicine to tubulin.

In an elegant series of experiments, Scherrmann's group has studied the pharmacokinetics and toxicokinetics of colchicine, its major metabolites, colchicine-specific antibodies and colchicine-specific Fab fragments. One milligram of colchicine requires 125 mg of Fab fragments for neutralization. Using antisera and Fab raised in goats (Sabouraud et al. 1991), studies have been carried out in mice, rats and rabbits. Colchicine-specific antibody has been shown to cross-react with the two major active metabolites of colchicine. The efficacy of specific goat polyclonal anti-colchicine IgG in reversing acute colchicine poisoning was first demonstrated in mice (Terrien et al. 1990). Further work with Fab fragments (Sabouraud et al. 1991) showed a clear dose–effect relationship: 80% of mice survived when using a half stoichiometrically equivalent dose (M/2) of Fab fragments and a 100% lethal colchicine dose; mortality with an M/4 and M/8 dose of Fab fragments was 50% and 80%. In a kinetic study in the rabbit, Sabouraud et al. (1992a) found that colchicine-specific Fab fragments at a half stoichiometrically equivalent dose increased total colchicine concentrations in plasma 10–16-fold within 15 min. As with digoxin, the free plasma fraction decreased and was undetectable over a 2 h period. There was a 24-fold and 17-fold decrease in V_d and systemic clearance, and a significantly greater amount of colchicine was excreted in the urine (45% versus 31%). In further work, the influence of colchicine-specific Fab fragments on colchicine plasma disposition and excretion routes in bile duct cannulated rats was studied (Sabouraud et al. 1992b). The effect of colchicine-specific Fab fragments on the V_d and systemic clearance of colchicine was confirmed, illustrating that during Fab treatment, colchicine follows the elimination kinetics of Fab fragments: in this study Fab fragments reduced the biliary excretion of colchicine.

One case of colchicine poisoning treated with colchicine-specific Fab fragments has been reported (Baud et al. 1992; Sabouraud et al. 1992c). A 25-year-old woman was treated with polyclonal, colchicine-specific Fab fragments 40 h after ingestion of 60 mg (a lethal dose) of colchicine. On admission, she had an ARDS and was in circulatory shock. Assuming bioavailability of 45% and a half-life of 27 h, it was calculated that the total body load of colchicine at the time of treatment was 9 mg. The dose of Fab fragments given was equivalent to one-eighth molar neutralization of the dose taken, or about 40% of the remaining total body load. The Fab was given by infusion over 7 h. A six-fold increase in total colchicine concentration in plasma was found 10 min after starting the infusion. There was a six-fold increase in the urinary excretion rate of colchicine after Fab; 98% was bound to Fab. The amount of Fab-bound colchicine excreted renally was equal to the binding capacity of the Fab fragment recovered in the urine. Thus, the neutralization yield of Fab fragments was almost 100%. About 3.7 mg of colchicine was neutralized, representing about 40% of the total body load of colchicine. The patient survived, although she had neutropenia and alopecia.

This case clearly shows that a stoichiometrically equivalent dose of Fab is not necessary to change the course of colchicine poisoning. Because colchicine poisoning is an infrequent cause of severe poisoning in most countries, it remains to be seen whether this important advance in clinical toxicology will be commercialized.

Tricyclic Antidepressants

Tricyclic antidepressant (TCA) overdose is a major cause of morbidity and mortality from self-poisoning in the industrialized world. The estimated number of hospital admissions ranges from 200 to 400/million inhabitants/year. Although several potentially less toxic antidepressants have been marketed over the last decade, the number of prescriptions of first-generation TCA continues to increase (Henry 1991, personal communication). Most deaths in hospital occur within a few hours of admission. In a hospital setting death is due to cardiac complications such as hypotension and ventricular arrhythmias rather than respiratory depression. Management is supportive (Frommer et al. 1987) and includes sodium bicarbonate, which has been shown to ameliorate cardiotoxicity (Pentel and Benowitz 1984). Haemodialysis and haemoperfusion do not significantly increase total body clearance of TCA and have not been shown to affect the course of intoxication (Heath et al. 1982). Although most TCA have an elimination half-life exceeding 24 h, typical features of overdose such as coma, respiratory depression, seizures and conduction disturbances present within 1 or 2 h and resolve rapidly, often within 12–14 h (Hultén and Heath 1983). Thus symptoms follow a time course that parallels the redistribution of TCA (the distribution, or α phase) where the TCA half-life is about 1–2 h in contrast to 25–30 h when in the elimination (or β) phase (Hultén et al. 1992). Since the V_d is smaller in the α phase less antidote may be required to lower plasma TCA concentrations and thereby effect a clinical response.

The success of digoxin-specific Fab fragments has stimulated interest in developing a similar product for TCA. Whole IgG antibodies (O'Callaghan et al. 1987; Sabouraud et al. 1990), monoclonal $F(ab')_2$ (Brunn et al. 1991), monoclonal Fab′ (Brunn et al. 1992) and polyclonal Fab (Sidki 1993, personal communication) have been raised against desipramine, imipramine, nortriptyline and amitriptyline. For anti-TCA antibodies to enter clinical practice, four major hurdles must be overcome. First, the clinical presentation of different tri- and tetracyclic TCA is quite similar. Therefore, the clinical value of an antidote in an emergency situation to a large extent depends on the degree to which the antidote, raised against one or more TCA, cross-reacts with another TCA and its major active metabolites. Cross-reactance between at least desipramine, imipramine, nortriptyline and amitriptyline is highly desirable. Sabouraud et al. (1990) have shown that whole antibodies raised against nortriptyline can significantly reduce amitriptyline-induced mortality in rabbits. In vitro studies have shown good cross-reactance between amitriptyline, nortriptyline, imipramine and desipramine with an ovine Fab raised against a combined nortryptyline–desipramine immunogen (Sidki 1993, personal communication).

Secondly, is stoichiometric equivalence a prerequisite for TCA antibodies or Fab to reverse TCA toxicity in vivo? If this is true, then enormous quantities of antibodies may be required. Even using a Fab fragment, complete neutralization of 4 g of amitriptyline would require more than 700 g of Fab. If, however, the severity of TCA poisoning (toxicodynamics) follows the kinetics of the distribution (α) phase, much less Fab will be required. A 2000 ng/ml decrease in the plasma concentration in the α phase (when the volume of distribution is smaller) may only require 20–50 g of Fab. Whole antidesipramine antibody (Pentel et al. 1987) and desipramine-specific Fab fragments (Hursting et al. 1989) have been shown to rapidly redistribute desipramine from tissue to plasma. The efficacy of the desipramine antibody appears to be dose related: a given dose of antibody binds more drug as desipramine concentrations increase (Pentel et al. 1991a; Pond et al. 1991). Consequently, in vivo binding studies should be carried out using toxic doses of TCA, even though this requires larger amounts of antibody. Earlier (Pentel et al. 1991b) and recent results from this group (Brunn et al. 1992) support the concept that less than equimolar doses of antibody can significantly reduce cardiac toxicity, although the quantity required will be more than the amount needed just to bind free (unbound) TCA in plasma (Pentel and Keyler 1988). Cross-reactive anti-TCA Fab′ has been shown to counteract desipramine-induced hypotension by redistributing desipramine. Concurrent treatment with sodium bicarbonate increases the efficacy of anti-TCA Fab′, and enhances urinary desipramine excretion by increasing anti-Fab′ excretion (Brunn et al. 1992). The authors conclude that desipramine toxicity can be substantially reduced by binding only a small fraction of the desipramine dose. In this study blood pressure increased and the QRS duration on the ECG shortened when only 11% of the calculated equimolar dose was given. If a Fab rather than a Fab′ is used the amount of protein administered could be reduced by 10%, further increasing the distribution volume and enhancing efficacy. Based on experimental evidence to date, some 50–100 g of Fab fragments may be required to treat human TCA poisoning.

Thirdly, cost. The large quantity of Fab required can most probably only be produced at an acceptable cost by using polyclonal technology. The fourth question to be answered before anti-TCA Fab fragments enter clinical practice concerns safety: is a rapid infusion of 50–100 g ovine Fab safe? In a study by Pentel et al. the mean total protein dose was 1–2.4 g/kg, a dose that has been found to be well tolerated in earlier work. However, Keyler et al. (1990) noted a transient increase in serum creatinine in dogs given up to 5.2 g/kg of non-specific human IgG Fab fragments.

Clinical trials are now planned with a polyclonal, ovine anti-TCA Fab. Only results from these trials can provide definitive answers to these questions. In the best case, an antidote to TCA poisoning should be available within the next 5 years.

It is now more than a decade since drug-specific Fab fragments were introduced into clinical practice. So far anti-digoxin Fab is the only product marketed, and anti-colchicine and anti-TCA Fab the only other products in clinical trials.

This slow development has several explanations. Anti-drug Fab can only be expected to have very narrow indications. Because of the small market and the very different production technology required (compared with conventional pharmaceutical medicine) to produce large quantities of polyclonal Fab, it is unlikely that more than a few products will become available. Nonetheless, the dose of Fab required may be less than that at first anticipated. Much less than molar quantities may be sufficient to effect a clinical response, and optimal dosing may ensure that no Fab is excreted before binding to its target drug.

References

Aeberhard P, Butler V-P, Smith TW et al (1980) Le traitement d'une intoxication digitalique massive (20 mg de digitoxine) par les anticorps anti-digoxine fractionnés (Fab). Arch Mal Coeur 12: 1471–1478

Allen NM, Dunham DG, Sailstad JM, Findlay JW (1991) Clinical and pharmacokinetic profiles of digoxin-immune Fab in four patients with renal impairment. Drug Intell Clin Pharm 25: 1315–1320

Antman EM, Wenger TL, Butler VP, Haber E, Smith TW (1990) Treatment of 150 cases of life-threatening digitalis intoxication with digoxin-specific Fab antibody fragments. Final report of a multicenter study. Circulation 81: 1744–1752

Baud FJ, Scherrmann JM, Sabouraud A, Taboulet P (1992) Clinical course of one life-threatening colchicine intoxication treated with colchicine-specific Fab fragments. Proceedings of the XV European Association of Poison Centres and Clinical Toxicology Congress, Istanbul, 1992

Bayer M (1991) Recognition and management of digitalis intoxication. Am J Emerg Med 9 (suppl 1): 29–32

Bismuth C, Baud F, Dally S (1986) Standardized prognosis evaluation in acute toxicology. Its benefit in colchicine, paraquat and digitalis poisonings. J Toxicol Clin Toxicol 6: 33–38

Bismuth C, Motte G, Conso F, Chauvin M, Gaultier M (1977) Acute digitoxin intoxication treated by intracardiac pacemaker: Experience in sixty-eight patients. Clin Toxicol 10: 443–456

Blum LM, Rieders F (1987) Oleandrin distribution in a fatality from rectal and oral *Nerium oleander* extract administration. J Anal Toxicol 11: 219–221

Bouffard Y, Bui Xuan B, Roux H et al. (1982) Intoxication à la digitoxine. Traitment par des fragments Fab d'anticorps anti-digoxine. La Nouvelle Presse Medicale 11(39): 2928

Brunn GJ, Keyler DE, Pond SM, Pentel PR (1992) Reversal of desipramine toxicity in rats using drug specific antibody Fab' fragment: Effects on hypotension and interaction with sodium bicarbonate. J Pharmacol Exp Ther 260(3): 1392–1399

Brunn GJ, Keyler DE, Ross CA, Pond SM, Pentel PR (1991) Drug specific $F(ab')_2$ fragment reduces desipramine cardiotoxicity in rats. Int J Immunopharmacol 13(7): 841–852

Butler VP, Chen JP (1967) Digoxin specific antibodies. Proc Natl Acad Sci USA 57: 71–78

Clark RF, Selden BS, Curry SC (1991) Digoxin specific Fab fragments in the treatment of oleander toxicity in a canine model. Ann Emerg Med 20(10): 1073–1077

Clifton GD, Mclntyre WJ, Zannikos PN, Harrison MR, Chandler MH (1989) Free and total serum digoxin concentrations in a renal failure patient after treatment with digoxin immune Fab. Clin Pharmacol 8: 441–445

Colburn WA (1980) Specific antibodies and Fab fragments to alter the pharmacokinetics and reverse pharmacologic/toxicologic effects of drugs. Drug Metab Rev 11(2): 223–262

Colucci RD, Chow M, Kluger J et al (1989) The pharmacokinetics of digoxin immune Fab, total digoxin and free digoxin in patients with renal impairment. Pharmacotherapy 9: 175 (abst)

Cummins RO, Haulman J, Quan L, Graves JR, Peterson D, Horan S (1990) Near-fatal yew berry intoxication treated with external cardiac pacing and digoxin-specific Fab antibody fragments. Ann Emerg Med 19: 38–43

Curd J, Smith TW, Jaton J (1971) The isolation of digoxin specific antibodies and its use in reversing the effects of digoxin. Proc Natl Acad Sci USA 68: 2401–2406

Ellenhorn MJ, Barceloux DG (1988) Medical toxicology. Diagnosis and treatment of human poisoning. Elsevier, New York

Erdmann E, Mair W, Knedel M, Schaumann W (1989) Digitalis intoxication and treatment with digoxin antibody fragments in renal failure. Klin Wochenschr 67: 16–19

Frommer DA, Kulig KA, Marx JA, Rumack B (1987) Tricyclic antidepressant overdose. JAMA 257: 521–526

Goodlin RC (1988) Antidigoxin antibodies in eclampsia. N Engl J Med 318(8): 518
Hamburger RN, Douglass JH (1969) Chloramphenicol-specific antibody. II. Reactivity to analogues of chloramphenicol. Immunology 17(4): 587–591
Heath A, Wickström I, Ahlmen J, Mårtensson E (1982) Treatment of antidepressant poisoning with resin haemoperfusion. Human Toxicol 1(4): 152–156
Hickey AR, Wenger TL, Carpenter VP et al. (1991) Digoxin immune Fab therapy in the management of digitalis intoxication: Safety and efficacy. Results of an observational surveillance study. J Am Coll Cardiol 17(3): 590–598
Hooker SB, Boyd WC (1940) Antibodies to strychnine. J Immunol 38: 479–490
Huang CT, Smith RM (1984) Lowering of blood pressure in chronic aortic coarctate hypertensive rats with antidigoxin antiserum. Life Sci 35: 115–118
Hultén B-A, Heath A (1983) Clinical evaluation of tricyclic antidepressant poisoning. Acta Med Scand 213: 275–278
Hultén B-A, Heath A, Knudsen K, Nyberg G, Starmark J-E, Mårtensson E (1992) Severe amitriptyline overdose: Relationship between toxicokinetics and toxicodynamics. J Toxicol Clin Toxicol 30(2): 171–179
Hursting MJ, Opheim KE, Raisys CA, Kenny MA, Metzger G (1989) Tricyclic antidepressant-specific Fab fragments alter distribution and elimination in the rabbit: A model for overdose treatment. J Toxicol Clin Toxicol 27: 53–66
Jaeger A, Berton C, Kopferschmitt J et al. (1992) Dosing with digoxin-Fab fragments. Proceedings of the XV European Association of Poison Centres and Clinical Toxicology Congress, Istanbul, 1992
Keyler DE, Murakami MA, Salerno DM, Ruth GR, Pentel PR (1990) Toxicity and pharmacokinetics of high doses of antibody Fab fragments in dogs. Vet Hum Toxicol 32(4): 341 (abstr)
Kirkpatrick CH (1991) Allergic histories and reactions of patients treated with digoxin immune Fab (ovine) antibody. Am J Emerg Med 9 (suppl 1): 7–10
Kunes J, Stolba P, Pohlova I, Jelinek J, Zicha J (1985) The importance of digoxin-like factors in rats with various forms of experimental hypertension. Clin Exp Hypertens 7: 707–720 (abstr)
Lewander WJ, Gauldreault P, Einhorn H, Henretig FM, Lacouture PG, Lovejoy FH (1986) Acute pediatric digoxin ingestion: A ten year experience. Am J Dis Child 140: 770–773
Lloyd BL, Smith TW (1978) Contrasting rates of reversal of digoxin toxicity by digoxin specific IgG and Fab fragments. Circulation 58: 280–283
Mahdyoon H, Battilana G, Rosman H, Goldstein S, Gheorghiade M (1990) The evolving pattern of digoxin intoxication: Observations at a large urban hospital from 1980–1988. Am Heart J 120(5): 1189–1194
Marchlinski FE, Hook BG, Callans DJ (1991) Which cardiac disturbances should be treated with digoxin immune Fab (ovine) antibody? Am J Emerg Med 9 (suppl 1): 24–28
Nuwayhid NF, Johnson GF (1989) Digoxin elimination in a functionally anephric patient after digoxin-specific Fab fragment therapy. Ther Drug Monit 11: 680–685
O'Callaghan AM, Phillips OM, Williams DC (1987) Antisera raised against the drug imipramine. J Neurochem 49(4): 1091–1095
Osterloh J, Herold S, Pond SM (1982) Oleander interference in the digoxin radioimmunoassay in a fatal ingestion. JAMA 247: 1596–1597
Owens SM, Mayersohn M (1986) Phencyclidine-specific Fab fragments alter phencyclidine disposition in dogs. Drug Metab Dispos 14: 52–58
Pentel PR, Benowitz NL (1984) Efficacy and mechanism of action of sodium bicarbonate in the treatment of desipramine toxicity in rats. J Pharmacol Exp Ther 230: 12–19
Pentel PR, Keyler DE (1988) Effect of high dose alpha-1-acid glycoprotein on desipramine toxicity in rats. J Pharmacol Exp Ther 246: 1061–1066
Pentel P, Pond SM, Schoof D (1987) Redistribution into plasma of tracer doses of desipramine by anti-desipramine antiserum in rats. Biochem Pharmacol 36(2): 293–295
Pentel PR, Keyler DE, Brunn GJ et al. (1991a) Redistribution of tricyclic antidepressants in rats using a drug-specific monoclonal antibody: Dose–response relationship. Drug Metab Dispos 19: 24–28
Pentel PR, Brunn GJ, Pond SM, Keyler DE (1991b) Pretreatment with drug specific antibody reduces desipramine cardiotoxicity in rats. Life Sci 48(7): 675–683
Persson H (1992) Initial experience with *V. berus* specific Fab antivenom. Proceedings of the XV European Association of Poison Centres and Clinical Toxicology Congress, Istanbul, 1992 (abstr)

Pond SM, Pentel PR, Keyler DE, Winzor DJ (1991) Determination of the in-vivo antigen–antibody affinity constant from the redistribution of desipramine specific monoclonal antibody. Biochem Pharmacol 41(3): 473–476

Rabetoy GM, Price CA, Findlay JWA, Sailstad JM (1990) Treatment of digoxin intoxication in a renal failure patient with digoxin specific antibody fragments and plasmapheresis. Am J Nephrol 10: 518–521

Sabouraud A, Denis H, Urtizberea M, Chappey O, Scherrmann J-M (1990) The effect of nortriptyline-specific active immunization on amitriptyline toxicity and disposition in the rabbit. Toxicology 62(3): 349–360

Sabouraud A, Urtizberea M, Grandgeorge JM, Gattel P, Makula MF, Scherrmann J-M (1991) Dose-dependent reversal of acute murine colchicine intoxication by specific goat anti-colchicine Fab fragments. Toxicology 68: 121–132

Sabouraud AE, Urtizberea M, Cano NJ, Grandgeorge JM, Rouzioux M, Scherrmann J-M (1992a) Colchicine specific Fab fragments alter colchicine disposition in rabbits. J Pharmacol Exp Ther 260(3): 1214–1219

Sabouraud AE, Urtizberea M, Benmoussa K, Cano NJ, Scherrmann J-M (1992b) Fab bound colchicine appears to adopt Fab fragment disposition in rats. J Pharm Pharmacol 44: 1015–1019

Sabouraud A, Urtizberea M, Scherrmann J-M, Caraux J, Baud F, Bismuth C (1992c) First pharmacokinetic investigation of colchicine specific Fab fragments in one case of human colchicine poisoning. Proceedings of the XV European Association of Poison Centres and Clinical Toxicology Congress, Istanbul, 1992

Schaumann W, Kaufmann B, Neubert P, Smolarz A (1986) Kinetics of the Fab fragments of digoxin antibodies and of bound digoxin in patients with severe digoxin intoxication. Eur J Clin Pharmacol 30: 527–533

Shumiak GM, Wu AW, Ping AC (1988) Oleander poisoning. Treatment with digoxin specific Fab antibody fragments. Ann Emerg Med 17: 732–735

Sinclair AJ, Hewick DS, Johnston PC, Stevenson IH, Lemon M (1989) Kinetics of digoxin and anti-digoxin antibody fragments during treatment of digoxin toxicity. Br J Clin Pharmacol 28: 352–356

Smith TW (1988) Digitalis: Mechanisms of action and clinical use. N Engl J Med 318: 358–365

Smith TW, Haber E (1970) Digoxin intoxication: The relationship of clinical presentation to serum digoxin concentration. J Clin Invest 49: 2377–2386

Smith TW, Butler VP, Haber E et al. (1982) Treatment of life threatening digitalis intoxication with digoxin-specific Fab antibody fragments. Experience in 26 cases. N Engl J Med 307: 1357–1362

Smith TW, Haber TE, Yeatman L, Butler VP Jr (1976) Reversal of advanced digoxin intoxication with Fab fragments of digoxin-specific antibodies. N Engl J Med 294: 797–800

Smolarz A, Roesch E, Lenz H, Neubert P, Abshagen U (1984) Erfahrungsbericht über die Behandlung von 16 schweren Glykosidvergiftungen mit digitalis-antikorper-Fragmenten (Fab). Z Kardiol 73(2): 113–119

Sullivan JB (1986) Immunotherapy in the poisoned patient. Overview of present applications and future trends. Med Toxicol 1: 47–60

Terrien N, Urtizberea M, Scherrmann JM (1990) Reversal of advanced colchicine toxicity in mice with goat colchicine-specific antibodies. Toxicol Appl Pharmacol 104(3): 504–510

Ujhelyi MR, Colucci RD, Cummings DM et al. (1991) Monitoring serum digoxin concentrations during digoxin immune Fab therapy. Drug Intell Clin Pharm 25: 1047–1049

Ujhelyi MR, Cummings DM, Green PJ, Robert S, Vlasses PH, Zarowitz BJ (1992) Free digoxin concentrations using three immunoassay methods in patients receiving digoxin Fab antibodies. 92nd Annual Meeting of the American Society for Clinical Pharmacology and Therapeutics, San Antonio. Clin Pharm Ther 49(2): 131

Wenger TL (1991) Experience with digoxin immune Fab (ovine) in patients with renal impairment. Am J Emerg Med 9 (suppl 1): 21–23

Wieland JM, Marchlinski FE (1986) Electrocardiographic response of digoxin toxic fascicular tachycardia to Fab fragments: Implications for tachycardia mechanism. PACE 9: 727–738

Woolf AD, Wenger T, Smith TW, Lovejoy FH (1992) The use of digoxin-specific Fab fragments for severe digitalis intoxication in children. N Engl J Med 326: 1739–1744

Zucker AR, Lacina SJ, DasGupta DS et al. (1982) Fab fragments of digoxin specific antibodies used to reverse ventricular fibrillation induced by digoxin ingestion in a child. Pediatrics 70(3): 468–471

6 Therapeutic Antibodies to Snake Venoms

R.D.G. Theakston and D.C. Smith

History

Studies on immunization against snake venoms began over 100 years ago when Sewall (1887) demonstrated that pigeons could be immunized against the venom of the pygmy rattlesnake (*Sistrurus catenatus tergeminus*) after treating the animals with gradually increasing amounts of the venom. These studies were followed closely by those of Calmette (1894a, 1895, 1898) and Phisalix and Bertrand (1894) who immunized horses against snake venoms. Calmette (1894a) recommended mixtures of hypochlorite and venom, and Phisalix and Bertrand (1894) used heat-treated venom in order to reduce the toxicity and retain the antigenicity of the immunogens. Subsequently, Fraser (1895), working in Scotland, produced a specific immune serum against cobra venom. Calmette's work resulted in the publication of a book on venoms which contained the first basic information on techniques for animal immunization against venoms. Later, Pasteur Institutes throughout the world started to produce and supply antivenoms on a commercial basis. Further detailed studies on antivenoms were made by Brazil (1911) in São Paulo; the Instituto Butantan subsequently initiated large-scale antivenom production, which has continued almost unchanged to the present day.

Standard Methods of Antivenom Production

Because of biochemical and immunological differences between snake venoms from different areas of the world, antivenoms are produced commercially by 63 different laboratories in 37 countries (Russell and Lauritzen 1966; Latifi 1978; Russell 1980; WHO 1981; Detrait 1982; Chippaux and Goyffon 1983; Theakston and Warrell 1991). Antivenoms are made by the gradual hyperimmunization of large animals against one or a group of medically important venoms present in either a country or in a specific geographical region.

Ideally, antivenoms should be capable of neutralizing all the toxic components in a venom, and to do this it is generally considered best to use unmodified venom for immunization rather than relying on detoxification using formaldehyde treatment and other methods, such as irradiation, glutaraldehyde or heat treatment, which may result in a reduction or complete loss of important antigens (Latifi 1978). In highly toxic venoms, such as those of some elapids and sea snakes, however, the use of formol toxoids (prepared under acid conditions, as alkalinity leads to loss of both toxicity and antigenicity) has been considered unavoidable. Venom used in the preparation of antivenoms is best presented combined with an adjuvant, such as Freund's complete adjuvant, which results in a decrease in toxicity because only gradual release of the venom is permitted (Christensen 1955; Latifi and Manhouri 1966; Sawai et al. 1972). Unfortunately, horses do not normally tolerate these adjuvants well, the reason for which will be discussed later. Other additives, which include substances such as bentonite (Christensen 1966a), aluminium hydroxide gel and sodium alginate (Amies 1959), also permit a relatively sustained low-level stimulation of the immune response.

In most cases antivenom is produced as a fluid or lyophilized ampouled preparation comprising either crude filtered horse serum or, in most cases, as an ammonium sulphate-precipitated, pepsin-digested, concentrated $F(ab')_2$ fraction of the IgG molecule (Christensen 1966a,b; Grasset and Christensen 1947; Latifi and Manhouri 1966). Ammonium sulphate is used to precipitate the globulins; the technique was based on the assumption that the albumin, rather than the globulin fraction, was responsible for most of the undesirable serum reactions obtained when large volumes of horse serum are injected into human victims of envenoming (Latifi 1978). The heat-labile fraction of the IgG molecule, the Fc fragment, has no direct immunological activity and is thought by some to be responsible for the early reactions induced by some antivenoms. The Fc portion may be removed by pepsin digestion; the ammonium sulphate, used for precipitation of the IgG, is removed by dialysis and lipids are eliminated by aluminium hydroxide gel agglutination. Filtration is carried out by molecular filtration using gels such as Sephadex. The final product is subsequently tested for pyrogenic activity (usually using rabbits), bacterial sterility, immunological specificity using electrophoresis or immunodiffusion and potency before the final procedure of ampouling under sterile conditions to produce either a lyophilized preparation or a straightforward fluid antivenom. It is remarkable that even today a few producers use crude filtered horse serum alone with all its additional attendant problems (Theakston and Warrell 1991).

Different Types of Available Antivenoms

If a single venom is used for immunization, the antiserum is termed monospecific (monovalent); if more than one venom is used the antiserum is polyspecific (polyvalent). It is assumed that polyspecific antisera should be produced by immunization of animals with a mixture of venoms rather than by mixing of monospecific antivenoms, as the latter method was thought to result in dilution of each component (Christensen 1966a); this, however, may not be true in all cases (see 'Antivenom composition', p. 123). A problem with immunizing animals with more than a single venom may be the production of a competitive effect or antigen-induced suppression, which could well result in an alteration or decrease in the response against one or more of the many antigens involved (Adler 1957). This may be due to competition for antigen-sensitive cells or to a range of other factors (Bouquet 1979), but would certainly apply to a greater extent with polyspecific as opposed to monospecific antivenoms. Generally clinicians prefer to use polyspecific antivenoms as this avoids the necessity for deciding which preparation to use for patient treatment; frequently the clinical signs of envenoming do not provide a clear indication as to which species is responsible for the bite. The advantage of using a monospecific preparation is that (a) it is usually more effective in that a lower volume is required for treatment, and (b) it is useful in areas where a single species of snake that exhibits readily identifiable clinical symptoms (e.g. non-clotting blood following bites by the carpet viper, *Echis ocelletus*, in West Africa) is involved. More detailed information on the advantages and disadvantages of the different types of antivenoms is given in the detailed section on antivenom composition.

Antivenom Reactions

All patients given antivenom should be regarded as likely to exhibit a reaction; in fact about 30% of patients receiving unrefined antivenom develop either early (anaphylactoid) or delayed serum sickness type reactions. According to Reid (1968), following purification (ammonium sulphate precipitation and enzyme digestion) the incidence is reduced to about 10%, but more recent studies suggest that levels far in excess of this are frequently obtained. For example, recent studies on victims of *Bothrops jararaca* (Jararaca) envenoming in Brazil (Cardoso et al. 1993) have indicated that even antivenoms comprising primarily $F(ab')_2$ fragments can produce 30%–84% incidence of early serum reactions. Malasit et al. (1986) stated that the reported incidence of early (potentially life-threatening) reactions ranges from 3% to 54%, the incidence being highest when larger doses of unrefined antivenom are given and related to the speed at which it is administered (Editorial 1980).

Sutherland (1977) reported that most commercial antivenoms are anti-complementary in vitro, and these results led to the recommendation that antivenom should be administered diluted and by slow intravenous infusion. However, more recently Malasit et al. (1986) found no significant differences in the incidence of immediate reactions when antivenom was administered by slow "push" injection or by slow intravenous infusion. Generally, complement activation (Sutherland 1977; Malasit et al. 1986; Pugh and Theakston 1987) and other mechanisms may be involved in addition to immediate (type I) hypersensitivity to equine serum, but the precise causes remain obscure. Of 28 Thai patients treated with unrefined antivenom, 11 suffered early reactions; complement components (C3, C4) were within the normal range and C3b and C3d were not detected (Malasit et al. 1986). Likewise results were inconclusive in six Nigerian patients in whom C3 levels were assayed (Pugh and Theakston 1987). Serum samples in the 11 Thai patients were assayed for immune complexes using Clq and protein A binding assays and no consistent changes in binding activity after antivenom treatment were recorded. There was no apparent association between the presence of complexes and the development of early reactions (Malasit et al. 1986). It is possible that aggregates of immunoglobulins or their components may be either partly or wholly responsible for early reactions.

Results of sensitivity testing proved that these have no predictive value for the occurrence of early reactions, including severe anaphylaxis, and they therefore appear to be a waste of time. Reactions to homologous immunoglobulins resemble reactions to antivenom in that they are not predicted by results of skin tests (Malasit et al. 1986). Anaphylactoid reactions are overcome, in the normal way, by stopping antivenom administration as soon as they occur, injecting subcutaneously 0.5 ml of 1:1000 adrenaline, and cautiously restarting the antivenom if necessary with antihistamine cover. In patients with severe systemic envenoming and a history of allergy, antivenom should still be given with the added precautions applied as described above.

Methods of Antivenom Potency Assessment

Conventional Methods

It is realized that antivenom producers have to make some estimation of neutralizing potency with respect to their products; usually this is presented as the number of lethal doses or the dry weight of a particular venom neutralized by a known volume of antivenom. Potency of an antivenom is generally measured by its ability to save the life of an experimental animal and this is assessed by the ED_{50} test, different doses of antivenom under test being mixed with, for example, five intravenous LD_{50}s (median lethal dose) incubated for 30 min, injected intravenously into mice of known weight, sex and strain, and the survival after 24 h recorded (Theakston and Reid 1983). Other laboratories use other animals such as pigeons and chickens for this assay, which is even more unrealistic than using mice. Christensen (1968) rightly stated that such measures of potency are pointless unless different laboratories use identical methods in relation to the test animal, route of injection and the composition of venom/antivenom mixtures. The intravenous route of injection is normally used in these assays; this is an artificial system because when a snake bites a human, venom is normally introduced via the intradermal, subcutaneous or occasionally the intramuscular route. Christensen (1968) also stressed that the same venom sample must be used in the assays. It is well established that considerable variation exists in venoms from the same species in different geographical areas, as well as between individuals from the same area (Taborska 1971). Venoms also change in biological characteristics as snakes age (Reid and Theakston 1978; Theakston and Reid 1978). In 1968 Christensen proposed that such problems may be avoided by expressing potencies of commercial products against a standard antivenom preparation. Earlier, Christensen (1962) first produced a proposed international standard antivenom from eight horses that had already been immunized against the venoms of *Naja nivea* (Cape cobra), *Hemachatus haemachatus* (ringhals) and *Bitis arietans* (puff adder) and which were subsequently immunized against *N. naja* venom. It was concluded that the proposed standard preparation behaved satisfactorily in tests with some venoms and less so with others.

In 1979 a WHO coordination meeting was held in Zurich to examine the work in progress throughout the world on the characterization of medically important venoms and the standardization of antivenom preparations (WHO 1981). Following this meeting, the Liverpool School of Tropical Medicine was designated as the WHO Collaborative Centre for the Control of Antivenoms and given the responsibility for organizing the collection of eight proposed WHO International Reference Venoms (IRVs) of medical importance – *N. kaouthia*, Thai cobra (Thailand); *N. scutatus*, tiger snake, (Australia); *E. carinatus* (Iran and Mali); *Daboia* (a.k.a *Vipera*) *russelli*, Russell's viper, (Thailand); *Crotalus atrox*, western diamondback rattlesnake, (Mexico); *B. atrox/asper*, barba amarilla, (Costa Rica); and *Trimeresurus flavoviridis*, Habu, (Japan) – and the production of proposed WHO International monospecific Standard Antivenoms (ISAs) against each of these. At the same time simple biological characterization tests, to be carried out by 13 different laboratories throughout the world, were proposed for assessing lethality (LD_{50} test), haemorrhagic and necrotizing activities (rat intradermal skin tests), coagulant activity (in vitro clotting test) and defibrinogenating activity (in vivo mouse test) of the venoms (WHO 1981; Theakston and Reid 1983). Currently, further simple tests for assessment of systemic neuromuscular paralytic activity and systemic myotoxic activity are being developed by Professor J.B. Harris, University of Newcastle, UK (Theakston 1986). The results of these assays on the eight venoms are currently being coordinated; the next stage will be the assessment of the neutralizing activity of the ISAs against the biological effects of the IRVs. Thus, for the first time, it should be possible to have a system whereby the potency of commercial antivenoms can be assessed comparatively. The development of reliable tests is necessary if antivenoms are to be graded easily and consistently in different laboratories in terms of their venom neutralizing abilities. As with all animal-based studies, however, great caution is urged when extrapolating the results of such tests to envenoming in humans.

New Methods for Screening Antivenoms

Christensen (1968) considered that eventually the use of animals could largely be replaced by in vitro methods for estimation of antivenom neutralizing activity. This is not simply of importance because of the difficulty of extrapolating between non-human species and humans; it is highly desirable to avoid the suffering and death of animals. If in vitro methods measure life-saving capability with a precision similar to that obtained with in vivo methods, a major reason for the continued use of animals would be eliminated. That such a system was possible was demonstrated by Theakston and Reid (1979), who investigated ELISA as a screen of antivenom potency. One batch of antivenom from each of three commercial sources (SAIMR, Behringwerke, Haffkine) and two research antisera raised in rabbits were used. These five sera were used as reference antivenoms, and the ED_{50} for neutralizing four venoms of medical importance in Africa – *E. carinatus, B. arietans, N. nigricollis* (spitting cobra), *N. haje* (Egyptian cobra) – were estimated in mice. Reference curves were prepared relating ED_{50} to ELISA optical densities. The ED_{50} of 38 different batches of test antivenom were estimated by ELISA and "ELISA ED_{50}" were then compared with in vivo mouse ED_{50}. Excellent correlation was obtained ($r = 0.96; p<0.001$) and the method proved to be rapid, cheap, simple, economical in amounts of venom used, and, most importantly, greatly reduced the need for live animals. If validated in an extended range of venoms and antivenoms, ELISA screening of antivenom potency could be a useful standard procedure. ELISA measures antibody (or antigen), and it is realized that antigen–antibody reactions of venoms and their degree of toxicity are two distinct and sometimes unrelated phenomena (Schottler 1951). Antigens may be non-toxic and toxins may be non-antigenic. Nevertheless, these preliminary studies suggest sufficient correlation between in vivo mouse ED_{50} and ELISA optical density readings to warrant further exploration of this system.

Current lethality assays for assessing antivenoms (and other drugs) involve the use of a large number of mice for each determination in order to obtain statistically significant results. Recently, Meier and Theakston (1986) described a method in which only eight to ten experimental animals were used to obtain a result instead of 30 or more. If proved to be satisfactory, this method may well replace the classical assay.

Clinical Trials

The most reliable and meaningful method of assessing antivenoms is of course by direct clinical trial in human victims of envenoming (Warrell et al. 1974, 1980, 1986; Daudu and Theakston 1988; Phillips et al. 1988; Cardoso et al. 1993). It is notable that very few well-controlled trials have been performed, and this reflects the logistic problems associated with organizing such trials in developing countries where snake bite is a problem (e.g. lack of basic facilities such as constant and stable electricity supply, reliable or existent water supply, etc.).

It is obviously necessary to conduct comparative trials on a randomized double-blind basis with a detailed protocol and clinical proforma available. There are usually two main aims of such studies: (i) potency comparison of different antivenoms in human patients (potencies as estimated in animal models are frequently unreliable), and (ii) the calculation of the optimum initial dosage of an antivenom in relation to the defined severity of envenoming (e.g. mild, moderate, severe). Both involve accurate monitoring of antivenom treatment using both clinical and laboratory parameters.

Ideally the species involved should be confirmed either by the taxonomic identification of the snake or by positive identification of venom in the blood, wound aspirate or other body fluids of the victim by either enzyme or radioimmunoassay (Theakston et al. 1977; Coulter et al. 1978, 1980; Ho et al. 1986). Patients who have already received antivenom prior to admission, are very young or very old, pregnant women or already infirm individuals should be excluded from the study. Informed consent by patients or relatives for inclusion into the study should be obtained.

Methods used in such studies should include recording the history of the patient and results of physical examination on a standard proforma. This should be divided into local signs (e.g. fang marks, evidence of pre-hospital treatment such as incisions, extent of swelling, local bleeding, bruising, blistering, signs of infection and necrosis) and systemic signs (e.g. evidence of spontaneous systemic bleeding, shock, cardiac arrhythmias, neurotoxic).

Laboratory studies should include, among others, the assessment of the kinetics of venom and antivenom using immunoassay techniques (Theakston et al. 1977, 1992; Ho et al. 1986) to estimate the half-lives of both venom and antivenom in the system, correction of haemostatic and blood coagulation abnormalities and reversal of neurological and myolytic effects depending on the type of snake involved. The effect of the antivenom on the resolution of local effects such as swelling and necrosis should be assessed as well as the side-effects of the antivenom/s (e.g. early anaphylactic, pyrogenic and late serum sickness type reactions).

Recent Developments in Antivenom Production

Choice of Host Animal

Antivenoms have been raised in a number of host species, notable examples being horses, donkeys (Calmette 1894b), goats (Mohamed et al. 1966; Russell et al. 1970; Kochalty et al. 1971), rabbits (Russell 1961), dogs (Theakston and Warrell 1991) and even llamas (Russell, personal communication). For manufacturing purposes, however, the choice has been largely restricted to the horse (Minton 1974) and there are currently over 60 centres throughout the world using this animal to raise antisera to a variety of venoms (Theakston and Warrell 1991). This situation is far from ideal.

The prevalence of horses as a source of immune serum is largely historical since serotherapy developed at the turn of the century when they were both plentiful and cheap. Commercially, therefore, these big docile animals seemed to be the ideal host. Large volumes of blood could be taken at regular intervals with no apparent detrimental effect on the animals' health making antivenom production a cost-effective enterprise, particularly in developing countries where large numbers of bites occur each year. In the last quarter of the twentieth century, however, horses and low-cost stabling are no longer readily available. Consequently, production of antiserum using these animals is more expensive today and represents a large investment for any potential antivenom producer. As a direct result of these increased costs, production methods have not changed radically since the advent of antivenoms (Christensen 1979).

Capital for product development is often unavailable for what is usually a low-profit enterprise and, tragically, this problem is most acute in the developing countries where the need for antivenom is often the greatest.

Horse-based therapies are also associated with an intrinsic problem. In the past, treatment of envenoming has been considered more art than science and for this reason, in order to ensure that sufficient antivenom was administered, large amounts of horse protein are often given to the victim. This, in conjunction with the fact that many people are sensitive to horse serum proteins, often results in patients exhibiting severe side-effects to treatment typified by both early and delayed sensitivity reactions (Russell et al. 1985); indeed it has been reported (Corrigan et al. 1978) that up to 75% of patients treated with crotalid antivenom in the USA develop serum sickness. This sensitivity is thought to be due, in part, to the well-documented immunogenicity (Weir and Porter 1966) of immune equine immunoglobulin containing, as it does, a high proportion of the IgG(T) subclass. IgG(T), when injected into mice, provokes a strong immune response, greater than that produced by either sheep or pig immunoglobulin (Cartledge et al. 1992) and it has also been found that only half the amount of IgG(T) was needed to elicit precipitating lapine antibodies as other equine subclasses (Buchowicz et al. 1969). However, as Christensen (1979) comments, anaphylactic shock is said to be observed more often after the first than after subsequent injections of horse serum, incriminating naturally acquired hypersensitivity to equine protein.

It is mainly for these reasons that alternative host animals have been investigated as a source of antivenom. Russell (1961) showed that rabbits could provide safe and effective antisera and no sensitivity reactions were seen in the small number of patients treated. This animal, although readily abundant in most countries and easy to handle, provides only a limited amount of blood, necessitating the use of large numbers of animals; one bleed from a horse will provide the equivalent of that from 200 rabbits. Russell et al. (1970) also produced a similar treatment in goats, which proved both safe and efficacious. Goats produce significant amounts of serum and are ubiquitous in developing countries where the need for such therapies is often greatest and they could well fit the role of alternative host animal. However, being particularly prone to tropical infections, this animal may not respond well to repeated and long-term immunization programmes in hot climates. Despite these advantages it is regrettable that, with one exception (Twyfords *C. rhodostoma* antivenom; Warrell et al. 1986; Theakston and Warrell 1991), no major effort has been made by the world's antivenom producers to use the goat as a source of antivenom. Even in North America, where it is estimated that over 8000 bites occur annually, resulting in an average of 12 deaths per year (Loprinzi et al. 1983), equine-based products often remain the only choice to the emergency department physician.

A third animal, which combines all these qualities and which is found in great abundance in both the Northern and Southern Hemispheres, is the sheep. These animals are comparatively cheap to buy and maintain, are resistant to disease and provide 500 ml of blood at each bleeding. Sheep immunoglobulin is not associated with any of the immunogenicity problems of equine IgG(T), and it is probably not coincidental that ovine serum has been chosen as the source of immunoglobulin for the successful cardiac glycoside treatment, Digibind. In trials conducted in the USA, this drug, a digoxin-specific immunoglobulin fragment, has been used successfully in the management of over 700 cases of overdose, almost all patients responding well to symptomatic treatment (Hickey et al. 1991).

Recently, experimental antivenoms against detoxified crotalid venoms (*C. durissus terrificus, C. atrox* and *Trimeresurus flavoviridis*) have also been produced by immunizing laying chickens (Carroll et al. 1992). The ready availability and low price of purchasing and maintaining hens makes this an attractive proposition. If the technique can be developed commercially, this animal provides a possible alternative to antivenoms raised in mammals.

Antivenom Production

Immunization

With over 60 producers of antivenom in operation, minor details of production are certain to exist. However, the overall strategy remains basically the same. The effectiveness of the antiserum depends on its antibody titre, its specificity and its degree of concentration. Conventional immunization of horses to produce antivenom follows a hyperimmunization schedule in which large amounts of venom are given in rapidly increasing sequential doses of up to 1200 mg per injection (Russell 1988; Table 6.1). Such protocols do not, however, result in equivalent, regular increases in serum antibodies. Initially, antibody levels increase progressively, but this may be followed by a decline in titre after further stimulation with large venom doses (Christensen 1966a; Bouquet 1979). Bouquet (1979) considered that a more satisfactory method was to give two subcutaneous injections of antigen at short intervals, allow the animals to rest and 3 weeks later repeat the process with booster injections, thus priming the secondary immune response, which confers an immunological memory to immunocompetent cells (Celada 1971; Miller et al. 1971).

The necessity for such large amounts of venom, which are almost certainly detrimental to the condition of the animal is, in part, due to the equine intolerance of oil-based adjuvants such as Freund's complete and incomplete adjuvants, which are known to enhance the immune response to immunogen. Theories on the mode of action of adjuvants have been outlined by Bouquet (1979). Briefly, macrophages are thought to process antigen and to present it to immunocompetent cells simultaneously with major histocompatibility antigens, causing these recipient cells to divide and differentiate. It is thought that adjuvants may facilitate contacts between macrophages and lymphocytes as well as exerting an enhancing effect on the antibody-producing cells (B lymphocytes) after uptake by macrophages; they also "turn on" T helper cells, which results in increased stimulation of B cells. According to Braun and Nakano (1967) and Johnson et al. (1968), the cell destruction induced by some adjuvants, such as Freund's complete adjuvant, causes the liberation of nucleic acid, which also enhances the immune response. Emulsions of venom in oil-based adjuvants such as Freund's also result in a toxicity reduction because venom is only gradually released into the host animal (Christensen 1955; Latifi and Manhouri 1966; Sawai et al. 1972).

Sheep, in which the response is predominantly humoral, do not demonstrate the severe local reactions manifested in horses when adjuvants such as these are used; also, the resulting circulating specific antibody concentrations in sheep, receiving a maximum of 4 mg venom per month (Table 6.1), are in the region of 7–10 g/l (Smith et al. 1992). This represents approximately 25% of the total immunoglobulin concentration and compares favourably with values of below 10% typically achieved with horses (DCS, unpublished results) where adjuvants such as silica gel and aluminium hydroxide are used. Such additives are also thought to permit a slow release of antigen allowing a relatively sustained low level stimulation of the immune response (Amies 1959; Christensen 1966a). The high levels of specific antibody achieved by immunizing sheep with low venom doses in conjunction with Freund's adjuvant reduce the number of animals required to produce commercial quantities of antivenom, while the low doses of immunogen save venom, which can be both costly and difficult to acquire. Higher circulating antibody levels in the serum also reduce the degree of concentration required to produce a potent product in a manageable form for administration.

Table 6.1. A comparison of hyperimmunization with low-dose protocols

Week no.	Hyper dose (mg/horse)	Low dose (mg/sheep)
0	3	0.5
1	6	
2	10	
3	24	
4	40	1.0
5	100	
6	200	
7	400	
8	600	2.0
9	750	
10	1000	Bleed
11	Bleed	
12	Rest	4.0
13	800	
14	1200	Bleed
15	Bleed	
16	Bleed	4.0
17	Rest	
18	Rest	Bleed
19	Rest	
20	500	4.0
21	750	
22	1200	Bleed
23	Bleed	

The low-dose ovine immunization protocol uses considerably less venom than the conventional protocol used, for example, by Wyeth Laboratories for the production of their crotalid polyvalent antivenom, even taking into account the size differences. (Modified from Russell 1988.)

The high doses of venom immunogen required for conventional immunization often result in a reliance on toxoids to overcome intrinsic venom toxicity. This is often the case when using elapid or sea snake venoms where toxicity is particularly high; in the past detoxification using glutaraldehyde, irradiation or heat treatment has been employed. These techniques alter, and in some cases completely destroy, the all-important secondary and tertiary structure of the proteins. Toxicity is thereby reduced, but in so doing the antigens required for raising neutralizing antibodies are also eliminated and ineffective antivenom is produced. More antivenom must then be given to treat the systemic envenoming thus increasing the probability of adverse reactions. Low-dose protocols in combination with a suitable host animal and judicious use of oil-based adjuvants overcome this problem because the amounts of venom used are usually well below the lethal dose of the venom.

Formaldehyde, glutaraldehyde or heat-treated crotalid venoms in Freund's complete and incomplete adjuvants have been used to immunize hens by the subcutaneous route. Although a relatively large amount of each venom was required for immunization due to the necessity to toxoid or partially inactivate the material because of the high level of sensitivity in the animals, potent experimental antivenoms were produced (Carroll et al. 1992), which were more active in mouse assays (Theakston and Reid 1983) than the proposed WHO standard antivenoms (WHO 1981).

The quality of the venom used for immunization is also of great importance. Owing to the well-documented variation in venom composition (see the excellent review by Chippaux et al. 1991), it is vital that venom pools used in production take account of seasonal, geographic, genetic and sex-related variation. Failure to do so may well result in an antivenom of limited use. Strict quality control measures must be employed to ensure that the venom used is of consistent composition, not always an easy task because antivenoms are also often manufactured using venoms from outside the countries in which they are intended for use. For example, the *E. carinatus* venoms used for the preparation of SAIMR (South African Institute for Medical Research), Pasteur and Behringwerke antivenoms used in West Africa originate in East Africa (Ethiopia and Sudan) (Warrell et al. 1974, 1980). The new Pasteur "Ipser Africa" antivenom, however, is prepared incorporating *E. carinatus* venom from Mali and a preliminary clinical trial has suggested that it may be more effective than the Behringwerke polyspecific preparation (Daudu and Theakston 1988). A more detailed trial is currently in progress in Nigeria.

Antivenom Collection

Some producers of antivenom still use serum as a raw material (Theakston and Warrell 1991); however, the majority now use plasma, bleeding into sodium citrate and separating erythrocytes by sedimentation (Latifi 1978). This process is very slow and several hours may be required for adequate separation. It also results in precipitation of large aggregates of fibrinogen, which again are both time consuming and difficult to remove. However, the process does allow the reinjection of the erythrocytes into the host animal. Serum collection, even allowing time for clot retraction, can be accomplished rapidly and results in a solution that can be salt precipitated to yield an IgG-rich fraction. Ammonium sulphate is commonly used for precipitation, although the sodium salt results in a pellet that is more easily reconstituted, contains lower levels of albumin and avoids the addition of potentially toxic ammonium ions. It has also been suggested that ammonium sulphate irreversibly denatures immunoglobulin, reducing the yield of viable antivenom (Sullivan 1987).

Serum Processing

In order to overcome the hypersensitivity reactions mentioned above, many antivenom manufacturers digest immune immunoglobulin using pepsin to produce bivalent $F(ab')_2$ fragments which lack the C terminal Fc domains (Latifi 1978; Fig. 6.1). It is this region of the IgG molecule that is responsible for cell binding and through which many of the hypersensitivity reactions are mediated. $F(ab')_2$ fragments retain the ability to bind antigen and reduce significantly the incidence of hypersensitivity reactions to equine proteins; however, despite this treatment side-effects are frequently seen in treated patients (Karlsson-Steiber and Persson 1994). These effects, which are most likely to be caused by complex-mediated or type III hypersensitivity reactions, because $F(ab')_2$ retains divalency and the ability to bind complement, are characterized by a rise in temperature, chills and swollen lymph nodes. Severe anaphylactic reactions to $F(ab')_2$-based products, however, unlike

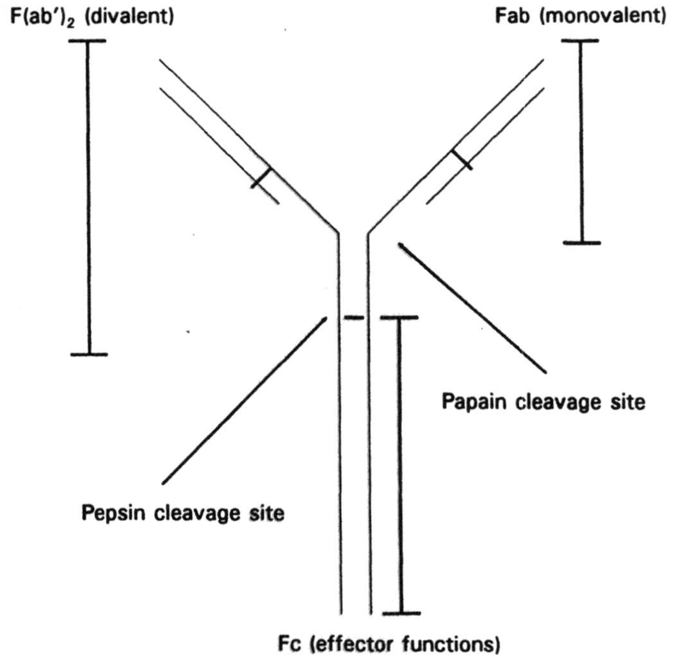

Fig. 6.1. Schematic representation of the IgG molecule highlighting both $F(ab')_2$ and Fc regions.

their intact IgG-based counterparts, are thankfully rare. One such product, produced by the Institute of Immunology, Zagreb, Croatia, has been used with considerable success in the treatment of systemic envenoming by the European adder, *Vipera berus* (Theakston and Reid 1976).

A recent development in immunotherapy is the use of Fab fragments produced by digesting IgG with the plant enzyme, papain. This enzyme, a thiol protease from the papaya plant, removes the Fc portion of the immunoglobulin molecule to yield two monovalent antibody binding sites (Fab) of approximately 50 000 molecular weight (Fig. 6.1). Fab fragments have a number of advantages over both IgG and $F(ab')_2$. First, they are not associated with type III hypersensitivity because, with only one antigen binding site, they do not form immune complexes of sufficient size, and secondly, lacking the Fc region, they do not bind complement or macrophages eliminating vasoactive amine release. Fab fragments have been shown to elicit a delayed and significantly smaller immune response in rabbits than intact IgG molecules; in a group of 16 test animals to which Fab was administered, none exhibited anaphylactic or anaphylactoid reactions (Smith et al. 1979).

Fab fragments also have greater volumes of distribution and faster kinetics than either IgG or $F(ab')_2$. IgG has a very small volume of distribution, which is similar to the plasma volume, while Fab fragments, because of extracellular space penetration, produce a value some eight to nine times greater (Smith et al. 1979; Sullivan 1987). Owing to their smaller size, Fab fragments also distribute around the body more rapidly; this, in conjunction with their greater distribution volume, indicates their importance as therapeutic agents. Clinical use of Fab fragments has up to now been centred on the use of Digibind for treatment of cardiac glycoside overdose; experience with over 700 patients has shown an incidence of allergic reaction in less than 1% of cases (Hickey et al. 1991).

Rapid distribution is of particular importance in the treatment of snake envenoming because of the very low molecular weights of some venom components. Elapid venoms, for example, contain a high proportion of neurotoxic polypeptides (molecular weight 7000–8000). These molecules are themselves distributed very rapidly through the tissues and the intravenous administration of Fab to the patient may prove more efficacious in treating these patients. Snake bites and bites by some types of spider (e.g. brown recluse spider, *Loxosceles reclusa*) are often associated with severe necrosis at the site of the bite, an effect as yet unalleviated by commercially available antivenoms (Reid 1964). Iddon et al. (1987) pointed out that this inefficiency was most probably due to late administration of antivenom rather than to any deficiency on the part of the neutralizing antibody, and, indeed, Ownby et al. (1983), using an antivenom to *Crotalus viridis viridis* myotoxin, showed that neutralization was achieved only when the antivenom was administered within 30 min of experimental envenoming. The more rapid effects of Fab may therefore be beneficial in this type of therapy where rapid treatment is vital.

Three recent papers report the use of Fab fragments in neutralization of venom activity (Al-Joufi et al. 1991; Bailey et al. 1991; Smith et al. 1992). Venom kininogenase, or arginine esterase, activity is responsible for the hypotensive shock and severe pain often associated with viperid and crotalid snake bites and therefore the ability of an antivenom to neutralize these effects would be beneficial. These enzymes, which are found predominantly in viperine and crotaline venoms, convert serum kininogen to kinin, a low molecular weight vasoactive peptide that also affects pain receptors. In a radioimmunoassay that measures the ability of a venom to produce kinin from purified kininogen, Fab fragments were shown to be highly effective in neutralizing enzyme activity and, indeed, proved more efficacious than similar $F(ab')_2$-based products.

The removal of the Fc region of the IgG molecule by papain digestion has the added beneficial effect of reducing the molecular weight of the therapeutic agent resulting in smaller amounts (in terms of weight) of antivenom being required for successful treatment. Theoretically, because Fab fragments are only two-thirds the size of intact IgG, then only two-thirds as much Fab-based antivenom need be given.

Chicken immunoglobulin (IgY) can be relatively easily extracted (Thalley and Carroll 1990; Carroll et al. 1992) and subsequently affinity purified as described below. An advantage of the avian product is that, because IgY does not fix mammalian complement (Benson et al. 1961; Rose and Orlans 1962; Carroll et al. 1992), the risk of side-effects is decreased. However, this benefit is reduced, and others gained, if papain is used to digest the Fc region and reduce molecular weight.

Affinity Purification

The total immunoglobulin fraction of any immune serum will, by definition, contain antibodies that are directed against molecules other than the immunogen. These antibodies comprise the background complement of immunoglobulins acquired by the animal during its lifetime and as such are of no therapeutic benefit to the patient. Such antibodies are, however, a component of all currently available commercial antivenoms. For example, sheep antisera typically contain 25–30 g of immunoglobulin per litre, of which only a quarter to a third can be expected to be specific to the antigen (Smith et al. 1992). Thus if the total immunoglobulin fraction is administered, these non-effective molecules simply increase the burden of foreign protein administered to the envenomed patient and the possible risk of side-effects.

It is for this reason that affinity chromatography techniques have been applied to antivenom research in recent years because they enable the isolation of antibodies specific only to the venom antigen. This process has been performed by a number of investigators using a number of methods; however, all are based on antigen (in this case a venom) bound to inert matrix material over which antiserum is passed, specific antibodies to the venom binding to the venom on the matrix, non-specific material passing through. The matrix may then be washed, usually with a low pH buffer, and the specific antibody harvested. Although affinity purification has long been used as a means of isolating antibodies to specific venom components, it was Russell et al. (1985) who first pointed to this technique as a means of reducing antivenom doses. Using polyacrylamide as a supportive matrix, Russell purified specific antibodies to a number of rattlesnake venoms – *C. adamanteus* (Eastern diamondback rattlesnake), *C. atrox, C. viridis helleri* (Southern Pacific rattlesnake) and *C. scutulatus scutulatus* (Mojave rattlesnake) – using, as a source material, the equine Antivenin (Crotalidae) Polyvalent produced by Wyeth Laboratories. He subsequently showed that material produced in this way was more effective in neutralizing lethal, haemorrhagic, coagulant, platelet-aggregating, necrotizing and neurotoxic activities than the starting material, and found no evidence that such antibodies produced anaphylaxis or anaphylactoid reactions in animals sensitized to horse serum. This material, however, was also shown to be predominantly comprised of the IgG(T) subclass (Sullivan and Russell 1983).

A more recent paper (Smith et al. 1992) reports the successful production of an ovine affinity-purified Fab-based antivenom that combines all the advantageous features mentioned above. The treatment uses specific Fab fragments that have been purified using agarose gels as a support matrix. Venom from a single snake species, *V. berus*, was coupled to the support and papain-digested immune ovine antibody then added. Affinity purification resulted in a four-fold increase in specific activity when compared with the original source serum; the material was also shown to have a greater neutralizing effect on paraspecific venoms such as *V. ammodytes* (Al-Joufi et al. 1991). More importantly, this antivenom was shown to have a nine- to ten-fold superiority over current commercially available antivenoms in protecting mice from the lethal effects of *V. berus* venom.

Avian venom antibodies (IgY) have been purified from 3.5% or 12% polyethylene glycol fractions of egg yolks from immunized hens by passage of individual *C. atrox, Tr. flavoviridis* or *C.d. terrificus* venom antigen matrices prepared by coupling 5–10 mg of venom/ml Actigel A affinity resin (Thalley and Carroll 1990; Carroll et al. 1992).

Antivenom Composition

When only one species of venomous snake occurs in a particular area, the choice of antivenom is simple; however, when more than one exists the manufacturer is faced with the question of how to provide adequate protection against all. Two choices are available: either to immunize individual animals with different venoms or to combine venoms and immunize with the mixture.

Products such as the *V. berus* antivenom described above are termed monospecific antivenoms because they are raised by immunizing an animal with a single venom. Monospecific antivenom will always be more effective than polyspecific antivenoms where a mixture of venoms has been used as an immunogen, because all antibodies are directed against one species. This could be described as 100% cross-reactivity. However, when there is more than one species in an area, the treating physician would ideally need to stock many monospecific antivenoms and rely on the victim to identify accurately the culprit snake in order to benefit from this advantage, in most cases not a feasible proposition. It is for this reason that the majority of antivenoms are polyspecific. A broad but reduced cross-reactivity is thereby provided against a number of snakes and difficult choices are avoided. However, there are a number of arguments against this approach.

With a limited number of antibodies in any one host animal, mixing complex antigens such as snake venoms may result in some venom components failing to elicit an immune response or, conversely, all antigens eliciting only a weak response. Also, because many venom components share elements of secondary structure, those of low molecular weight that are weakly immunogenic or in low concentration may be selected against, their larger more immunogenic brethren binding in preference to immunoglobulin on the surface of B cells. Finally, the large number of possible antigens may also severely immunocompromise the host animal, all antibodies being directed against the venoms, leaving few to provide protection against environmental pathogens. This method, if four venoms were mixed to form the immunogen, should provide only 25% of the protection afforded by a similar monospecific antivenom against any one snake venom; however, because the venoms used usually show a high degree of cross-neutralization, this figure is often much higher.

A second approach is to mix monospecific antisera, each produced in separate animals. This method maximizes the possible number of available antibody-producing cells and, in theory, should provide a wider range of specific antibodies. However, because these antisera are then mixed, a dilution effect is produced, the magnitude of which is dependent on the number of monospecific antisera included in the product. Such dilution should, in theory, reduce the effectiveness of such a product, but because many venoms are highly cross-reactive (for the reasons given above) the dilution effects are again much reduced. Experiments to monitor the ability of both poly-, monospecific and mixed monospecific antivenoms to neutralize the phospholipase activity of crotalid venoms have shown that, as anticipated, monospecific products often offer the best protection, while mixed monospecific antivenoms are in general better than polyspecific antivenoms (Fig. 6.2).

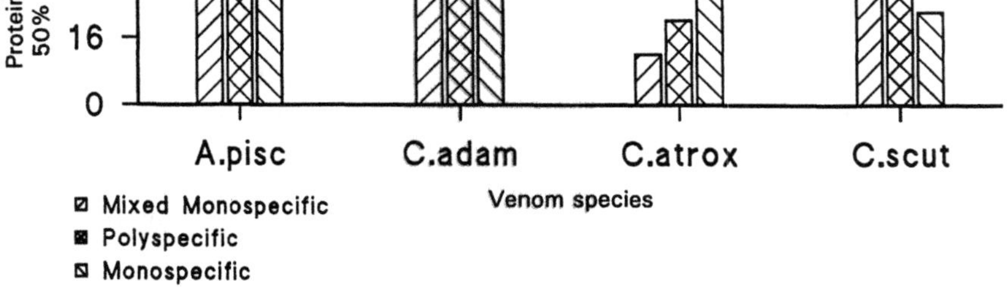

Fig. 6.2. Phospholipase activity neutralization. Monospecific, mixed monospecific and polyspecific ovine antisera were used to neutralize the venom phospholipase activity of four crotalid venoms. The amount of antivenom required to reduce the activity in each by 50% was determined using a chromagenic indicator to monitor fatty acid release.

Liposomal Immunization

New methods of animal immunization are currently being developed, one of which involves the use of specially treated membrane-stabilized reverse evaporation phase (REV) liposomes for stimulating a rapid and sustained high-titre protective antibody response in experimental animals following a single immunizing injection (New et al. 1984, 1985). The study has been extended from mice and rabbits into sheep (Theakston et al. 1985) where preliminary results have proved encouraging. The immune response using this procedure can be intensified by incorporating immunostimulants such as *Escherichia coli* endotoxin or lipid A into the venom/liposome system (Laing et al. 1986, 1988). Antivenoms developed using this or related methods should result in cheaper, more avid antivenoms, which would be greatly welcomed in developing countries where snake bite is a serious problem.

The liposome technique also has potential application as a screening test for horses suitable for immunization. For example, antivenom producers in Brazil have problems over selection of suitable horses for immunization against the venoms of *C. durissus* subspecies; many animals either do not respond at all or are poor responders to standard immunization procedures, possibly due to some form of immunosuppression (Freitas et al. 1988). Horses could be screened by inoculating them with a test dose of this venom incorporated into liposomes. Animals that show ELISA positivity 2 weeks after the injection should be suitable for the full immunization protocol. Preliminary studies have indicated that this system works well in experimental mice (Freitas et al. 1988).

Active immunization of man has been attempted with some degree of success in the past (Haast and Winer 1955; Wiener 1960, 1961; Flowers 1963), but Rosenfeld (1971) reported that it did not provide real protection due mainly to the short-lived antibody titres conferred; immunization would not work unless the challenge bite occurred soon after the end of the immunization procedure. Investigations are in progress to study the possibility of active immunization of man using venom/liposomes administered orally to experimental animals. Laing et al. (1988) have demonstrated a raised serum IgG response in experimental mice following oral administration of *E. carinatus* venom incorporated into REV liposomes following a post-immunization sublethal subcutaneous boost of whole venom. This indicated a priming of the immune system following oral immunization. New et al. (1985) also reported a direct serum IgG response in mice following oral administration of venom liposomes. These workers concluded that although the serum antibody titre was not high enough to confer direct protection, the observation of such a response suggests the generation of a considerable degree of intestinal-mediated immunity. Further studies are currently in progress.

Monoclonal Antibody Technology

The development of avid monoclonal antibodies active against pathological venom fractions may have application in future programmes for antivenom production. The mode of action of antivenom (i.e. how antibodies neutralize venom toxins) is not known, and is probably variable from one toxin to another. To improve antivenom serotherapy, it is critically important to determine whether antibodies interact at the toxic or enzymatic site of the molecule or at an unrelated antigenic site, and which isotype of immunoglobulin is most effective in its neutralizing activity. Recent work by Boulain et al. (1982) and Boulain and Menez (1982) in France suggests that in the case of the α-neurotoxin of *N. nigricollis* venom, a monoclonal antibody with an epitope localized at a distance from the acetylcholine (ACH)-binding site can effectively interact with venom–ACH binding, either by inhibition of binding or by dislocation of the association when binding has already occurred (Menez et al. 1986). The latter mode of action is consistent with the kinetics of antivenom therapy after neurotoxic envenoming in humans, when the serum remains beneficial for several days after snake bite. The major implication of the results obtained in this model system (the venom of *N. nigricollis* is one of the few elapid venoms that apparently produces no neurotoxic signs in man owing to the unique configuration of the human ACH receptor; Low and Corfield 1988) is that a well-chosen polypeptide fraction of a toxin could, when linked to a suitable carrier/adjuvant, be used for immunization to prepare antivenom without the usual toxic side-effects. Such a molecule could possibly be used for preventive immunization of individuals at high risk.

In the future it may thus be possible to produce a monoclonal antibody for use as an antivenom against elapid neurotoxins. Current studies are concentrating on the development of "useful" monoclonal antibodies against the α-neurotoxin of *N. kaouthia* venom (Karlsson et al. 1971), but real problems have been encountered. For example, initial difficulties arose in immunization of animals against the low molecular weight α-neurotoxin. These were overcome, but it is frequently found that potentially useful antibody-secreting hydridomas are unstable (Sells, unpublished observations), although they were initially capable of actively reversing the systemic effects of neuromuscular paralysis induced by the neurotoxin. Current studies include the use of Balb-c/Biozzi cross-bred mice for immunization instead of Balb-c mice (Sells, unpublished data) and the use of in vitro immunization techniques involving the immunization of mouse spleen cells with the neurotoxin followed by hybridization of the immunized cells with a mouse plasmacytoma cell line (Luben and Mohler 1980). Currently, an in vitro assay system is being developed for the study of elapid venoms and neurotoxins isolated from them, which will be useful for studying the neutralization by both monoclonal antibodies and antivenoms in general. The system involves the use of non-solubilized human ACH receptors instead of the more conventional technique, which uses *Torpedo* ACH receptors (Weber and Changeux 1974).

Preliminary studies on sera from Thai previous snake bite victims using ELISA indicated that all 23 sera had high antibody titres when assayed against whole *N. kaouthia* venom, but only two of these contained detectable antibody against the purified α-neurotoxin (Sells, unpublished data). This is not really surprising as the neurotoxin is a low molecular weight polypeptide, and is not therefore highly immunogenic. This study therefore emphasizes the need for a therapeutic monoclonal antibody active against the main pathological component of the venom, the α-neurotoxin (either as a supplement to the currently available antivenom, or as a separate therapeutic entity). The use of such an avid monoclonal antibody could have real application in envenoming by elapids such as *N. kaouthia* where up to 450 ml of antivenom is often necessary to reverse or eliminate the symptoms of systemic envenoming (Virivan et al. 1986). Indeed, a total of 1150 ml of antivenom was given in one case of poisoning by the king cobra, *Ophiophagus hannah*, in Thailand (Ganthavorn 1971). An avid antineurotoxin monoclonal antibody may result in much smaller volumes of antivenom being required for treatment of neurotoxic envenoming.

Commercial antivenoms used for treatment of envenoming by viperine species are generally polyspecific preparations, which, although they leave a great deal to be desired in terms of neutralizing potency, are relatively well established in the countries of use. The application of monoclonal antibodies for treatment of viperine envenoming is therefore less hopeful; also a multiplicity of toxins are involved in the production of systemic signs. A "cocktail" of monoclonal antibodies would therefore be necessary if such a system were to be used. Additionally, because of the derivation of monoclonal antibodies from myeloma cells, there may well be ethical objections to their use for therapeutic treatment. In this case it is thought that the main potential of monoclonal antibodies may be in the isolation of pathological venom fractions from whole venom by affinity chromatography or by recovery of recognized protein bands from electrophoresed gels (Iddon et al. 1988). These fractions could then be used for the subsequent production of highly specific antitoxins probably by incorporating them into the liposomal immunization system. According to Menez (1985) another approach may be the chemical analysis of the toxin fragments that correspond to the antigenic areas that bind specifically to efficiently neutralizing antibodies.

Menez (1985) considers that in the case of elapid venoms one monoclonal antibody is capable of neutralizing the main neurotoxin. In the case of viperine and crotaline venoms the situation, as mentioned above, may be somewhat different. A monoclonal antibody specific for the haemorrhagic fraction present in *C. atrox* venom has been found to be weakly neutralizing. Perez et al. (1984) considered that haemorrhagic factors probably have several antigenic determinants and it is unlikely that a single antibody directed to one of them could neutralize their activity. Conversely, Iddon et al. (1985) found that the haemorrhagic and necrotizing activities of West African *E. carinatus* venom were neutralized effectively by a monoclonal antibody raised against the haemorrhagin of the venom; likewise, Pukrittayakamee et al. (1983) reported that one monoclonal antibody neutralized the coagulant activity of the factor X activator of *D. russelli* venom.

Recombinant DNA Technology

Taylor et al. (1986) used monoclonal antibodies (Iddon et al. 1988) raised against components of *E. carinatus* venom, polyclonal antibodies raised against the procoagulant fraction (ecarin) and against whole venom to screen venom secretion by the venom gland cells of this species by the direct immunofluorescent antibody technique. The study indicated that each venom gland secretory cell produces all the venom constituents as a single package and that different constituents are produced at different times and at different rates throughout the secretory cycle. It was therefore determined that the optimum time to remove gland tissue for extraction of RNA for use in the production of a cDNA library was on the third day following milking for this particular species; at this time maximum synthesis of venom proteins was occurring. Currently, work is in progress on the production and characterization of cDNA libraries to determine whether useful antigens (e.g. haemorrhagins, procoagulants, etc.) have been produced. Recently, Tamiya et al. (1985) cloned the cDNA encoding a curaremetric toxin with the aim of producing mutant proteins with single mutations by means of site-directed mutagenesis (Pielak et al. 1985).

Conclusions

As stressed earlier, methods of antivenom production have not altered significantly since their conception almost a century ago. One of the main reasons for this is probably the conservatism that exists among antivenom manufacturers who are not willing, possibly because of financial constraints, to invest in improving the existing methodology. The fact that antivenoms are sold to many developing countries, who cannot afford the high prices, means that quality control probably suffers and the resulting product is therefore inefficient, large volumes being required to reverse the symptoms of envenoming. This in turn leads to a high incidence of serum reactions. Conversely, in many countries who produce government-subsidised products of high neutralizing efficacy, excessively high amounts of antivenom are often administered to the patients, which again results in an unacceptably high incidence of early anaphylactic reactions. Patients may also be treated with antivenom even in the absence of signs of systemic envenoming, which obviously puts them unnecessarily at risk.

Another major problem is the frequent lack of availability of antivenoms. For example, in Nigeria at present, Pasteur and Behringwerke antivenoms are virtually unobtainable unless the patients themselves, their families or their villages can afford to pay high prices for the drugs; many people are dying simply because they cannot afford the antivenom or enough of it to have adequate therapeutic value.

There is a real need to adapt modern technology to antivenom production in order to produce cheaper, more effective and less reactive therapeutic agents. There are indications that this may be happening as demonstrated by the use of more suitable animals for immunization and the use of affinity purification. Other possibilities for the future include research into methods of active immunization of man in areas of high snake bite incidence and mortality, and the study of possible alternatives to antivenom therapy.

References

Adler FL (1957) Antibody formation after injection of heterologous immunoglobulin – II. Competition of antigens. J Immunol 78: 201–210

Al-Joufi A, Bailey GS, Reddi K, Smith DC (1991) Neutralisation of kinin-releasing enzymes from viperid venoms by antivenom IgG fragments. Toxicon 29: 1509–1512
Amies CR (1959) The use of topically formed calcium alginate as a depot substance in active immunization. J Path Bact 77: 435–442
Bailey GS, Al-Joufi A, Rawat S, Smith DC (1991) Neutralisation of kinin-releasing enzymes from crotalid venoms by monospecific and polyspecific antivenoms. Toxicon 29: 777–781
Benson HN, Brumfield HP et al. (1961) Requirement of avian C1 for fixation of guinea pig complement by avian antibody–antigen complexes. J Immunol 87: 616–622
Boulain J-C, Menez A (1982) Neurotoxin-specific immunoglobulins accelerate dissociation of the neurotoxin–acetylcholine receptor complex. Science 217: 732–733
Boulain J-C, Menez A, Couderc J, Faure G, Liacopoulos P, Fromageot P (1982) Neutralizing monoclonal antibody specific for *Naja nigricollis* toxin: Preparation, characterization and localization of the antigenic binding site. Biochemistry 21: 2910–2915
Bouquet P (1979) Immunological properties of snake venoms. In: Lee C-Y (ed) Snake venoms. Springer, Berlin, pp 751–824 (Handbook of experimental pharmacology, vol 52)
Braun W, Nakano M (1967) Antibody formation: Stimulation by polyadenylic acids. Science 157: 819–821
Brazil V (1911) La defense contre l'ophidisme. Instituto Butantan, São Paulo, Brazil
Buchowicz I, Goch H, Zakrzewski K (1969) Equine immunoglobulins: A comparison of molecular properties. Acta Biochem Polon 16: 279–294
Calmette LCA (1894a) Contribution a l'etude du venin des serpents (immunization des animaux et traitement de l'envenimation). Ann Inst Pasteur 8: 275–291
Calmette LCA (1894b) Proprietes du serum des animaux immunises contre le venin des serpentes, et therapeutique de l'envenomation. C R Acad 68: 720–725
Calmette LCA (1895) Contribution a l'etude des venins, des toxins et des serums antitoxiques. Ann Inst Pasteur 9: 225–251
Calmette LCA (1898) Sur la mechanisme de l'immunisation contre les venins. Ann Inst Pasteur 12: 343–353
Cardoso JLC, Fan HW, Franca FOS et al. (1993) Randomized comparative trial of three antivenoms in the treatment of envenoming by lance-headed vipers (*Bothrops jararaca*) snakes in São Paulo, Brazil. J Med 86: 315–325
Carroll SB, Thalley BS, Theakston RDG, Laing G (1992) A comparison of the purity and efficacy of affinity purified avian antivenoms with commercial equine crotalid antivenoms. Toxicon
Cartledge C, Maclean C, Landon J (1992) Production of polyclonal antibodies in ascitic fluid of mice – time and dose relationships. J Immunoass 13: 339–353
Celada F (1971) The cellular basis of immunologic memory. Prog Allergy 15: 223–267
Chippaux J-P, Goyffon M (1983) Producers of antivenomous sera. Toxicon 21: 739–752
Chippaux J-P, Williams V, White J (1991) Snake venom variability: Methods of study, results and interpretation. Toxicon 29: 1279–1303
Christensen PA (1955) "South African snake venoms and antivenoms". The South African Institute for Medical Research, Johannesburg
Christensen PA (1962) Antivenom standardization. Progress report, WHO Expert Committee on Biological Standardization, Geneva, 10–15 December
Christensen PA (1966a) The preparation and purification of antivenoms. Mems Inst Butantan Simp Internac 33: 245–250
Christensen PA (1966b) Venom and antivenom potency estimation. Mems Inst Butantan 33: 305–326
Christensen PA (1968) The venoms of Central and South African snakes. In: Bucherl W, Buckley EE, Deulofeu V (eds) Venomous animals and their venoms. Vol I, Venomous vertebrates, Ch 16. Academic Press, New York, pp 437–461
Christensen PA (1979) Production and standardisation of antivenin. In: Lee CY (ed) Snake venoms. Springer-Verlag, Berlin, pp 825–846 (Handbook of experimental pharmacology, vol 52)
Corrigan P, Russell FE, Wainschel J Jr (1978) Clinical reactions to antivenin. In: Rosenberg P (ed) Toxins: Animal, plant, microbial. Pergamon Press, Oxford
Coulter AR, Cox JC, Sutherland SK, Waddell CJ (1978) A new solid-phase sandwich radioimmunoassay and its application to the detection of snake venom. J Immunol Methods 23: 242–252
Coulter AR, Harris RD, Sutherland SK (1980) Enzyme immunoassay for the rapid identification of snake venom. Med J Aust 1: 433–435

Daudu I, Theakston RDG (1988) Preliminary trial of a new polyspecific antivenom in Nigeria. Ann Trop Med Parasitol 82: 311–313
Detrait J (1982) Repertoire des instituts et laboratoires producteurs de serum antivenimeux. Bull Soc Herpet Fr 21: 44–56
Editorial (1980) Antivenom therapy and reactions. Lancet i: 1009–1010
Flowers HH (1963) Active immunisation of a human being against cobra (*Naja naja*) venom. Nature 200: 1017–1018
Fraser TR (1895) The rendering of animals immune against the venom of the cobra and other serpents, and on the antidotal properties of the blood serum of the immunised animals. Br Med J 1: 1309–1312
Freitas TV, Tavares AP, Theakston RDG, Laing G, New RRC (1988) Use of liposomes for protective immunisation against *Crotalus durissus* (tropical rattlesnake) venom. Toxicon 27: 341–347
Ganthavorn S (1971) A case of king cobra bite. Toxicon 9: 293–294
Grasset E, Christensen PA (1947) Enzyme purification of polyvalent antivenine, South and Equatorial African colubrine and viperine venoms. Trans R Soc Trop Med Hyg 41: 207–211
Haast WE, Winer ML (1955) Complete and spontaneous recovery from the bite of a blue krait snake (*Bungarus caeruleus*). Am J Trop Med Hyg 4: 1135–1137
Hickey AR, Wenger TL, Carpenter VP et al. (1991) Digoxin immune Fab therapy in the management of digitalis intoxication: Safety and efficacy results of an observational surveillance study. JACC 17: 590–598
Ho M, Warrell MJ, Warrell DA, Bidwell D, Voller A (1986) A critical reappraisal of the use of enzyme-linked immunosorbent assays in the study of snake bite. Toxicon 24: 211–221
Iddon D, Hommel M, Theakston RDG (1988) Characterization of a monoclonal antibody capable of neutralizing the haemorrhagic activity of West African *Echis carinatus* (carpet viper) venom. Toxicon 26: 167–179
Iddon D, Theakston RDG, Hommel M (1985) A monoclonal antibody active against the "haemorrhagin" of Nigerian *Echis carinatus* venom. Toxicon 23: 576
Iddon D, Theakston RDG, Ownby CL (1987) A study of the pathogenesis of local skin necrosis induced by *Naja nigricollis* (spitting cobra) venom using simple histological staining techniques. Toxicon 25: 665–672
Johnson AG, Schmidtke J, Mreitt K, Han I (1968) Enhancement of antibody formation by nucleic acids and their derivatives. In: Plescia OJ, Braun W (eds) Nucleic acids in immunology. Springer-Verlag, Berlin, p 379
Karlsson E, Arnberg H, Eaker D (1971) Isolation of the principal neurotoxins of two *Naja naja* subspecies. Eur J Biochem 21: 1–16
Karlsson-Steiber C, Persson H (1994) Antivenom treatment in 30 cases of *Vipera berus* evenomation in Sweden 1985–1989. J Intern Med, in press
Kochalty WF, Bowles-Ledford E, Daly JG, Billings TA (1971) Preparation of coral snake antivenom from goat serum. Toxicon 9: 297–298
Laing G, Theakston RDG, New RRC (1987) Use of liposomes incorporating immunostimulant for parenteral and oral immunization against snake venom. In: Gopalkrishnakone P, Tan CK (eds) Progress in venom and toxin research, Faculty of Medicine, University of Singapore, pp 283–295
Laing G, Theakston RDG, New RRC (1988) Use of liposomes incorporating immunostimulants for immunisation against snake venom. Toxicon 26: 29
Laing G, Theakston RDG, New RRC, Zumbuehl O, Parsley A (1986) Use of liposomes incorporating immunostimulants for immunization against snake venom. Trans R Soc Trop Med Hyg 80: 338
Latifi M (1978) Commercial production of commercial anti-snakebite serum (antivenin). In: Gans C, Gans KA (eds) Biology of the reptilia. Vol 8, Physiology. Academic Press, London, p 561
Latifi M, Manhouri H (1966) Antivenin production. Mems Inst Butantan 33: 893–897
Loprinzi CL, Hennessee J, Tamsky L et al. (1983) Snake antivenin administration in a patient allergic to horse serum. South Med J 76: 501–502
Low BW, Corfield PWR (1988) The acetyl choline receptor: Identification of prime alpha-toxin binding site. In: Dolly JO (ed) Neurotoxins in neurochemistry. Ellis Horwood, Chichester, pp 13–26
Luben RA, Mohler MA (1980) In vitro immunization as an adjunct to the production of

hybridomas producing antibodies against the lymphokine osteoclast activating factor. Mol Immunol 17: 635–639
Malasit P, Warrell DA, Chanthavanich P et al. (1986) Prediction, prevention and mechanism of early (anaphylactic) antivenom reactions in victims of snake bites. Br Med J 292: 17–20
Meier J, Theakston RDG (1986) Approximate LD_{50} determinations of snake venoms using eight to ten experimental animals. Toxicon 24: 395–401
Menez A (1985) Molecular immunology of snake toxins. Pharmacol Ther 30: 91–113
Menez A, Boulain J-C, Grognet J-M et al. (1986) The use of monoclonal antibodies to elucidate the antigenic structure and the mechanisms of neutralization of snake toxins. In: Harris JB (ed) Natural toxins. Animal, plant and microbial. Clarendon Press, Oxford, pp 332–346
Miller JFAP, Basten A, Sprent J, Cheers C (1971) Interaction between lymphocytes in immune responses. Cell Immunol 2: 469–495
Minton SA (1974) Venom diseases. Charles C Thomas, Springfield, Illinois, p 171
Mohamed AH, Bakr IA, Kamel A (1966) Egyptian polyvalent anti-snake-bite serum: Technique of preparation. Toxicon 4: 69–72
New RRC, Theakston RDG, Zumbuehl O, Iddon D, Friend J (1984) Immunization against snake venoms. N Engl J Med 311: 56–57
New RRC, Theakston RDG, Zumbuehl O, Iddon D, Friend J (1985) Liposomal immunization against snake venoms. Toxicon 23: 215–219
Ownby CL, Odell GV, Woods GV, Colberg TR (1983) Ability of antiserum to myotoxin from a prairie rattlesnake (*Crotalus viridis viridis*) venom to neutralise local myotoxicity and lethal effects of myotoxin a and homologous crude venom. Toxicon 21: 35–41
Perez JC, Garcia VE, Huang SY (1984) Production of a monoclonal antibody against the hemorrhagic activity of *Crotalus atrox* (western diamondback rattlesnake) venom. Toxicon 22: 967–973
Phillips RE, Theakston RDG, Warrell DA et al. (1988) Paralysis, rhabdomyolysis and haemolysis caused by bites of Russell's viper (*Vipera russelli*) in Sri Lanka: Failure of Indian (Haffkine) antivenom. Q J Med 68: 691–716
Phisalix C, Bertrand G (1894) Sur la propriete antitoxique du sang des animaux vaccines contre le venin de vipere. C R Acad Sci 118: 356–358
Pielak GJ, Mauk AG, Smith M (1985) Site-directed mutagenesis of cytochrome c shows that an invariant Phe is not essential for function. Nature 313: 152–154
Pugh RNH, Theakston RDG (1987) Antivenom reactions and complement depletion in snake bite. Ann Trop Med Parasitol 81: 73–75
Pukrittayakamee S, Esnouf MP, McMichael AJ (1983) Purification and inactivation of the factor X activator of Russell's viper venom with monoclonal antibodies. Mol Biol Med 1: 123–135
Reid HA (1964) Cobra bites. Br Med J 2: 540–544
Reid HA (1968) Symptomatology, pathology and treatment of land snake bite in India and Southeast Asia. In: Bucherl W, Buckley EE, Deulofeu V (eds) Venomous animals and their venoms. Vol I, Venomous vertebrates. Academic Press, New York, pp 611–642
Reid HA, Theakston RDG (1978) Changes in coagulation effects by venoms of *Crotalus atrox* as snakes age. Am J Trop Med Hyg 27: 1053–1057
Rose ME, Orlans E (1962) Fowl antibody IV. The estimation of haemolytic fowl complement. Immunology 5: 642–648
Rosenfeld G (1971) Symptomatology, pathology and treatment of snake bites in South America. In: Bucherl W, Buckley EE (eds) Venomous animals and their venoms. Vol II, Venomous vertebrates. Academic Press, New York, pp 345–384
Russell FE (1961) Use of Crotalus monovalent antivenom from rabbit serum. C Ther Res 3: 438–440
Russell FE (1980) Snake venom poisoning. Lippincott, Philadelphia, pp 797–810
Russell FE (1988) Snake venom immunology: Historical and practical considerations. J Toxicol 7: 1–82
Russell FE, Lauritzen L (1966) Antivenins. Trans R Soc Trop Med Hyg 60: 797–810
Russell FE, Sullivan JB, Egan NB, Markland FS, Wingert WA, Bar-Or D (1985) Preparation of a new antivenom by affinity chromatography. Am J Trop Med Hyg 34: 141–150
Russell FE, Timmerman WF, Meadows P (1970) Clinical use of antivenin prepared from goat serum. Toxicon 8: 63–65
Sawai Y, Chinzei H, Kawamura Y, Fukuyama T, Okonogi T (1972) Studies on the improvement of treatment of Habu (*Trimeresurus flavoviridis*) bites. IX. Studies on the immunogenicity of the purified Habu venom toxoid by alcohol precipitation. Jpn J Exp Med 42: 155–164

Schottler WHA (1951) Antigen–antibody relations in the present antivenin production of Brazil. Am J Trop Med 31: 500–509
Sewall H (1887) Experiments on the preventive inoculation of rattlesnake venom. J Physiol 8: 203–210
Smith DC, Reddi KR, Laing G, Theakston RDG, Landon J (1992) An affinity purified ovine antivenom for the treatment of *Vipera berus* envenoming. Toxicon 30: 865–871
Smith TW, Lloyd BL, Spicer N, Haber E (1979) Immunogenicity and kinetics of distribution and elimination of sheep digoxin-specific IgG and Fab in the rabbit and baboon. Clin Exp Immunol 36: 384–396
Sullivan JB (1987) Past, present and future immunotherapy of snake venom poisoning. Ann Emerg Med 16: 35–41
Sullivan JB, Russell FE (1983) Isolation, quantitation and subclassing of IgG antibody to Crotalidae venom by affinity chromatography and protein electrophoresis. Toxicon suppl 3: 429–432
Sutherland SK (1977) Serum reactions: An analysis of commercial antivenoms and the possible role of anticomplementary activity in de novo reactions to antivenoms and antitoxins. Med J Aust i: 613–615
Taborska E (1971) Intraspecies variability of the venom of *Echis carinatus*. Physiol Bohemoslov 20: 307–318
Tamiya T, Lamouroux A, Julien J-F et al. (1985) Cloning and sequence analysis of the cDNA encoding a snake neurotoxin precursor. Biochimie 67: 185–189
Taylor D, Iddon D, Sells P, Semoff S, Theakston RDG (1986) An investigation of venom secretion by the venom gland cells of the carpet viper (*Echis carinatus*). Toxicon 24: 651–659
Thalley BS, Carroll SB (1990) Rattlesnake and scorpion antivenoms from the egg yolks of immunized hens. Bio/Technology 8: 934–938
Theakston RDG (1986) Characterization of venoms and standardization of antivenoms. In: Harris JB (ed) Natural toxins. Animal, plant and microbial. Clarendon Press, Oxford, pp 287–303
Theakston RDG, Reid HA (1976) Effectiveness of Zagreb antivenom against envenoming by the adder, *Vipera berus*. Lancet i: 121–123
Theakston RDG, Reid HA (1978) Changes in the biological properties of venom from *Crotalus atrox* with ageing. Periodicum Biologorum 80: 123–135
Theakston RDG, Reid HA (1979) Enzyme-linked immunosorbent assay (ELISA) in assessing antivenom potency. Toxicon 17: 511–515
Theakston RDG, Reid HA (1983) Development of simple standard assay procedures for the characterization of snake venoms. Bull WHO 61: 949–956
Theakston RDG, Warrell DA (1991) Antivenoms: A list of hyperimmune sera currently available for the treatment of envenoming by bites and stings. Toxicon 29: 1419–1470
Theakston RDG, Fan HW, Warrell DA et al. (1992) Use of enzyme immunoassays to compare the effect and assess dosage regimens of three Brazilian *Bothrops* antivenoms. Am J Trop Med Hygl, in press
Theakston RDG, Lloyd-Jones MJ, Reid HA (1977) Micro-ELISA for detecting and assaying snake venom and venom antibody. Lancet ii: 639–641
Theakston RDG, Zumbuehl O, New RRC (1985) Use of liposomes for protective immunization in sheep against *Echis carinatus* snake venom. Toxicon 23: 921–925
Virivan C, Veeravat U, Warrell MJ, Theakston RDG, Warrell DA (1986) ELISA confirmation of acute and past envenoming by the monocellate Thai cobra (*Naja kaouthia*). Am J Trop Med Hyg 35: 173–181
Warrell DA, Davidson NMcD, Ormerod LD et al. (1974) Bites by the saw-scaled or carpet viper (*echis carinatus*): trial of two specific antivenoms. Br Med J 4: 437–440
Warrell DA, Looareesuwan S, Theakston RDG et al. (1986) Randomised comparative trial of three monospecific antivenoms for bites by the Malayan pit viper (*Calloselasma rhodostoma*) in southern Thailand: Clinical and laboratory correlations. Am J Trop Med Hyg 35: 1235–1247
Warrell DA, Warrell MJ, Edgar W et al. (1980) Comparison of Pasteur and Behringwerke antivenoms in envenoming by the carpet viper (*Echis carinatus*). Br Med J 1: 607–609
Weber M, Changeux J-P (1974) Binding of *Naja nigricollis* [3H]α-toxin to membrane fragments from *Electrophorus* and *Torpedo* electric organs. II. Effect of cholinergic agonists and antagonists on the binding of the tritiated neurotoxin. Mol Pharmacol 10: 15–34

Weir RC, Porter RR (1966) Comparison of the structure of the immunoglobulins from horse serum. Biochem J 100: 53–58
WHO (1981) Progress in the characterization of venoms and standardization of antivenoms. Offset Publication No. 58. World Health Organisation, Geneva, p5
Wiener S (1960) Active immunization of man against the venom of the Australian tiger snake (*Notechis scutatus*). Am J Trop Med Hyg 9: 284–292
Wiener S (1961) Snake bite in a subject actively immunized against snake venom. Med J Aust 1: 658–659

7 Therapeutic Antibodies to Tumours

J.A. Ledermann

Introduction

Many tumours initially respond to systemic drug therapy, but, because of drug resistance, treatment is rarely curative. The specificity of most such agents is low, and attempts to overcome drug resistance by increasing the dose are limited by side-effects. Obviously, the efficacy of therapy could be much improved by using potent agents that selectively attack tumour cells. One such approach is to use antibodies that recognize antigens on the surface of tumour cells; this would target therapy to the tumour site and spare normal host tissues from excess toxicity.

Since Behring and Kitasato first described the therapeutic use of antibodies, there has been much interest in developing these molecules to attack cancer cells. Héricourt and Richet (1895) used serum from dogs and donkeys that had been immunized with extracts of human tumours to treat patients with sarcomas. Tumour responses were reported, but further studies were curtailed owing to side-effects of repeated injections of animal antisera. The concept of using antibodies as a vehicle to target tumours was promoted by Ehrlich (1913), who suggested that tumours, like the toxins of microorganisms, might be suitable targets for antibodies. Forty years later, Pressman and Korngold (1953) and Bale et al. (1955) showed that injection of radiolabelled antisera raised against the transplantable Wagner osteogenic sarcoma tumour or Walker carcinoma led to specific localization of antibodies in these tumours. Nothing was known about the tumour antigen: the antibodies were partially purified by absorption with normal tissues.

In the last 20 years there has been a great increase in knowledge of the nature of antigens on the surface of tumour cells. This has been partly due to the development of hybridoma technology, which is a powerful tool that can be used to probe the cell surface. A pure and virtually limitless supply of monoclonal antibodies to tumour antigens can then be produced for targeted cancer therapy.

Human tumours can now be grown as a xenograft in rodents and enable preclinical studies of the targeting potential of antitumour antibodies. Quinones et al. (1971) showed that radiolabelled antibodies to human chorionic gonadotrophin, a glycoprotein known for many years to be produced by choriocarcinoma, localized specifically in the tumour when grown as a xenograft in the hamster cheek pouch. Similar experiments have been performed using radiolabelled antibodies to carcinoembryonic antigen (CEA). Antibodies to this tumour-related oncofetal glycoprotein, expressed in gastrointestinal and other epithelial tumours, localized specifically in colon cancers growing in the hamster cheek pouch or in congenitally T cell deficient "nude" mice (Primus et al. 1973; Mach et al. 1974). By 1974 it became possible to identify radioiodinated antibodies in tumours by external gamma scintigraphic imaging (Goldenberg et al. 1974; Mach et al. 1974) and this technique was soon extended to image deposits of colon cancer in patients who had been given an intravenous injection of radiolabelled antibodies to CEA (Goldenberg et al. 1978). These results have established a firm basis for developing antibodies for localization and therapy of cancer.

Cell Surface Targets for Antibody Therapy

Using monoclonal antibodies to probe the surface of tumour cells, several glycoproteins and glycolipids other than CEA and alphafetoprotein (AFP) have been identified as possible targets for antibody-directed therapy. However, apart from lymphoproliferative disorders that express tumour-specific idiotypes, none of these antigens is tumour specific. Instead, they should be regarded as tumour-related molecules, often expressed in greater concentrations in tumours than in normal tissues. The search for more specific antigens continues with current work focusing on oncogene products. Despite these limitations, antibodies to tumour-related products are regularly used to assist histological and serological diagnosis of many types of cancer. Several are also being investigated as potential targets for therapy (Table 7.1).

Biodistribution of Antibodies

The success of tumour detection and therapy depends on the ability of antibodies to localize specifically in a tumour. The tumour to normal tissue uptake ratio should be high and for therapy an adequate dose of antibody needs to be delivered to the tumour. Clinical studies to localize tumours using external scintigraphic imaging of radiolabelled antibodies, together with investigations in animals, have provided important information that has been used to develop targeted therapy.

Studies with radiolabelled antibodies in animals have shown that the concentration of antibody in blood, following intravenous injection, remains high for several days. Specific accumulation of polyclonal or monoclonal antibody in the tumour occurs within the first few hours and may persist for some days, or at least for as long as high levels of antibody remain in the blood. As antibody is cleared from blood, the tumour to blood and normal tissue ratios increase but the absolute amount of antibody remaining in a tumour decreases owing to its loss from the tumour. The clearance of antibody from blood is related to

Table 7.1. Clinical studies with therapeutic antibodies

Tumour-associated antigen	Tumour target
Oncofetal products	
Carcinoembryonic antigen (CEA)	Colorectal cancer
Alphafetoprotein (AFP)	Testicular teratoma
Hormones	
Human chorionic gonadotrophin (hCG)	Testicular teratoma Choriocarcinoma Ovarian germ cell tumours
Tumour-associated glycoproteins	
TAG-72 (tumour-associated glycoprotein)	Colorectal cancer
CA125	Ovarian cancer
Melanoma-associated glycoproteins	Melanoma
Breast-associated mucins (e.g. HMFG)	Ovarian cancer
Increased expression of normal products	
Ferritin	Hodgkin's disease Hepatoma Cholangiocarcinoma
Epidermal growth factor receptor	Glioma
Neuronal antigens	Neuroblastoma
B or T cell antigens	Non-Hodgkin's lymphoma Cutaneous T cell leukaemia
Tumour-specific products	
Idiotypic antibody	Non-Hodgkin's lymphoma

its physicochemical properties. Murine monoclonal antibodies are cleared much more rapidly in man than in mice. Antibody uptake is also affected by the presence of circulating tumour antigen, which may accelerate its clearance from blood and reduce its ability to accumulate in the tumour (Pedley et al. 1989a).

The delivery of antibody to the tumour site is affected by local factors such as the concentration gradient between antibody in blood and in the interstitial fluid, and its ability to permeate into interstitial spaces. Small immunoglobulin fragments, such as Fab′ or $F(ab')_2$ penetrate better into tumour nodules (Sutherland et al. 1987), but are cleared more rapidly from the blood than intact immunoglobulin. Other factors are important, including the permeability of the vascular endothelium, which varies in different normal tissues, and the affinity of the antibody for its antigen. Mathematical models based on experiments in mice showed that the permeability of the fenestrated liver endothelium is 50 times that of the gut (Covell et al. 1986). Little is known about the permeability of endothelium supplying tumours, though the studies of Clauss and Jain (1990) using the rabbit ear chamber model showed better permeability of antibodies into tumours than into normal tissues. These studies also demonstrated that diffusion was not solely a function of molecular size: 150 kDa dextrans diffused through the endothelium more readily than immunoglobulins and the vascular permeabilities to sheep and rabbit IgG were different. Tumours usually have a disorganized growth pattern with hypoxic and necrotic areas towards their centre; this might offset any benefit from increased permeability of the tumour endothelium. Furthermore, the hydrostatic pressure in central areas is high and this is likely to hinder the diffusion of macromolecules (Jain 1988).

The accumulation of antibody within a tumour also depends on its interaction with antigen. Animal studies have repeatedly confirmed that specific antibody is retained longer by tumours than is non-specific immunoglobulin. The relative importance of affinity for antigen is unclear, particularly as saturation of antigen has not been shown to occur in animal models. Theoretical arguments have been advanced in favour of using both low- and high-affinity antibodies, but a recent study demonstrated that uptake of antibody is greatest with high-affinity antibodies (Schlom et al. 1992). The therapeutic effect of an immunoconjugate also depends on the time it is resident in the tumour. Catabolism of the immunoconjugate is poorly understood, but is obviously an important determinant of biological half-life.

The complex inter-related factors affecting the distribution of antibodies determine the effectiveness of antibody-targeted therapy. Mathematical models have been developed in an attempt to predict the behaviour of antibodies and immunoglobulin fragments in vivo (Covell et al. 1986; Thomas et al. 1989), but it is difficult to extrapolate these results to man. For example, accumulation of antibody in mice bearing a xenograft is 1000 times greater than the highest uptake of antibody seen in tumours in man. Thus, the therapeutic ratio in man is lower; this may explain the less favourable results of antibody therapy in man (Dykes et al. 1987). Nevertheless, antitumour activity continues to be reported in man and this provides an incentive for further research into antibody-directed therapy.

Therapeutic Strategies

There are two general approaches to the treatment of tumours with antibodies. One uses the host's natural immune system to interact with the antitumour antibody to kill tumour cells. The other and more frequently used approach is to conjugate antibody to a cytotoxic agent, which then acts as a vehicle to carry the cytotoxic compound to the site of the tumour. Several agents have been used to target therapy, as summarized in Table 7.2 and discussed more fully below.

Natural Effector Mechanisms

Naturally occurring antibodies are most effective at combating infection, but there is little evidence to suggest that this system is active in cancer, perhaps because tumours are poorly immunogenic in the host. However, antibodies to human tumours can be raised in animals and it has often been suggested that injection of these antibodies in man might activate complement or antibody-dependent cell-mediated cytotoxicity. Serotherapy has been used for nearly a century, but, until recently, there has been little evidence that

Table 7.2. Mechanism of action of therapeutic antibodies

Natural effector mechanisms	
Cytotoxic T cells, antibody-dependent cellular cytotoxicity, complement	
Immunoconjugates	
Cytotoxic drugs:	methotrexate, vinca alkaloids, daunomycin
Plant or bacterial toxins:	ricin, abrin, diptheria toxin
Radioisotopes:	*β emitters* – iodine-131, yttrium-90, copper-67, phosphorus-32, rhenium-186; *α emitters* – astatine-211
Enzymes to activate prodrugs:	nitrogen mustard derivatives, etoposide phosphate

it has any useful effect. The ability to make large quantities of monoclonal antibodies has led to renewed enthusiasm for this form of treatment and initial therapeutic trials have been encouraging. For example, a patient with a non-Hodgkin's lymphoma has been treated with a monoclonal antibody raised against an idiotypic antibody expressed on the surface of a B cell tumour. This therapy was effectively "tailor-made" for the individual and led to complete remission of the tumour for more than 5 years (Miller et al. 1982). Further attempts to develop anti-idiotypic antibody therapy have been less successful, but responses continue to be reported, particularly in lymphoma. The results of therapy in solid tumours, such as colorectal cancer or melanoma, have been disappointing. Anti-idiotype therapy is very labour intensive and work is proceeding on a more generic therapy, using either a single antibody or cocktail of antibodies.

Little is known about the mechanism of action of "serotherapy". The amount of antibody reaching a tumour is small and its residence in the tumour is likely to be short. Koprowski et al. (1984) have suggested that the effect of antibody therapy may be mediated through the idiotypic network. The network hypothesis, proposed by Jerne (1974), states that determinants on antibodies give rise to further antibody responses. In this way an anti-idiotypic response (AB2), against the binding region of an antitumour antibody, would act as a substitute for a tumour antigen and give rise to an anti-anti-idiotypic antibody (AB3). This would provide a constant supply of antibody capable of combining with the tumour antigen. AB2 responses have been seen in some patients with colorectal cancer who responded to therapy with 17-1A, an antibody that reacts with an antigen on colorectal cancers. Herlyn et al. (1991) have used a monoclonal anti-idiotype antibody (AB2) to immunize patients with the aim of stimulating an AB3 response. As ability to manipulate the immune response increases, it may become possible to extend this approach to the development of idiotypic vaccines.

Radioimmunotherapy

Targeted radiation therapy using a radioisotope conjugated to an antibody has attracted most attention over the last 20 years. Most experience has been gained using iodine-131 for tumour localization and therapy. This isotope emits β and γ radiation and is easily conjugated to proteins. Much is known about the toxicity of this isotope as therapeutic doses have been used for many years to treat thyroid cancer.

For the treatment of solid tumours, radioimmunotherapy has several advantages over drug and toxin conjugates. Autoradiography of tissues resected after injection of radiolabelled antibody has shown a heterogeneous micro-distribution of radiolabelled antibody. This is due to heterogeneous expression of antigen and the presence of poorly vascularized and thus inaccessible regions. The "radiation field" of radioimmunoconjugates helps to overcome the disadvantage of unequal distribution of antibody within a tumour. Furthermore, if gamma-emitting isotopes are given, external scintigraphy can be used to demonstrate tumour localization and examine the distribution of antibody (Fig. 7.1).

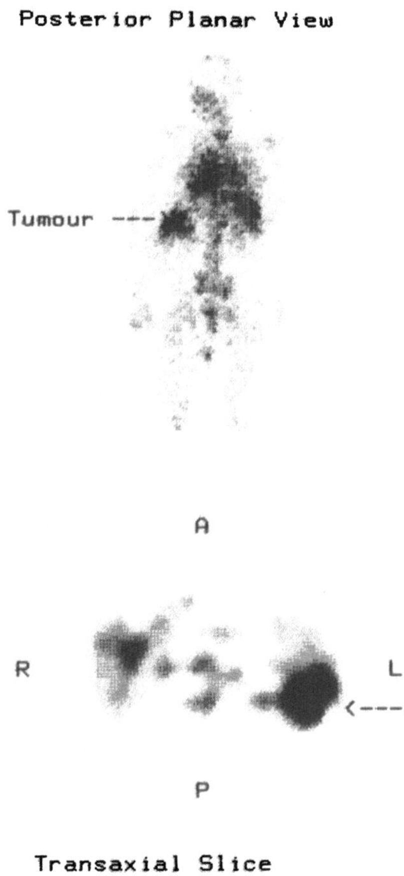

Fig. 7.1. Gamma camera images of a patient 70 h after injection of 36 mCi of ^{131}I-labelled anti-CEA (A5B7). The patient had a recurrent colorectal cancer in the splenic flexure. Localization of radioactivity in this area is seen on the posterior planar view and transaxial images. (Courtesy of Professor R. Begent.)

Many practical and theoretical considerations affect the choice of radionuclide. The antitumour effect of the conjugate depends on the concentration in the tumour, the energy emission spectrum and the half-life. The microscopic distribution within the tumour is important because the range of cell damage varies between α and β emitting isotopes. Most clinical experience has been gained with iodine-131. This emits β radiation that can penetrate to a depth of about 1 mm, about 40 cell diameters. Studies have also been performed with antibody conjugated to yttrium-90, which has a greater β energy than iodine-131 and can penetrate 100–1000 cell diameters. However, the biodistribution of these two conjugates is very different. Yttrium-90 is a metal that has to be linked to an antibody by a chelating agent and the conjugate accumulates in liver and bone to a greater extent than iodine-131 conjugates. Alpha emitters, such as astatine-211 or bismuth-212 have a very high energy, but a short path length. They are likely to be most effective in treating small clumps or single cell suspensions of tumour. The half-life of the isotope and the biological half-life of the conjugate must be such that most of the energy is expended during the time the antibody is attached to the tumour.

Animal Models of Radioimmunotherapy

Models to study radioimmunotherapy have been established in immunodeprived "nude mice" bearing human tumour xenografts. Intravenous injections of antibodies conjugated to β-emitting isotopes, such as iodine-131 (Badger et al. 1986; Cheung et al. 1986; Sharkey et al. 1988a; Buchegger et al. 1989) and yttrium-90 (Sharkey et al. 1988b), have produced a delay in growth of many types of xenograft tumour. A therapeutic effect has also been seen with astatine-211, an α emitter, in lymphoma (Harrison and Royle 1987). Small tumours derived from colon, kidney and small cell lung cancers have been eradicated by large doses of iodine-131 (Cheung et al. 1986; Buchegger et al. 1989; Smith et al. 1991). While it has been useful to perform preclinical studies with new conjugates in mice, animal models have many limitations. The amount of antibody that localizes in a mouse xenograft tumour is two or three orders of magnitude greater than that in man. This may be due to differences in the circulating half-life of the antibody, the dose in relation to body weight, and the permeability of the mouse endothelium supplying the tumour. In addition, mice are more tolerant to the effects of radiation damage to bone marrow than man. Partly because of these limitations, clinical trials have been instituted at an early stage in the development of radioimmunotherapy.

Clinical Trials

There is now more than 20 years of clinical experience with targeted radiation therapy. The group at the Johns Hopkins Hospital, Baltimore, have treated large numbers of patients with radioiodinated polyclonal antibodies to ferritin. Radiolabelled antibody has been used to treat patients with hepatoma in a protocol that included external beam radiation and surgery; 48% of patients responded with a complete remission in 7% (Order et al. 1985). Over 100 patients have been treated, but it is difficult to know how much of the therapeutic effect could be attributed to the radiolabelled antibody. Using iodine-131 antiferritin, the same group has reported a 40% response rate to Hodgkin's disease (Lenhard et al. 1985). Antiferritin radiolabelled with yttrium-90 has also been used successfully in some patients with Hodgkin's disease (Vriesendorp et al. 1989). Tumour responses following intravenous therapy with iodine-131 monoclonal antibodies to non-Hodgkin's lymphoma, resistant to conventional therapy, have been reported by several other groups (DeNardo et al. 1988; Zimmer et al. 1988; Press et al. 1989). Trials have been performed in colorectal cancer, melanoma and neuroblastoma. Tumour responses have been seen in some patients, but it is unusual for these to be sustained.

The distribution of radiolabelled antibody can be studied by external imaging, and the activity in tumours and normal tissues can be measured. From these data, the radiation dose delivered to the tumour and normal tissues can be estimated (Fig. 7.2) and used to assess the therapeutic index of radiolabelled antibodies, to compare the activity of different conjugates and to design methods of improving the therapeutic potential of radioimmunotherapy. Begent at al. (1989) have made serial observations on the distribution of iodine-131 anti-CEA antibody given to patients with recurrent colorectal cancer. The maximum concentration of radioactivity was found in the tumour 8 h after injection of iodine-131 anti-CEA. There was as much as a nine-fold variation in radioactivity in the tumour of different patients. Higher levels of radioactivity were found in the tumour than any

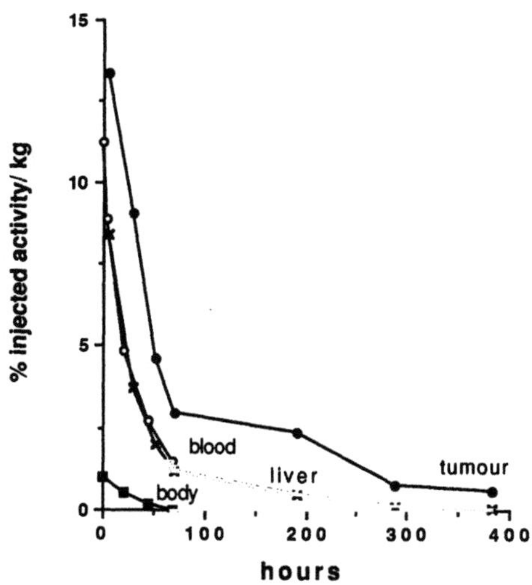

Fig. 7.2. Distribution of ^{131}I-labelled anti-CEA (A5B7) in a patient with colorectal cancer. The amount of radioactivity in the tumour situated in the left upper abdomen is greater than in the liver, blood or body. Activity is measured in relation to tissue mass calculated from computed X-ray tomography. From these data an estimate of the radiation dose to tissues can be made. (Courtesy of Professor R. Begent.)

other tissue, though antibody also accumulated in the liver, lung and blood relative to the rest of the body. The best tumour response was seen in a patient who had the greatest concentration of radioactivity in the tumour, and the most favourable ratio of radioactivity in the tumour relative to other tissues. In this patient the β radiation dose to tumour was estimated to be 5.1 cGy/mCi injected with a whole body dose of 0.25 cGy/mCi, a ratio of 20:1. These results are encouraging as theoretical predictions from mathematical models have suggested that a ratio of 30:1, assuming that a whole body dose of 200 cGy is tolerable, is needed for effective therapy (Dykes et al. 1987).

Calculations of tumour dose from external imaging have suggested that responses in lymphoma, colon cancer and hepatoma occur following the delivery of between 500 and 1000 cGy to the tumour. These doses, given by external beam therapy, would not normally be associated with significant tumour destruction. The results suggest that current methods of measurement underestimate the dose of radiation delivered to the nuclei of cancer cells. This may be due to non-uniform distribution of radioactivity within the tumour. Autoradiographic studies also show a preferential distribution of radioactivity around tumour cells relative to stromal cells (Esteban et al. 1987; Boxer et al. 1992).

Some improvement in the therapeutic effect may be gained by increasing the dose of antibody. However, large single doses of iodine-131 or yttrium-90 produce myelosuppression. Studies in thyroid cancer have shown that a radiation dose of 200 cGy to blood will produce myelosuppression from which recovery is predictable. The situation is similar when intravenous iodine-131 antibodies are given to treat tumours. A higher dose to the bone marrow might be acceptable provided autologous bone marrow support or haematopoietic growth factors are given.

Efforts have also been directed at improving the therapeutic ratio – the proportion of the dose reaching the tumour relative to the dose to normal tissues.

Cytotoxic Drug Conjugates

Immunoconjugates have been prepared with many different drugs including methotrexate, chlorambucil, adriamycin, daunorubicin, vindesine and mitomycin C. They have been shown to be active in vitro and in animal tumour models (Arnon and Hurwitz 1985; Embleton 1987). However, the potency of these drugs is low in comparison to toxins (Table 7.2). Large doses are likely to be required in order to overcome the drug resistance that occurs very readily with cytotoxic agents. It is difficult to deliver large quantities of conjugate to the tumour as conjugation of large amounts of drug reduces immunoreactivity of the antibody. Carrier molecules such as albumin and dextran can be linked to the antibody: these increase the number of drug molecules that can be conjugated. However, it is uncertain whether these conjugates will persist in the circulation sufficiently long to target satisfactorily in man. A very high specific uptake of drug conjugate could offset these disadvantages, but there is no evidence to suggest that the uptake ratio of a drug conjugate in tumour relative to normal tissues is any greater than for a radioimmunoconjugate or an immunotoxin. Internalization of the cytotoxic drug conjugate is also necessary. This depends on the expression of antigen on the cell surface and the ability of the antibody conjugate molecule to cross the cell membrane. Despite these limitations, small increases in the therapeutic ratio may be useful in clinical practice. This is supported by the results of a clinical trial with an antibody to colorectal carcinoma linked to neocarzinostatin given via the hepatic artery to patients with liver metastases. Three of eight patients had a reduction of tumour volume on an imaging scan (Takahashi et al. 1988). Favourable localization of the conjugate by comparison with normal colon was also demonstrated.

Immunotoxins

Various toxins of plant and bacterial origin have a potency several orders of magnitude greater than conventional chemotherapeutic drugs. Those toxins can be linked to antibodies, which can be used to target tumour cells (Vitetta et al. 1983). The high potency of toxins results from enzymatic inhibition of protein synthesis; this action depends on internalization. Ricin, found in beans of *Ricinus communis*, has been extensively studied. The molecule has a lectin B chain that binds non-specifically to many cell types. Following internalization the cytotoxic A chain exerts its effect by inactivating the 60s ribosomal subunit of eukaryotic cells by modifying nucleoside residues of the 28s ribosomal RNA (Endo and Tsurugi 1987). For antibody therapy the isolated A chain can be linked to antibody or the linkage arranged so that the B chain is chemically "blocked" and is inactive. The conjugate will then localize specifically to tumours. In vitro ricin A chain immunoconjugates can be 10^3–10^4 times as toxic to tumour cells as ricin A chain alone. Press et al. (1988) have shown that, once internalized, immunoconjugates may vary in their effectiveness according to the epitope on the antigen molecule with which the targeting antibody reacts. Reaction with an epitope close to the cell membrane resulted in longer retention in the cell and slower metabolism and expulsion than reaction with an epitope more distant from the cell membrane. The route of internalization may also affect the action of immunotoxins. Some are internalized via endosomal membranes; others enter lysosomes and undergo proteolysis.

Lymphomas and leukaemias may be particularly well suited to immunotoxin therapy. In contrast to most solid tumours, antigen expression is fairly homogeneous and cells are accessible to antibody; circulating tumour cells are often present and tumour masses are rarely avascular and necrotic. Animal models show that immunotoxins can prevent the establishment of leukaemia. These models have been used to study the kinetics of immunotoxins and to devise ways of reducing rapid clearance from the circulation. For example, deglycosylation of the ricin A chain removes the mannose-terminating oligosaccharides, reducing the rate of uptake by Kupffer cells in the liver. Chemical deglycosylation is now being replaced by the use of unglycosylated recombinant ricin A chain.

One clinical study with ricin A chain linked to an antimelanoma antibody showed responses (Spitler et al. 1987), but it is not clear whether these were mediated directly by the ricin A chain or by natural effector mechanisms.

Table 7.3. Strategies to improve antibody therapy

Tumour targeting	
	Increase antigen expression
	Improve vascular access
	Use immunoglobulin fragments
Therapeutic ratio	
	More potent conjugates
	Local therapy
	Clearance of unbound immunoconjugate
	Two-phase amplification of targeting
Host immune response	
	Immunosuppression of antiglobulin response
	Human monoclonal antibodies with low immunogenicity
	Induction of immunological tolerance

A clinical trial with deglycosylated ricin immunotoxin in non-Hodgkin's lymphoma is in progress and the results are eagerly awaited. Preliminary reports indicate that the immunotoxins cause a reduction in tumour burden and side-effects are in general mild and reversible. Studies with immunotoxins in colorectal cancer are also in progress.

Limitations of Antibody Therapy

Initial expectations about antibody-directed therapy were too optimistic. Clinical trials have established major limiting factors. The therapeutic dose reaching the tumour is too small and the therapeutic ratio of the conjugate is not sufficiently high to overcome the inadequate delivery of immunoconjugate to the target. Furthermore, it is often difficult to build on responses, as repeated therapy is prevented by the host's immune response to the immunoconjugate. Considerable effort is now being directed towards overcoming these difficulties (Table 7.3).

Delivery of Immunoconjugate

Study of the local tumour environment has shown areas with weak or heterogeneous antigen expression. In some tumours it has been possible to increase the expression of tumour antigen by pretreatment with alpha interferon. The selection of an isotope of sufficient energy to reach areas inaccessible to antibodies may also improve results. Alternatively, a cocktail of antibodies, reacting with different epitopes, can be given: in a xenograft model this has been shown to lead to a greater delivery of radionuclide to the tumour. However, it is unclear to what extent this approach will be clinically useful.

Delivery of antibody to the site of the tumour is a more important factor. Solid tumours are often poorly vascularized; this reduces the ability of molecules, particularly intact immunoglobulin with a molecular weight of about 150 000 Da, to reach the tumour. The use of smaller molecules, such as divalent or monovalent immunoglobulin fragments, might increase delivery provided that a high enough dose is given to offset the more rapid clearance of immunoglobulin fragments. Pharmacological agents such as vasodilators and interleukin-2 have been shown to improve the perfusion or vascular permeability of tumours and have increased the delivery of immunoconjugate to mice bearing human tumour xenografts (Smyth et al. 1987; LeBerthon et al. 1991). The benefit of these manoeuvres is likely to be greatest in small tumours without areas of necrosis and with a relatively small supporting stroma. As the proportion of antibody accumulating in small tumours is much higher than in large masses, the effect of therapy is likely to be greatest when given as an adjuvant to the treatment of micrometastatic disease.

Improvements in Therapeutic Ratio

Some of the toxicity of immunoconjugates can be reduced by local injection of an antibody into the body cavity containing the tumour. Alternatively, systemic toxicity can be reduced by arterial infusion as the tumour is exposed to a higher concentration. Both approaches would increase the accumulation of antibody in a tumour relative to systemic exposure and so increase the therapeutic ratio. Tumour remissions have been reported following intracavity radioimmunotherapy in ovarian cancer, malignant pleural effusions and malignant meningitis (Pectasides et al. 1986; Epenetos et al. 1987; Lashford et al. 1988). Intra-arterial therapy has also been used in gliomas (Epenetos et al. 1985). In ovarian cancer it has been shown that intraperitoneal therapy is only advantageous in very small tumours, or malignant ascites (Ward et al. 1988). Regional therapy is still limited by myelosuppression as antibody and its conjugate diffuse into the circulation.

The toxicity of iodine-131 and radioiodinated antibody is related to its persistent circulation in blood. Patients who clear antibody slowly from blood have a greater degree of myelosuppression (Ledermann et al. 1990). Radiolabelled antibody can be cleared from the circulation by injecting a second antibody, directed against the first antibody, which leads to the formation of an immune complex that is cleared rapidly from the blood. Animal studies have shown that a clearing antibody produces a significant decrease in circulating antibody, a reduction in the radiation dose to bone marrow and only a small reduction in the dose to a tumour (Pedley et al. 1989b). Similar findings were seen in one study in man (Begent et al. 1989). It may be possible to increase the benefit of this approach by altering the time at which the clearing antibody is given.

Amplification of a therapeutic effect using a dual-phase approach to increase the specificity of targeted therapy is an area of active research. Bispecific antibodies have been constructed with one arm that binds to the tumour and the other directed against a drug or receptors on host cytotoxic lymphocytes (Corvalan et al. 1987; Titus et al. 1987). A more generic approach, developed by Fodstad et al. (1988), uses a toxin linked to an antimouse antibody. This can be targeted to any previously administered mouse antitumour antibody. In vitro and animal studies are being performed, but the increase in therapeutic ratio being achieved by this approach is not yet clear.

Bagshawe (1988) has used an antitumour antibody linked to carboxypeptidase G_2, a non-mammalian enzyme. The antibody localized in the tumour. After the conjugate cleared from blood, a prodrug was given which was activated by carboxypeptidase to form a benzoic acid mustard, released at the tumour site. In nude mice this approach can eradicate xenografts of human choriocarcinoma. ADEPT (antibody directed enzyme prodrug therapy) is now being investigated in patients with colon cancer using an antibody to CEA. The generation of large quantities of active drug with a short half-life at the site of the tumour should lessen systemic toxicity and therefore increase the therapeutic index.

Repeated Therapy with Monoclonal Antibodies

Cancer is rarely cured by a single treatment with a drug or radiation, and it is likely that successful treatment with antibodies will require the administration of repeated courses. Repeated therapy with immunoconjugates is limited both by the toxicity of the conjugate and by the host immune response to the antibody. Immunization to polyclonal or rodent monoclonal antibodies generally occurs after one or two injections. The administration of further courses of antibody in the presence of a human anti-antibody leads to hypersensitivity reactions, rapid removal of conjugate from the body and failure to localize in a tumour (Carrasquillo et al. 1984; Shawler et al. 1985). The antiglobulin response is particularly evident in patients with solid tumours. It is less often seen in patients receiving antibody therapy for B cell lymphoma as they are immunosuppressed.

There has been much interest in using drugs and monoclonal anti-T cell antibodies that suppress cell-mediated rejection of organ and bone marrow allografts to prevent the human anti-antibody response. However, most of these agents do not prevent the humoral immune response to murine monoclonal antibodies. The immunosuppressive drug cyclosporin A is an exception: this also inhibits humoral immunity. It can delay the development of an antiglobulin response to murine iodine-131 anti-CEA and reduce the magnitude of the immune response (Ledermann et al. 1988). Even in the presence of small amounts of anti-antibody, further injections of monoclonal antibody could be given, provided that cyclosporin A therapy was continued. The distribution of antibody and tumour localization was unaltered by repeated injections of antibody and therapy was limited only by host toxicity to the conjugate (Ledermann et al. 1990). However, the drug is unable to suppress a secondary immune response and is of no value if started after an antibody response has developed. There is no evidence that cyclosporin A accelerates tumour growth, but its use is associated with side-effects.

Much work is directed towards modifying the structure of immunoglobulins to reduce their immunogenicity. $F(ab')_2$ fragments are less immunogenic than intact antibody, but human antimouse activity still occurs sufficiently often to prevent repeated use. Chemical modification of antibodies with polyethylene glycol reduces their immunogenicity in animals (Wilkinson et al. 1987), but this approach has not yet been tried in man. Advances in molecular engineering are being applied to develop antibodies with low immunogenicity. Examples include the construction of human–mouse hybrid antibodies, or an immunoglobulin with a mouse variable region and a human constant region (Morrison 1985; Reichmann et al. 1988). Some of these constructs have been given to patients. Intact human monoclonal antibodies have a longer circulatory half-life than murine antibodies. Although they are less immunogenic, an immune response can occur to sequences in the small amount of mouse framework that remains, or to idiotypic determinants (LoBuglio et al. 1989; Khazeli et al. 1991). Using molecular engineering techniques it is possible to construct small molecules such as single domain antibodies and Fv fragments that have a much shorter half-life in the circulation than intact humanized antibody. The latter persist in the circulation longer than murine monoclonal antibodies; this may increase delivery of a conjugate to tumour, but can also increase toxicity to normal tissues. It is not yet clear which type of construct will be most suitable for clinical use.

A method for inducing immunological tolerance to antitumour antibodies would be desirable. The use of high doses of immunoglobulin to produce "high zone" tolerance has yielded inconsistent results. Inactivation of antibody-forming clones has many attractions and has been achieved in animals by the use of radiolabelled antigen or antibody–drug conjugates (Ada and Byrt 1969; Durrant et al. 1989). Waldmann (1989) has used specific anti-T cell antibodies to induce tolerance to immunoglobulin in animals. As understanding of the T cell regulatory responses to B cell activation increases, it may become possible to use antibodies to provide a signal to the immune system that leads to tolerance rather than immunization.

Conclusions

It is now abundantly clear that antibodies can be targeted specifically to tumour cells. These antibodies can be put to therapeutic use in a variety of tumours and in some cases this has led to a significant reduction in tumour burden. In other cases, the therapeutic ratio of antibody-targeted therapy is still too small. Successful therapy is most likely when antibodies are used to eliminate a small tumour burden. Clinical experience with therapeutic antibodies has demonstrated the need to develop ways of increasing the therapeutic index of these agents, such as local amplification of the therapeutic effect or protection of systemic toxicity by clearing mechanisms. Further improvements are likely to come from the application of more potent conjugates, such as recombinant plant and bacterial toxins and radionuclide conjugates with high-energy β emission. As our understanding of the factors controlling the immune system increases, it may become possible to exploit the more general use of natural effector mechanisms, as already shown in the therapy of lymphoma. Progress is slow, but present results justify an optimism that therapeutic antibodies will eventually be used more extensively to treat common malignancies.

References

Ada GL, Byrt P (1969) Specific inactivation of antigen reactive cells with 125-I-labelled antigen. Nature 222: 1291–1292

Arnon R, Hurwitz E (1985) Monoclonal antibodies as carriers for immunotargeting of drugs. In: Baldwin RW, Byers VS (eds) Monoclonal antibodies for cancer detection and therapy. Academic Press, London, pp 365–383

Badger CC, Krohn KA, Shulman H, Flournoy N, Bernstein ID (1986) Experimental radioimmunotherapy of murine lymphoma with 131-I labelled anti-T-cell antibodies. Cancer Res 46: 6223–6228

Bagshawe K (1988) Antibody directed enzymes revive anticancer prodrugs concept. Br J Cancer 56: 531–532

Bale WF, Spar IL, Goodland RL, Woolfe DE (1955) In vivo and in vitro studies of labelled antibodies against rat kidney and Walker carcinoma. Proc Soc Exp Biol Med 89: 564–568

Begent RHJ, Ledermann JA, Green AJ et al. (1989) Antibody distribution and dosimetry in patients receiving radiolabelled antibody therapy for colorectal cancer. Br J Cancer 60: 406–412

Boxer GM, Begent RHJ, Kelly AMB et al. (1992) Factors influencing variability of localisation of antibodies to carcinoembryonic antigen (CEA) in patients with colorectal carcinoma – implications for radioimmunotherapy. Br J Cancer 65: 825–831

Buchegger F, Pfister C, Fournier K et al. (1989) Ablation of human colon carcinoma in nude mice by ^{131} I-labeled monoclonal anti-carcinoembryonic antigen antibody $F(ab')_2$ fragments. J Clin Invest 83: 1449–1456

Carrasquillo JA, Krohn KA, Beaumier P et al. (1984) Diagnosis of and therapy for solid tumours with radiolabelled antibodies and immune fragments. Cancer Treat Rep 68: 317–328

Cheung NV, Landmeier B, Neely J et al. (1986) Complete tumour ablation with iodine 131-radiolabelled disaloganglioside GD2-specific monoclonal antibody against human neuroblastoma xenografted in nude mice. JNCI 77: 739–745

Clauss MA, Jain RK (1990) Interstitial transport of rabbit and sheep antibodies in normal and neoplastic tissues. Cancer Res 50: 3487–3492

Corvalan JRF, Smith W, Gore VA, Brandon DR, Ryde PJ (1987) Increased therapeutic effect of vinca alkaloids targeted to tumour by hybrid-hybrid monoclonal antibody. Cancer Immunol Immunother 24: 138–143

Covell DG, Barbet J, Holton OD et al. (1986) Pharmacokinetics of monoclonal immunoglobulin G1, $F(ab')_2$ and Fab′ in mice. Cancer Res 46: 3969–3978

DeNardo SJ, DeNardo GL, O'Grady LF et al. (1988) Treatment of B cell malignancies with 131-I lym-1 monoclonal antibodies. Int J Cancer suppl 3: 96–101

Durrant LG, Robins AR, Marksman RA et al. (1989) Abrogation of antibody responses in rats to murine monoclonal antibody 791T/36 by treatment with daunomycin-cis-aconityl 791T/36 conjugates. Cancer Immunol Immunother 28: 37–43

Dykes PW, Bradwell AR, Chapman CE Vaughan ATM (1987) Radioimmunotherapy of cancer: Clinical studies and limiting factors. Cancer Treat Rev 14: 87–106

Ehrlich P (1913) In: Himmelweit F(ed) Collected papers, vol III. Pergamon Press, London, pp 505-518

Embleton MJ (1987) Drug-targeting by monoclonal antibodies. Br J Cancer 55: 227–231

Endo Y, Tsurugi K (1987) RNA N-glycosidase activity of ricin A chain. J Biol Chem 260: 12035–12041

Epenetos AA, Courtenay-Luck N, Pickering D et al. (1985) Antibody-guided irradiation of brain glioma by arterial infusion of radioactive monoclonal antibody against epidermal growth factor receptor and blood group A antigen. Br Med J 290: 1463–1466

Epenetos AA, Munro AJ, Stewart S et al. (1987) Antibody-guided irradiation of advanced ovarian cancer with intraperitoneally administered radiolabelled antibodies. J Clin Oncol 5: 1890–1899

Esteban JM, Colcher D, Sugarbaker P et al. (1987) Quantitative and qualitative aspects of radiolocalization in colon cancer patients of intravenously administered Mab B72.3. Int J Cancer 39: 50–59

Fodstadø, Kvalheim G, Pihl A, Godal A, Funderund S (1988) A new indirect approach to the therapeutic use of immunotoxins. JNCI 80: 439–443

Goldenberg DM, DeLand F, Kim E et al. (1978) Use of radiolabelled antibodies to CEA for

the detection and localisation of diverse cancers by external photoscanning. N Engl J Med 298: 1384–1386
Goldenberg DM, Preston DF, Primus FJ, Hansen HJ (1974) Photoscan localization of GW-39 tumours in hamsters using radiolabelled anti-carcinoembryonic antigen immunoglobulin G. Cancer Res 34: 1–9
Harrison A, Royle L (1987) Efficacy of astatine-211 labelled monoclonal antibody in treatment of murine T-cell lymphoma. Natl Cancer Inst Monogr 3: 157–158
Héricourt J, Richet C (1895) Traitement d'un cas de sarcome par la sérothérapie. C R Acad Sci 20: 948–950
Herlyn D, Caton A, Koprowski H (1991) Anti-idiotypes in cancer immunotherapy. In: Epenetos AA (ed) Monoclonal antibodies. Applications in clinical oncology. Chapman and Hall, London, pp 283–290
Jain RK (1988) Determinants of tumor blood flow: A review. Cancer Res 48: 2641–2658
Jerne NK (1974) Towards a network theory of the immune system. Ann Immunol (Inst Pasteur) 125C: 373–389
Khazeli MB, Saleh MN, Liu TP et al. (1991) Pharmacokinetics and immune response of ^{131}I-chimeric mouse/human B72.3 (human γ4) monoclonal antibody in humans. Cancer Res 51: 5461–5466
Koprowski H, Herlyn D, Lubeck M, DeFreitas E, Sears HF (1984) Human anti-idiotype antibodies in cancer patients: Is the modulation of the immune response beneficial for the patient? Proc Natl Acad Sci 81: 216–219
Lashford LS, Davies AG, Richardson RB et al. (1988) A pilot study of 131–I monoclonal antibodies in the therapy of leptomeningeal tumours. Cancer 61: 857–868
LeBerthon B, Khawli LA, Alauddin M et al. (1991) Enhanced tumour uptake of macromolecules by a novel vasoactive interleukin 2 immunoconjugate. Cancer Res 51: 2694–2698
Ledermann JA, Begent RHJ, Bagshawe KD et al. (1988) Repeated antitumour antibody therapy in man with suppression of the host response by cyclosporin A. Br J Cancer 58: 654–657
Ledermann JA, Begent RHJ, Massof C et al. (1990) A phase I study of repeated therapy with radiolabelled antibody to carcinoembryonic antigen using intermittent or continuous administration of cyclosporin A to suppress the immune response. Int J Cancer 47: 659–664
Lenhard RE, Order SE, Spunberg JJ, Asbell SO, Leibel SA (1985) Isotopic immunoglobulin: A new systemic therapy for advanced Hodgkin's disease. J Clin Oncol 3: 1296–1300
LoBuglio AF, Wheeler RH, Trang J et al. (1989) Mouse/human chimeric monoclonal antibody in man: Kinetics and immune response. Proc Natl Acad Sci USA 86: 4220–4224
Mach J-P, Carrel S, Merenda C, Sordat B, Cerottini J-C (1974) In vivo localisation of radiolabelled antibodies to carinoembryonic antigen in human colon carcinoma grafted into nude mice. Nature 248: 704–706
Miller RA, Maloney DG, Warnke R, Levy R (1982) Treatment of B cell lymphoma with a monoclonal anti-idiotype antibody. N Engl J Med 306: 517–522
Morrison SL (1985) Transfectomas provide novel chimeric antibodies. Science 229: 1202–1207
Order SE, Stillwagon GB, Klein JL et al. (1985) Iodine 131 antiferritin, a new treatment modality in hepatoma: A Radiation Oncology Group study. J Clin Oncol 3: 1573–1582
Pectasides D, Stewart S, Courtney-Luck N et al. (1986) Antibody guided irradiation of malignant pleural and pericardial effusions. Br J Cancer 53: 727–732
Pedley RB, Boden JA, Boden RW et al. (1989a) The effect of serum CEA on the distribution and clearance of anti-CEA antibody in a pancreatic tumour xenograft model. Br J Cancer 60: 549–554
Pedley RB, Dale R, Boden JA et al. (1989b) The effect of second antibody clearance on the distribution and dosimetry of radiolabelled anti-CEA antibody in a human colonic tumour xenograft model. Int J Cancer 43: 713–718
Press OW, Eary JF, Badger CC et al. (1989) Treatment of refractory non-Hodgkin's lymphoma with radiolabelled MB-1 (anti-CD37) antibody. J Clin Oncol 7: 1027–1038
Press OW, Martin PJ, Thorpe PE, Vitetta ES (1988) Ricin A-chain containing immunotoxins directed against different epitopes on the CD2 molecule differ in their ability to kill normal and malignant T cells. J Immunol 141: 4410–4417
Pressman D, Korngold L (1953) The in vivo localisation of anti-Wagner osteogenic sarcoma antibodies. Cancer 6: 619–623
Primus FJ, Wang RH, Goldenberg DM, Hansen HJ (1973) Localization of human GW-39

tumours in hamsters by radiolabelled heterospecific antibody to carcinoembryonic antigen. Cancer Res 33: 2977–2982
Quinones J, Mizejarski G, Beierwaltes WH (1971) Choriocarcinoma scanning using radiolabelled antibodies to chorionic gonadotrophin. J Nucl Med 12: 69–75
Reichmann L, Clark M, Waldmann H, Winter G (1988) Reshaping human antibodies for therapy. Nature 332: 323–327
Schlom J, Eggensperger D, Colcher D et al. (1992) Therapeutic advantage of high-affinity anticarcinoma radioimmunoconjugates. Cancer Res 52: 1067–1072
Sharkey RM, Kaltovich FA, Shih LB et al. (1988a) Radioimmunotherapy of human colon cancer xenografts with 90Y-labelled monoclonal antibodies to carcinoembryonic antigen. Cancer Res 48: 3270–3275
Sharkey RM, Primus FJ, Shochat D, Goldenberg DM (1988b) Comparison of tumour targeting of mouse monoclonal and goat polyclonal antibodies to carcinoembryonic antigen in the GW-39 human tumour-hamster model. Cancer Res 48: 1823–1828
Shawler DL, Bartholomew RM, Smith LM, Dillman RO (1985) Human immune response to multiple injections of murine monoclonal IgG. J Immunol 135: 1530–1535
Smith A, Waibel R, Stahel RA (1991) Selective immunotherapy of small cell cancer xenografts using ^{131}I-labelled SWA11 antibody. Br J Cancer 64: 263–266
Smyth MJ, Pietersz GA, McKenzie IFC (1987) Use of vasoactive agents to increase tumour perfusion and antitumour efficacy of drug–monoclonal antibody conjugates. JNCI 79: 1367–1373
Spitler LE, Rio M, Khentigan A et al. (1987) Therapy of patients with malignant melanoma using a monoclonal antimelanoma antibody-ricin A chain immunotoxin. Cancer Res 47: 1717–1723
Sutherland R, Buchegger F, Schreyer M, Vacca A, Mach J-P (1987) Penetration and binding of radiolabelled anti-carcinoembryonic antigen monoclonal antibodies and their antigen binding fragments in human colon multicellular spheroids. Cancer Res 47: 1627–1633
Takahashi H, Yamaguchi T, Kitamura K et al. (1988) Clinical application of monoclonal drug–antibody conjugates for immunotargeting chemotherapy of colorectal cancer. Cancer 61: 881–888
Thomas GD, Chappell MJ, Dykes PW et al. (1989) Effect of dose, molecular size, affinity, and protein binding on tumour uptake of antibody or ligand: A biomathematical model. Cancer Res 49: 3290–3296
Titus JA, Garrido MA, Hecht TT et al. (1987) Human T cells with anti-T3 cross-linked to antitumour antibody prevent tumour growth in nude mice. J Immunol 138: 4018–4022
Vitetta ES, Krolick KA, Miyama-Inaba M, Cushley W, Uhr JW (1983) Immunotoxins: A new approach to cancer therapy. Science 219: 644–650
Vriesendorp HM, Herpst JM, Leichner PK, Klein JL, Order SE (1989) Polyclonal 90 yttrium labelled antiferritin for refractory Hodgkin's disease. Int J Radiat Oncol Biol Phys 17: 815–821
Waldmann H (1989) Manipulation of T-cell responses with monoclonal antibodies. Ann Rev Immunol 7: 407–444
Ward B, Mather S, Shepherd J et al. (1988) Treatment of intraperitoneal malignant disease with monoclonal antibody guided 131-I radiotherapy. Br J Cancer 58: 658–662
Wilkinson I, Jackson C-JC, Lang GM, Holdford-Strevens V, Sehon AH (1987) Tolerance induction in mice by conjugates of monoclonal immunoglobulins and monomethoxypolyethylene glycol. J Immunol 139: 326–331
Zimmer AM, Rosen ST, Spies SM et al. (1988) Radioimmunotherapy of patients with cutaneous T-cell lymphoma using an iodine-131-labelled monoclonal antibody: Analysis of retreatment following plasmapheresis. J Nucl Med 29: 174–180

8 Therapeutic Antibodies to Microorganisms

P. L. Yap

Introduction

Immunoglobulin preparations against microorganisms are used currently for the prevention and treatment of a wide variety of infections. Initially, intramuscular immunoglobulin (IM IgG) preparations were given, but there has been renewed interest following the development of intravenous immunoglobulin (IVIG) preparations (Yap 1992). The use of antibody preparations for the prevention and treatment of various infectious diseases has a long history (Table 8.1), dating back to 1891, when sheep serum was used by Von Behring and Kitasato for the successful treatment of diphtheria in a child (Behring 1893). This work had followed the experimental use of equine antitoxin raised against diphtheria toxin and was a landmark in the history of antibody therapy because it was the first time that passive immunization had ever been performed successfully in humans.

This research aroused great interest at the time, but the use of animal antisera in patients was accompanied by many side-effects, particularly febrile reactions and serum sickness. Research was conducted on the use of serotherapy against viral infections and there was also particular interest in the use of equine antiserum to treat pneumococcal pneumonia. Finland (1930) and others published their considerable experience in pneumococcal serotherapy following the identification of the polysaccharide capsule as a virulence determinant. Because of the problems of serum sickness, an attempt was made to purify the antiserum for clinical use, and salt fractionation was introduced (Felton 1930). Although the incidence of serum sickness was considerably reduced, the recognition that human plasma could transmit hepatitis and the development of effective chemotherapy (in the form of the sulphonamides, followed by the penicillin antibiotics) for the treatment of infectious diseases discouraged further research and development in this area until the 1940s.

The next important development occurred during the Second World War, when adequate supplies of blood and blood products were needed for the

Table 8.1. History of passive antibody prophylaxis and treatment

Sheep serum – diphtheria protection	1891
Calf serum – vaccinia protection	1895
Dog serum – diphtheria protection	1889
Human serum – measles protection	1907
Salt fractionation of horse serum introduced for pneumococcal pneumonia	1930
Cold ethanol fractionation of human plasma to produce fraction II & III	1945
IM IgG shown to be protective for hepatitis	1945
Treatment of hypogammaglobulinaemia	1952
IVIG preparations introduced (UK)	1982
Mouse monoclonals used in virus infections	1986
Human monoclonals used in Gram-negative bacterial infection	1991

treatment of wartime casualties. In particular, a purified albumin fraction was needed for the resuscitation of soldiers with major injuries and shock. The cold ethanol fractionation procedure for human plasma was developed for the production of albumin, and a plasma fraction (called fraction II & III), which was rich in IgG, was also identified as a byproduct of albumin purification (Cohn et al. 1946). This fraction transformed antibody therapy for infectious diseases, because it was shown that serum hepatitis and other infections could be prevented by the prophylactic administration of this fraction (Cohn 1945). This fraction did not transmit serum hepatitis, even when icteric plasma was fractionated (Murray and Ratner 1953), and immunoglobulin concentrates for intramuscular administration, particularly "specific" preparations (see below), soon became standard therapy for the prophylaxis of a number of viral infections including measles, hepatitis A and B, varicella zoster and rabies.

The ability to administer immunoglobulin concentrates by the intravenous route for the prophylaxis of infection was the next objective because only limited amounts of such concentrates could be administered by the intramuscular route. Initially, severe adverse reactions accompanied attempts at intravenous immunoglobulin administration (Barandun et al. 1962; Janeway 1970), but it was observed that treatment of IgG at pH 4 could render the IgG molecule free of serious adverse reactions when administered intravenously (Barandun and Isliker 1986). Subsequently, other biochemical methods were discovered that rendered immunoglobulin preparations safe for intravenous use (McClelland and Yap 1984).

Antibody Preparations Available for Prophylaxis and Treatment of Infections

Antibody preparations can be classified into four different types:

1. *Human normal immunoglobulin and standard IVIG.* These are antibody preparations derived from human plasma donations that are not selected in any way. Such preparations contain the full spectrum of IgG antibodies that might be present in any randomly chosen healthy blood or plasma donor.

The levels of specific antibodies in individual blood or plasma donors may differ from area to area, or country to country, and minor differences can be observed between specific antibody levels against various pathogens in different antibody preparations, but, in general, these differences are not important. Such preparations can be for intramuscular (IM IgG) or intravenous (IVIG) use.

2. *Hyperimmune antibody preparations*. These are derived from human plasma donations selected on the basis of higher than normal antibody levels against a particular infectious agent compared with random plasma donations. Examples are the various specific (i.e. hyperimmune) intramuscular and intravenous preparations, e.g. CMV-IVIG, that are described below. It should be noted that it is not always necessary to formulate a specific hyperimmune IVIG preparation from selected plasma donations, because batches of IVIG can sometimes be identified that may contain higher levels than expected of a specific antibody against particular viruses (Preiksaitis et al. 1982) or bacteria (Harper et al. 1986). Alternatively, higher doses can be given of an IVIG preparation to achieve the same raised level of specific antibody.

3. *Animal antisera*. These can be used with or without some form of purification, but their administration may be accompanied by serum sickness and other adverse reactions. In general, animal antisera are little used today, although equine antitetanus toxin is still used in some parts of the world and, for some infections, e.g. *Clostridium welchii* (gas gangrene), animal antisera may be the only source of neutralizing antibodies against the toxin (see also Chapter 9).

4. *Rodent or human monoclonal antibody preparations*. Such preparations against microorganisms are now available, but there are few clinical trial data except for monoclonal antibodies against endotoxin (Greenman et al. 1991; Wenzel et al. 1991; Ziegler et al. 1991); these are considered in detail in Chapter 9.

It should also be noted that in the treatment of infectious disease, antibody preparations have hitherto been restricted to those that contain specific antibodies against the pathogen, or the toxin from the pathogen. However, blocking antibodies against the receptor for the pathogen or its toxin could theoretically be effective and it is conceivable that rodent or human monoclonal antibodies with such specificity could be developed for therapy in human infectious diseases. In some infections, the symptoms observed may be due to the liberation of toxic mediators; monoclonal antibodies against these mediators or their receptors are either being developed or in early clinical trials (Table 8.2). It is likely that such preparations will be evaluated in the future, but this review will be restricted to polyclonal IM

Table 8.2. Antibody therapy in infectious disease: options

Antibody against pathogen itself
Blocking antibody against receptor for pathogen
Antibody against toxin from pathogen, e.g. LPS, tetanus toxin
Blocking antibody against receptor for toxin
Antibody against humoral mediators involved in the pathogenesis of symptoms following infection, e.g. TNF, IL-6
Blocking antibody against receptor for mediator

NB: A comparison of efficacy between immunological and pharmacological approaches is needed.

IgG and IVIG preparations against bacteria and viruses; details of antibody preparations against endotoxins and cytokines are found in Chapters 9 and 10 respectively.

Applications of IM IgG Preparations for Prophylaxis of Viral Infection

Intramuscular immunoglobulin preparations have been used for the prophylaxis of infection for nearly half a century and are either used in the form of human normal immunoglobulin or hyperimmune specific intramuscular immunoglobulin preparations. These preparations are described below, but further details are available elsewhere (McClelland and Yap 1984; Joint Committee on Vaccination and Immunisation 1990).

Human Normal Immunoglobulin

Human normal immunoglobulin (HNI; also called immune serum globulin (ISG) in the USA) is manufactured from the plasma of unselected donors and contains the full spectrum of antibody specificities against microoganisms that might be expected in the normal population. However, in practice, HNI is only used for the prophylaxis of hepatitis A and measles because other hyperimmune ("specific") IM IgG preparations are available for the treatment of other infectious diseases.

Hepatitis A Prophylaxis

Pre-exposure Prophylaxis. Travellers to endemic areas and close contacts of hepatitis A cases may be given passive protection for a period of up to 6 months with HNI. Recommended dosages are given in Table 8.3.

Post-exposure Prophylaxis. HNI can also be administered to close contacts of all ages in order to control outbreaks of hepatitis A in households and institutions. Recommended dosages are 250 mg for individuals aged under 10 years and 500 mg for those aged 10 years and over.

For frequent travellers, measurement of circulating antibody levels against

Table 8.3. Recommended dosages for pre-exposure prophylaxis

Period abroad	Age	Dose (mg)
2 months or less	Under 10 years	125
	10 years and over	250
3–5 months	Under 10 years	250
	10 years and over	500

hepatitis A is preferable to repeated HNI injections, because up to half the adult population may already be immune. Alternatively, the recently developed hepatitis A vaccine provides long-term immunity of up to 10 years (Weidermann et al. 1990). If active immunization is combined with passive immunization, HNI and hepatitis A vaccine should be injected into separate sites.

HNI may interfere with the development of active immunity from other live virus vaccines and, preferably, such vaccines should be administered at least 3 weeks before the administration of HNI. If HNI is administered first then 3 months should elapse before the administration of a live virus vaccine, other than for yellow fever vaccine (as HNI does not contain antibody to the virus). For travellers, if there is insufficient time, the recommended intervals may have to be ignored, especially where oral polio vaccine is concerned.

Measles Prophylaxis

HNI may be used for the prophylaxis of measles in immunocompromised children and susceptible adult patients following contact with measles. The recommended dosages are 250 mg for individuals aged under 1 year, 500 mg for those aged 1–2 years, and 750 mg for those aged 3 years and over. An interval of at least 3 months should elapse before subsequent vaccination with measles vaccine, either on its own or in combination with mumps and rubella vaccine.

Immunodeficiency

In patients with a quantitative or qualitative deficiency of IgG, such as X-linked agammaglobulinaemia or common variable immunodeficiency, HNI may be administered as replacement therapy. However, doses are limited to 25–50 mg/kg per week (due to the injection volume) and more effective therapy may be attained using the higher doses of IgG available in IVIG preparations (see below).

Hyperimmune IgG Preparations

Hepatitis B Prophylaxis

Specific hepatitis B immunoglobulin (HBIG) is used for the post-exposure prophylaxis of hepatitis B infection in individuals who are inoculated with blood or secretions containing HBsAg because HBsAg-positive material is presumed to contain hepatitis B virus. HBIG is normally used in combination with hepatitis B vaccine to confer passive/active immunity and indications for the use of this product are:

1. *Parenteral exposure*. This consists of any subcutaneous or other injection, needle prick or blood transfusion. Other indications for HBIG are

skin-breaking bites by individuals infective for hepatitis B and cases in which there is clear evidence of contamination of a wound or the conjunctiva with hepatitis B contaminated material. Simultaneous administration of the first dose of hepatitis B vaccine should be considered, into a separate site.

2. *Sexual exposure.* HBIG may be administered to recent sexual contacts of individuals infected with hepatitis B. Limited evidence suggests that more effective protection is obtained by simultaneous administration of the first dose of a licensed hepatitis B vaccine into a separate site.

3. *Newborns.* HBIG is indicated for a neonate whose mother has had acute hepatitis B in the last trimester of pregnancy or is an HBsAg-positive carrier. A single dose of 200 i.u. HBIG is given within 4 h of birth (and not later than 48 h after) combined with the administration of the first dose of hepatitis B vaccine into a separate site. The hepatitis B vaccine course is then completed according to the manufacturer's instructions.

The adult dose is 500 i.u., but some authorities recommend a further injection of 500 i.u. a month later unless there is a fresh exposure incident. Alternatively, a 1000 i.u. dose can be administered following exposure. For children aged under 5 years and 5–9 years, the dose is 200 i.u. and 300 i.u. respectively. For children aged over 10 years, the dose is 500 i.u. HBIG must be administered as soon as possible after the exposure, ideally within 4 h and always within 7 days. Healthcare workers who have been successfully vaccinated should be given a booster dose of vaccine unless they are known to have adequate protective levels of hepatitis B antibodies. HBIG is not appropriate for prophylaxis of hepatitis A, hepatitis C or hepatitis non-A, non-B.

Rabies Prophylaxis

Rabies immunoglobulin must only be used in conjunction with rabies vaccine for prophylaxis in individuals exposed to suspected rabies and who are not considered to be adequately vaccinated. Rabies immunoglobulin gives temporary passive immunity until the vaccine induces an active immune response against the virus. In general, expert advice should be obtained regarding the need for rabies prophylaxis, but guidance has been published by the WHO Expert Committee (1983) and by the USA Centers for Disease Control (1984).

The recommended dose of rabies immunoglobulin is 20 i.u./kg and should be administered as soon as possible after exposure. Up to half the dose may be infiltrated round the wound if this is anatomically feasible. The remainder should be administered by deep intramuscular injection, in a separate site from that used for the rabies vaccine. Active and passive immunization should be combined with thorough cleansing of the wound. If more than 8 days have elapsed since the start of a course of human diploid cell vaccine, immunoglobulin will be unnecessary.

Rubella Prophylaxis

Maternal rubella infection in the first 10 weeks of pregnancy results in fetal damage. Some authorities consider that post-exposure prophylaxis does not prevent infection in non-immune contacts. However, limited evidence (reviewed in McClelland and Yap 1984) suggests that rubella immunoglobulin may reduce the likelihood of clinical symptoms and possibly the risk to the fetus. Rubella immunoglobulin may therefore be used for prophylaxis in early pregnancy in women with significant exposure to rubella who are known to be non-immune or whose immune status is in doubt, in whom rubella exposure occurred within the preceding 5 days, and in whom subsequent termination of pregnancy is not an acceptable option.

The recommended dose is 125 000 i.u. However, it should be noted that following the administration of rubella immunoglobulin, serological diagnosis of rubella infection may be hampered by the delayed onset of rubella infection and by levels of passively acquired IgG anti-rubella antibodies, which may mask true seroconversion unless an IgM-specific assay is used for detecting rubella antibodies. Careful serological follow-up after administration of rubella immunoglobulin is therefore essential over a 12-week period following injection.

Varicella Zoster Prophylaxis

Varicella zoster infection is a serious disease in immunocompromised patients. Varicella zoster immunoglobulin (VZIG) should therefore be used for prophylaxis in non-immune individuals exposed to varicella or zoster. VZIG should be used for the following groups of patients:

1a. Patients receiving corticosteroid or immunosuppressive treatment, including general radiation.
1b. Patients suffering from malignant conditions such as lymphoma, leukaemia, congenital or primary immunodeficiency or in whom the normal immunological mechanism may be impaired.
1c. Premature infants whose mother does not have a prior history of varicella, or those less than 28 weeks' gestation, or who weigh less than 1000 g regardless of maternal history.
1d. Newborn babies or mothers who have had onset of varicella within 5 days before the 48 h after delivery.
1e. Pregnant contacts of cases of varicella zoster.

In addition such patients should have had significant exposures to varicella or zoster, such as:

2a. Continuous household contact.
2b. Playmate contact (> 1 h play, indoors).
2c. Hospital contact (shared two- or four-bedded room, adjacent beds or prolonged face to face contact).
2d. Newborn contact (see 1d above).

It should be noted that VZIG is not indicated for the following groups of patients:

1. Patients with established varicella or zoster infections, or for the prevention of zoster dissemination.
2. Non-immunodeficient patients.

3. Patients whose exposure occurred more than 96 h previously.

The recommended dose of VZIG for prevention of infection in all at-risk individuals is 0.2 ml VZIG per kg body weight with a minimum dosage of 1 ml and a maximum dosage of 15 ml. VZIG must only be given by deep intramuscular injection as soon as possible after the presumed exposure and always within 96 h. The duration of protection after ZVIG administration is unknown, but if re-exposure occurs more than 3 weeks after a previous dose of VZIG the patient should receive an additional full dose.

Other Specific IM IgG Preparations

Hyperimmune antivaccinia immunoglobulin was previously available for the protection of contacts of smallpox cases, for the prevention and treatment of some of the complications of smallpox vaccination, and for the protection of eczematous children accidently exposed to smallpox vaccine or vaccination sites. However, in 1979, smallpox was eradicated globally and with the discontinuation of smallpox vaccination, antivaccinia immunoglobulin is no longer available.

There is limited evidence (reviewed by Seeff and Hoofnagle 1979) that HNI may provide passive immunity against icteric non-A, non-B hepatitis (NANBH) following transfusion. However, a newly discovered virus, the hepatitis C virus (HCV), has recently been identified as a major cause of transfusion-associated NANBH (Choo et al. 1989). Some preparations of HNI contain anti-HCV antibody, but there is no evidence currently available for the efficacy of HNI after needlestick injuries. Piazza (1990) reported an anecdotal study in which HNI (4 ml) was administered every 2 months to HCV-negative sexual partners of HCV-infected individuals and observed an absence of HCV seroconversion; it has been suggested by Alter (personal communication) that HNI could be administered after a needlestick injury involving hepatitis C. Firm recommendations regarding the use of HNI or a hyperimmune anti-HCV immunoglobulin preparation will need to await identification of HCV epitopes that elicit, or are associated with, protective immunity, and alpha interferon therapy should be considered for needlestick injuries.

HNI has in the past been suggested for the prophylaxis of mumps, but its efficacy has not been definitively shown and HNI is no longer recommended. Various other experimental human specific immunoglobulin preparations have also been developed to influenza and to various bacteria, but efficacy has not been clearly demonstrated; such preparations are not generally available.

Applications of IVIG Therapy

IVIG preparations contain a wide range of polyclonal antibodies against various microorganisms, reflecting the antibody spectrum of the human plasma from which they are derived. They allow the painless administration of large quantities of antibody, so that specific antibody levels can be raised quickly. They are used for the prophylaxis and treatment of infections in patients with primary and secondary immunodeficiency, where there is an increased susceptibility to various infections, and also in some specific infections.

Patients with Primary Immunodeficiency

Patients with primary hypogammaglobulinaemia (e.g. X-linked agammaglobulinaemia, common variable immunodeficiency, IgG subclass deficiency) suffer from recurrent bacterial infections, usually caused by Gram-positive encapsulated bacteria such as *Streptococcus pneumoniae* and *Haemophilus influenzae*. They were originally treated with IM IgG at a dose of 25–50 mg/kg/week, but such injections were painful and only low serum IgG levels were usually achieved. Following the availability of IVIG therapy, higher serum IgG levels could be achieved and a marked reduction in bacterial infections and a prevention or delay in the progression of structural lung damage could be demonstrated. Such patients may also suffer from *Giardia* and echovirus infections, and these are reduced with regular IVIG therapy (Williams et al. 1992).

Similarly, patients with combined immunodeficiencies involving antibody deficiency, such as severe combined immunodeficiency, ataxia-telangiectasia or the Wiskott–Aldrich syndrome, benefit from IVIG therapy if they suffer from recurrent bacterial infections (Table 8.4). However, it should be noted that patients who may have hypogammaglobulinaemia but who do not suffer from recurrent infections of Gram-positive encapsulated bacteria (e.g. selective IgA deficiency, patients with renal disease) do not normally benefit from IVIG therapy.

The exact dosage and frequency of IVIG treatment varies, but the objective of IVIG therapy in this group of patients is to attain a "trough" (pre-infusion) serum IgG concentration at or near the lower end of the normal range. This can be achieved with an IVIG dose of 200 mg/kg, initially every 3 weeks and subsequently at intervals of 4–5 weeks if this still ensures that trough serum IgG levels are maintained at or above 5 g/1. Patients with severe bronchiectasis or with co-existent loss of IgG through the gut may need higher doses

Table 8.4. Primary immunodeficiencies in which IVIG may be beneficial

Primary antibody deficiency
X-linked agammaglobulinaemia
Common variable immunodeficiency
IgG subclass deficiency
Transient hypogammaglobulinaemia of infancy (rarely)
Antibody deficiency with normal immunoglobulin levels (very rare)
Combined immune deficiencies
Severe combined immune deficiency
Wiskott–Aldrich syndrome
Ataxia-telangiectasia
X-linked lymphoproliferative syndrome

Table 8.5. Secondary immunodeficiencies in which IVIG may be beneficial

Haematological malignancies, e.g. CLL, multiple myeloma
Immunocompromised states, e.g. following major surgery, trauma or chemotherapy
Severe thermal injury
After transplantation
Premature birth
HIV infection especially in children

(400 mg/kg) given as often as every 2 weeks to maintain satisfactory trough serum IgG levels (Leen et al. 1986). If recurrent infections persist, despite IVIG therapy, high-dose antibiotics should be considered before increasing the dose of IgG, because high-dose antibiotic regimens are less expensive and do not require admission to hospital (Williams et al. 1987).

Patients with Secondary Immunodeficiency

Many forms of secondary immunodeficiency exist; in some of them, bacterial or viral infections may occur. The role of IVIG therapy in patients with secondary immune deficiencies has been evaluated in many of these conditions (Table 8.5) (Yap 1990). It is important to determine whether the patient suffers from bacterial or viral infections suggestive of antibody deficiency. Patients with primary hypogammaglobulinaemia typically suffer from recurrent upper respiratory tract infections or otitis media due to encapsulated organisms such as *Haem. influenzae* or *Strep. pneumoniae*. Thus patients with secondary immunodeficiency who suffer from the same range of infecting organisms are also likely to benefit whether or not they have hypogammaglobulinaemia.

Haematological Malignancies

Patients with haematological malignancies such as chronic lymphatic leukaemia (CLL) and multiple myeloma suffer from infections suggestive of antibody deficiency (Twomey 1973). In addition, such malignancies are sometimes accompanied by reduced serum immunoglobulin levels (other than that of the paraprotein, where present) and defects in the synthesis of specific antibodies can be demonstrated in vitro. Evidence for the value of IVIG therapy in CLL was recently reported in a study of 84 patients who were randomized to receive either IVIG (400 mg/kg) or placebo, every 3 weeks for a year. There was a decreased incidence of total bacterial infections, mainly in the moderate and trivial category (i.e. infections that could be treated with oral antibiotics (Cooperative Group 1988). Not surprisingly, there was no significant difference between the two groups with regard to non-bacterial infections, or in mortality. Further studies are required to establish which subgroups of patients with CLL benefit most from IVIG therapy.

This study was extended by Griffiths et al. (1989). Twelve patients who completed the trial continued in a crossover, double-blind study using the same dose of IVIG and the same infusion schedule. During treatment with IVIG, there was a significant reduction in life-threatening bacterial infections compared with the period while receiving placebo. Bacterial infections that were not life threatening but required antibiotic therapy also were reduced. In this study, it was possible to relate concurrent serum IgG levels and serious bacterial infections and such infections tended to occur when the serum IgG level was below normal.

There are also data that suggest IVIG therapy may be of benefit in multiple myeloma, although Salmon et al. (1967) failed to show any benefit from immunoglobulin administered in low doses by the intramuscular route. Schedel (1986) performed a crossover study of patients with an IgG or IgA myeloma, randomized to receive either 10 g of IVIG during the treatment phase or no immunoglobulin therapy during the control phase. This study showed that the incidence of infections (acute or chronic febrile bronchitis and pneumonia) was significantly lower during the treatment phase. The therapeutic response was unexpected as only a relatively modest dose of IVIG was used. Preliminary results from a further study suggest that IVIG therapy is not associated with a significant reduction in pyogenic infections in multiple myeloma (Bradwell, personal communication). It should be noted that in this group of patients, pyogenic infections mainly occur before and during the initial stages of cytotoxic therapy, suggesting that IVIG therapy would be most useful during this period rather than later. The choice of subgroup for investigation is important and data from further studies are awaited.

In the study of patients with CLL described above, patients were selected on the basis of an increased susceptibility to infection, as defined by either serum IgG levels less than 50% of the lower limit of the normal range, or the occurrence of one or more serious infections. Thus the role of IVIG therapy is not yet clear in patients with lesser degrees of hypogammaglobulinaemia or infection, or a more benign disease course, as in some elderly patients with CLL. Furthermore, the role of IVIG therapy, compared with antibiotic treatment, which is much cheaper, and of combinations of IVIG and antibiotic therapy needs to be investigated. Finally, the optimal dose of IVIG needs to be further investigated: we have found, in a small group of patients with CLL, that a dose of 200 mg/kg IVIG administered every 3 weeks was associated with a significant reduction in the number of infections as judged by a reduction in both the number of days taking antibiotics and in the days of hospitalization. IVIG therapy is therefore cost effective (Williams et al. 1991a).

HIV Infection

Infection with the human immunodeficiency virus (HIV) is characterized by a severe deficit of cellular immunity associated with progressive depletion of CD4-positive helper-inducer lymphocytes. As a result, HIV-infected patients suffer from a variety of opportunistic infections; attempts at immunotherapy have mostly focused on treating the cellular immunodeficiency. However, such patients may also have various abnormalities of B lymphocyte function. Some of the abnormalities may be due to the lack of adequate CD4 helper lymphocyte function, associated with the decline in the CD4 helper lymphocyte numbers. Although a hypergammaglobulinaemia is present there are more frequent infections of the respiratory tract due to encapsulated Gram-positive organisms, a pattern suggestive of antibody deficiency. Early studies in children (reviewed by Yap et al. 1991) suggested that IVIG therapy might be beneficial in reducing the number of recurrent infections. It should be emphasized that the IVIG preparations used in patients with HIV infection do not contain anti-HIV antibodies, because they are derived from donors who have been screened for HIV infection.

More recently two studies, by Schaad et al. (1988) and Hague et al. (1989), indicated that children with HIV infections had a significant reduction in the incidence of recurrent respiratory tract infections and hospitalization and an increase in weight when treated with IVIG. These studies were not randomized or controlled with a placebo. However, the results from a large multicentre study by the National Institute of Child Health and Human Development Intravenous Immunoglobulin Study Group (1991), involving 372 HIV-infected children randomized to receive either IVIG or placebo, have shown a significant benefit from IVIG therapy. In children with a CD4 lymphocyte count of over $200 \times 10^6/l$ and a prior history of an AIDS-defining infection, IVIG was associated with an increase in the time free of bacterial infections, and also with a reduction in the number of infections. There was no significant benefit from IVIG therapy in HIV-infected children with CD4 lymphocyte counts less than $200 \times 10^6/l$, and IVIG therapy was not associated with any differences in mortality in any study group.

In HIV-infected adults, by contrast, the situation is less clear; most suffer from a variety of opportunistic infections. However, some adult patients infected with HIV, especially intravenous drug abusers, whether or not they have progressed to AIDS, suffer from more frequent bacterial infections of the respiratory tract. The organisms include encapsulated Gram-positive bacteria (Polsky et al. 1986; Selwyn et al. 1988). The spectrum of infection is similar to that of the primary antibody deficiency syndromes described above and it is therefore possible that replacement therapy with IVIG may be beneficial. However, studies evaluating the efficacy of IVIG therapy in HIV-infected adults are difficult to perform. Only a minority of such patients suffer from recurrent bacterial infections, and they may be very heterogeneous with regard to symptoms and laboratory indices. Furthermore, it is difficult to adjust for the effects of other factors such as cigarette smoking and continued drug misuse, which may have an effect on the incidence of respiratory tract infections.

Brunkhorst et al. (1990) demonstrated a decrease in mortality in HIV-infected adults treated with IVIG, but there was no significant reduction in the number of bacterial or viral infections. However, in a double-blind, placebo-controlled study of high-dose IVIG given to individuals with AIDS-related complex who met the Walter Reed 5 classification (WR5) of symptomatic HIV disease, IVIG did not change the rate of progression to AIDS. Nonetheless, IVIG did appear to decrease the incidence of fevers and fatigue in the treated group, although it did not alter any of the virological or immunological parameters measured during or after the IVIG treatment (Schrappe-Bächer et al. 1990).

Further data are available from a pilot study of IVIG therapy in a group of six HIV-infected adult patients with recurrent bacterial infections (Williams et al. 1991b). To evaluate the efficacy of IVIG therapy, two relatively simple indices – days in hospital and days of antibiotic therapy – were used (Hague et al. 1989). Each patient suffered from recurrent infections that did not respond satisfactorily to antibiotic treatment prior to IVIG therapy. There was a significant reduction in in-patient hospitalization and antibiotic consumption in the period after IVIG therapy at a dose of 200 mg/kg every 3 weeks compared with the preceding 6-month period.

In summary, IVIG therapy is clearly indicated for children with HIV infection, although further research is required to compare it with zidovudine and other forms of therapy. In adults, there is evidence that a minority of HIV-infected patients with recurrent bacterial infections may benefit, but further data are required before IVIG therapy can be recommended.

Premature Neonates

Premature neonates may be born with hypogammaglobulinaemia, as most of the transplacental transfer of maternal IgG occurs in the last few weeks of gestation. Furthermore, there is a physiological reduction of serum IgG levels after birth and serum IgG levels can be similar to those observed in patients with primary hypogammaglobulinaemia, prior to IgG replacement therapy. This immunodeficiency is accentuated by the fact that such children have an immature complement and phagocytic system, and have an increased incidence of various bacterial infections.

There have been various attempts at preventing bacterial infections using IVIG therapy. However, most studies have reported relatively small numbers of patients as reviewed in detail by Cross (1992). Of the studies that were of particular interest, Haque et al. (1986) studied pre-term infants with a birth weight less than 2.5 kg. A dose of 120 mg/kg IVIG was administered prophylactically on day 1 or days 1 and 8; there was a 50% reduction compared with the control group (8/50). In another controlled but non-blind study from Italy (Chirico et al. 1987), IVIG was administered at a dose of 500 mg/kg/week to high-risk infants for 1 month or for the duration of intensive care. A significant reduction in the incidence of infection was seen only in the group of infants weighing less than 1500 g. Treated infants had a 51% incidence of infection and a 5% incidence of septicaemia, while the control group had a 77% incidence of infection and 20% incidence of septicaemia. However, the number of infants with septicaemia was small – only ten in a total of 133 neonates studied.

Conway et al. (1990), in a further randomized, non-blind small study of a particularly high-risk group of infants (<30 weeks gestation), also showed a significant reduction in infection at a dose of 200 mg/kg of IVIG at 3-weekly intervals. Eight infants (28%) in the treatment group and 17 (65%) in the control group had infections, although the difference was not significant when only blood-culture-positive episodes were considered.

More recently, the preliminary results of a large multicentre trial in the USA under the auspices of the Neonatal IVIG Study Group have been reported by Baker (1990). Pre-term neonates with birth weights of 500–1750 g were randomized to receive IVIG 500 mg/kg or placebo at 3–7 days, 1 week later and every 14 days thereafter for a total of five doses. There were 284 evaluable patients in the IVIG group and 293 in the placebo group. Late infections (onset after 7 days) were detected on the basis of clinical findings supported by laboratory isolates. IVIG-treated patients with a birth weight of less than 1500 g had a significantly reduced incidence of late infection, although this was not seen in infants of birth weight greater than 1500 g. The incidence of severe necrotizing enterocolitis and the duration of hospital stay were reduced in the IVIG group. However, there was no difference in mortality between the two groups, being approximately 4% in each in the first 2 months.

In summary, results from a large multicentre study, and a number of smaller studies, suggest that IVIG may be associated with a reduction in morbidity in premature neonates weighing less than 1500 g. However, the cost of IVIG therapy, its efficacy in comparison with antibiotics and the practical problems associated with IV therapy in small neonates need to be considered before a general recommendation for IVIG therapy in this group of patients can be made. Future studies will probably focus on the effect of IVIG on laboratory markers of infection or on clinical symptoms because the mortality is now very low in this group.

IVIG Therapy in Gram-Negative Septicaemia

In recent years much interest has been shown in the immunotherapy of immunocompromised patients, particularly after major surgery or trauma, or following a prolonged period within intensive care units with the risk of infection associated with invasive procedures such as mechanical ventilation. The infections include Gram-positive bacterial infections due to indwelling catheters, and septic shock due to Gram-negative bacteria. However, despite the availability of potent, broad-spectrum antibiotics, the mortality of patients with Gram-negative septicaemia still remains high, possibly due in part to the lysis of bacteria by antibiotics with the release of endotoxin (also called lipopolysaccharide or LPS), a major component of the outer cell wall of Gram-negative bacteria (Shenep and Mogan 1984). Exposure to LPS can lead to septic shock, organ failure and death, often in a matter of hours.

The LPS molecule is composed of three major parts. The hydrophobic part, lipid A, is the structure responsible for the toxic effects of LPS and is attached to the core region. The outer part of LPS, the side-chain, O polysaccharide (or O antigen), is responsible for antigenic specificity and differs between serotypes. The core of LPS is a highly conserved structure among the different enterobacteria and has therefore been the main target for antibody treatment of patients suffering from Gram-negative bacterial septicaemia, particularly with the advent of monoclonal antibody technology (see Chapter 9). However, O antigen-specific antibodies can protect against infections caused by the homologous bacterial strain. Unfortunately, these type-specific antibodies do not protect against challenge with strains of other serotypes. Since several hundreds of serotypes of Gram-negative bacteria may cause infections in humans, species-specific O antibodies might initially appear to be of limited value for treatment of patients with a sepsis-like syndrome. Nonetheless, human polyclonal IVIG preparations, derived from the plasma of many thousands of donors, have been shown to contain a wide variety of antibodies against surface antigenic determinants of Gram-negative bacteria and endotoxin. The use of IVIG has therefore been investigated in patients at risk of, or suffering from, Gram-negative septicaemia.

There have been a number of trials in which IVIG has been used for prophylaxis. Duswald et al. (1980) randomized 180 patients undergoing elective major surgery to receive either IVIG (2.5 g after surgery), high-dose IVIG (10 g after surgery and 24 h later), or no IVIG. The only benefit of IVIG was a reduction in the incidence of local infection in a subgroup of patients defined as low risk. In a randomized non-blind study, Schmidt et al. (1984) reported a reduction in the infection rate after IVIG therapy when 10 g was administered on three occasions to 32 patients during chemotherapy for small cell carcinoma of the lung. The control group did not receive IVIG therapy and the benefit was most marked in the neutropenic patients. However, all of the infections in this study were treatable with antibiotics and there was no placebo group. The role of IVIG was therefore difficult to define.

In a double-blind study by Glinz et al. (1985), 157 severely injured patients requiring artificial ventilation were randomized to receive either 12 g of IVIG or placebo, on three occasions over 2 weeks. There was a significant reduction in the incidence of pneumonia, but no significant difference in the incidence of septicaemia or mortality. In another study by Just et al. (1986), either 12 g of IVIG every 2 days or placebo was administered to 104 patients in an Intensive Care Unit. Although there was a reduction in the duration of artificial ventilation and length of stay with IVIG therapy, there was no significant reduction in mortality.

These studies were followed by attempts to prepare a hyperimmune IVIG preparation from the plasma of donors immunized with the J5 strain of *Escherichia coli* (see Chapter 9). Unfortunately, the results of a study by Callandra et al. (1988) using a hyperimmune anti-LPS IVIG preparation did not show any benefit compared with "standard" IVIG (i.e. not derived from specially immunized donors) in the treatment of septic shock. This led to the suggestion that the relevant protective antibody in the trials of Ziegler et al. (1982) and Baumgartner et al. (1985) were due to an antibody of the IgM isotype because IVIG preparations consist almost entirely of IgG. An alternative hypothesis was that standard IVIG itself had a protective effect and could not be considered similar to a placebo.

The results are similar to those of Cometta et al. (1990) who evaluated the prophylactic efficacy of standard IVIG, IVIG prepared from the plasma of donors with naturally high titres of antibody to core glycolipid, and albumin in 329 surgical patients at high risk of infection. Like Glinz et al. (1985), they observed a significant reduction in acquired pneumonia compared with placebo among patients receiving the standard IVIG, but not among those receiving IVIG enriched with anti-core glycolipid-enriched antibody. There was no difference in the number of episodes of sepsis, Gram-negative sepsis or mortality among the three groups.

More recently, Dominioni (1991) reported on a prospective double-blind placebo-controlled study of IVIG therapy in severely septic, high-risk surgical and trauma patients with an increased sepsis score on admission. Patients were randomized to receive either IVIG, 0.4 g/kg on days 0, 2 and 5, or an albumin placebo. The two study groups were similar in age, initial sepsis score and Apache II score. There was a significantly lower mortality in the

Table 8.6. Summary of clinical trials using antibody preparations in Gram-negative infections

Reference	Preparation[a]	Trial number	Outcome
Duswald et al. (1980)	IVIG	150 (P)	No placebo: modest effect only
Schmidt et al. (1984)	IVIG	32 (P)	No placebo: data not evaluable
Glinz et al. (1985)	IVIG	150 (P)	Modest effect on pneumonia
Just et al. (1986)	IVIG	104 (T)	No placebo: reduction in ICU stay
Ziegler et al. (1982)	J5 serum[b]	212 (P)	Significant reduction in mortality
Baumgartner et al. (1985)	J5 serum[b]	262 (P)	Reduction of incidence and mortality due to Gram-negative shock
Callandra et al. (1988)	J5-IVIG[c]	71 (T)	No significant effects observed
Cometta et al. (1990)	J5 Re-IVIG[d]	329 (P)	Significant reduction in IVIG pneumonia in IVIG arm only
Dominioni (1991)	IVIG	72 (T)	Significant reduction in mortality

P, prophylactic; T, therapeutic, ICU, intensive care unit.
[a] All studies use an inactive albumin placebo, unless otherwise stated. Studies using monoclonal antibody preparations against endotoxin are excluded (see Chapter 9).
[b] Serum collected before J5 vaccine immunization used as control.
[c] IVIG used as control. J5-IVIG manufactured from plasma collected from J5-immunized donors.
[d] IVIG preparation enriched with anti-Re antibodies, by selection of donors with naturally high anti-Re levels. Three-arm study (including placebo).

IVIG-treated group (11/29; 38%) compared with the placebo-treated group (22/33; 67%). Septic shock was the cause of death in 7% of the IVIG-treated group and in 33% of the placebo-treated patients. By contrast, the incidence of mortality due to multiple organ failure was the same in both groups.

In summary, these results indicate that IVIG therapy with polyclonal antibodies may be an alternative to monoclonal antibody therapy against endotoxin (Table 8.6). The higher doses used in the study by Dominioni (1991) compared with earlier studies may be critical, and results of further randomized double-blind placebo-controlled trials using higher doses of IVIG therapy on larger numbers of patients are awaited before final conclusions can be drawn about the efficacy of IVIG therapy.

IVIG in Other Immunodeficiency Disorders

The use of IVIG has been investigated in other immunodeficiency disorders. After bone marrow transplantation (BMT) there may be a persistent antibody deficiency, particularly in the IgG_2 subclass, and a depressed ability to synthesize anti-polysaccharide antibody, for up to 6 months (Aucouturier et al. 1987). This is associated with an increased incidence of bacterial infections, especially in children. IVIG therapy is therefore sometimes administered for the first 6 months after paediatric allogeneic BMT, together with prophylactic antibiotics to prevent serious bacterial infections. Similarly, IVIG has been shown to have an impact on the incidence of post-BMT septicaemia in adult patients. In a double-blind randomized trial, Sullivan et al. (1990) found a significantly reduced incidence of Gram-negative septicaemia and local infection associated with IVIG therapy.

Patients with severe burns may also have a demonstrable immunodeficiency, including depression of serum immunoglobulin levels and impaired cell-mediated immunity. The physical damage to the skin increases the likelihood of entry, colonization and invasion by various pathogens, including *Pseudomonas*. Because of the persistent hypogammaglobulinaemia, and the presence of antibodies against various Gram-negative bacteria and endotoxin in IVIG preparations, attempts have been made to "correct" the hypogammaglobulinaemia and reduce the incidence of septicaemia by regular IVIG administration. However, in a trial of IVIG in severely burned patients by Waymack et al. (1989), no reduction in mortality or morbidity was observed. This may have been due to the effective antibiotic prophylaxis available and a residual ability (despite the hypogammaglobulinaemia) to synthesize specific antibodies following bacterial invasion.

Use of IVIG Preparations for Prevention and Treatment of Specific Infection

There are three possible approaches to the use of IVIG preparations in the prevention and treatment of specific infections. First, there is the use of "standard" IVIG, i.e. unselected IVIG preparations. Such preparations contain a wide spectrum of antiviral antibodies; high doses should contain adequate amounts of a particular antiviral antibody even if this is present in low concentrations in the IVIG batch. This approach, although technically feasible, is expensive. Secondly, batches of IVIG can be screened, and those with high titres of antibody against the relevant virus used for prophylaxis and therapy. Thirdly, plasma from donors with high levels of antibody against the virus can be fractionated to produce a hyperimmune IVIG preparation. Levels of the specific antibody in the plasma donor can be raised, if necessary, by immunization as described for hepatitis B (Samuel et al. 1991), to produce hyperimmune plasma for fractionation.

Cytomegalovirus

Cytomegalovirus (CMV) causes severe infections in immunosuppressed patients and the virus itself has a profound effect on the host's immune system. CMV may be isolated from patients with fatal interstitial pneumonia after BMT and also causes death or graft rejection after renal transplants. Infection may be a result of reactivation of latent CMV infection or of primary infection.

The role of humoral and cellular factors in immunity against CMV is poorly characterized, but various antibody preparations (hyperimmune anti-CMV plasma; standard IVIG administered in higher doses; or hyperimmune anti-CMV IVIG preparations) have been assessed in patients at risk of CMV disease after transplantation.

Bone Marrow Transplantation

Antibodies against CMV have been used in six controlled trials in BMT patients, five of which were randomized (Table 8.7). In the two trials by Winston's group (Winston et al. 1982, 1987) the incidence of both interstitial pneumonia, CMV-associated pneumonia and graft-versus-host disease was reduced. The trials had significant differences in terms of antibody preparation, doses used, conditioning schedules and outcome. Taken together however, they concluded that immunoglobulin prophylaxis may reduce the incidence of CMV pneumonia in BMT recipients, but may not affect CMV infection rates. This conclusion was supported in a recent study by Sullivan et al. (1990) who demonstrated a decrease in interstitial pneumonia associated with IVIG therapy, after BMT, despite the lack of effect of IVIG on the incidence of CMV infection.

Table 8.7. Summary of clinical trials using antibody preparations for CMV prophylaxis in bone marrow transplantation

Reference	Preparation	Recipient CMV serological status[a]	Outcome
Winston et al. (1982)	Hyperimmune anti-CMV plasma	Negative and positive	Decreased CMV disease and CMV interstitial pneumonia
Meyers et al. (1983)	CMV-IVIG	Negative[b]	Decreased infection with screened blood
Condie and O'Reilly (1984)	CMV-IVIG	Negative and positive	Decreased CMV infection, interstitial pneumonia, mortality
Bowden et al. (1986)	CMV-IVIG	Negative	Decreased CMV infection for CMV-seronegative marrow donor
Winston et al. (1987)	Standard IVIG	Negative and positive	Decreased CMV disease, decreased CMV pneumonia, decreased GVHD
Ringden et al. (1987)	Hyperimmune anti-CMV plasma	Negative and positive	No benefit

GVHD, graft-versus-host disease.

[a] All studies were randomized except for that of Condie and O'Reilly (1984).

[b] CMV-screened blood was used by Meyers et al. (1983).

Organ Transplants

CMV disease may be severe and even fatal after kidney transplantation. The first randomized clinical trial of CMV-IVIG was a study of renal transplant recipients who were CMV-seronegative, and who received a kidney from a CMV-seropositive donor. The incidence of CMV-associated disease was reduced with CMV-IVIG therapy (Snydman et al. 1987). Studies of CMV prophylaxis using antibody preparations (CMV-IVIG or standard IVIG) have also been undertaken in other kidney (Gregor et al. 1985; Steinmuller et al. 1989), heart (Preiksaitis et al. 1982; Schafers et al. 1987) and liver (Bell et al. 1989; Saliba et al. 1989) transplant patients. However, the results have been difficult to interpret as many of the trials involved small numbers of patients and different anti-CMV antibody preparations.

Other Patients

Patients with HIV infection may suffer from severe CMV infection, particularly CMV retinitis. CMV-IVIG has been recommended in combination with ganciclovir. However, Jacobson et al. (1990) demonstrated no benefit from the combined regimen. Snydman et al. (1990) have also reported a randomized placebo-controlled double-blind trial of CMV-IVIG for the prevention of CMV disease in multiple-transfused premature neonates. CMV-IVIG was associated with a reduced incidence of the CMV syndrome.

In summary, standard IVIG, IVIG with a high titre against CMV or CMV-IVIG have been used in attempts to prevent CMV. Unfortunately, different dosages, different treatment schedules and different patient groups have been studied, and it is not possible to conclude that antibody preparations definitively protect transplant patients from CMV. CMV antibody titres also differ markedly between the available products and between successive lots of a single product. Various doses have been used in prophylaxis, and the incidence of CMV varies between countries and patient groups. There is little conclusive evidence that any antibody preparation is efficacious in the treatment of established CMV disease in transplant patients, although anecdotal evidence suggests that patients treated with CMV-IVIG may improve compared with historical controls (Blacklock et al. 1985). However, as with studies of prophylaxis, data from randomized controlled trials on larger groups of patients are needed before firm recommendations can be made.

Parvovirus B19

Parvovirus B19 infection is generally a mild or subclinical infection in childhood. However, in the presence of immunodeficiency or a haemolytic state, chronic red cell aplasia may occur due to virus persistence in the erythroid progenitor cells. IVIG preparations have high titres of neutralizing antibody to parvovirus B19 (Takahashi et al. 1991) and this therapy has been successful in the treatment of a child with hereditary spherocytosis and aplastic crisis secondary to parvovirus B19 infection. IVIG therapy has also been associated with a "cure" in a patient with a 10-year history of aplastic anaemia due to defective antibody response to parvovirus B19 (Kurtzmann et al. 1989).

Recently, parvovirus B19 infection has been recognized as a rare cause of chronic anaemia in HIV infection. Six patients with HIV infection and red cell aplasia due to parvovirus B19 infection responded to IVIG at a dose of 0.4 g/kg for 5 or 10 days; responses could be obtained in those who relapsed with further IVIG (Frickhofen et al. 1990). A similar patient was also successfully treated with IVIG by Mitchell et al. (1990). It is clear that IVIG should be considered standard therapy in all HIV-infected patients with proven parvovirus B19 infection and anaemia.

Other Viral Infections

Selected IVIG batches with high titres of a specific antibody have been used in the prevention and treatment of respiratory syncytial virus (RSV) infection. A high titre anti-RSV IVIG preparation was selected by screening various batches of IVIG. When administered to young infants this was well tolerated, with a significant reduction in RSV shedding and improvements in oxygenation (Hemming et al. 1987). Preliminary data in cotton rats (Prince et al. 1985), monkeys (Hemming et al. 1985) or young infants (Hemming et al. 1987) have shown that this is a promising approach.

IVIG preparations contain neutralizing antibody against enteroviruses. Selected batches of IVIG with high titres of antibodies against echovirus 11 have been used successfully in the therapy of echovirus meningoencephalitis associated with X-linked agammaglobulinaemia (Mease et al. 1981). Additionally, IVIG therapy may have a role in the occasional epidemics of echovirus infections in neonatal intensive care units and nurseries. However, owing to the rarity of echovirus infections (except during epidemics) the role of IVIG preparations for prevention and therapy will be difficult to assess.

IVIG preparations also contain specific neutralizing antibody against herpes simplex virus (HSV). Humoral and cellular mechanisms are involved in protection and recovery from HSV infection. Ehrlich et al. (1987) have shown that a standard IVIG preparation can be used to protect against death in a murine model of HSV infection. Unfortunately, there are few data about IVIG preparations in the prevention and treatment of human HSV infections. As acyclovir is effective against HSV (and to a lesser extent VZV) infections, the role of IVIG preparations might be in patients with HSV (or VZV) strains resistant to acyclovir, or in combination with acyclovir, for increased efficacy.

Conclusion

A century has elapsed since the first demonstration of the effectiveness of antibody therapy by Behring and Kitasato. In the last two decades a number of uses of antibody therapy (in the form of IVIG preparations) has been identified in infectious diseases. There are many clinical indications as well as possibilities for future development (Table 8.2), some of which are described elsewhere in this volume. Comparison of immunological and pharmacological approaches is needed; combination of IVIG preparations with various monoclonal antibody preparations could be synergistic. This approach could be used in patients at risk of severe Gram-negative infection because the monoclonal antibody may only be effective against a limited range of infections, while the IVIG preparation is polyspecific (albeit at low concentrations) against a number of different bacteria. Unfortunately, assessing the efficacy of such combinations may be very difficult in view of the large number of factors that can affect the outcome of a major infection in immunocompromised patients. In addition, there is the high cost of performing large clinical trials. It seems likely that, in the next decade, only a limited number of new indications for IVIG therapy will be identified.

References

Aucouturier P, Barra A, Intrator L et al. (1987) Long lasting IgG subclass and anti-bacterial polysaccharide antibody deficiency after allogeneic bone marrow transplantation. Blood 70: 779–785

Baker CJ (1990) New uses of intravenous immune globulin in newborn infants. J Clin Immunol 10: 47S–52S

Barandun S, Isliker H (1986) Development of immunoglobulin preparations for intravenous use. Vox Sang 51: 157–160

Barandun S, Kistler P, Jennet F, Isliker H (1962) Intravenous administration of human gammaglobulin. Vox Sang 7: 157–174

Baumgartner J-D, Glauser MP, McCutchan JA et al. (1985) Prevention of Gram-negative shock and death in surgical patients by antibody to endotoxin core glycolipid. Lancet 1: 59–63

Behring E (1893) Zur Behandlung der Diphtherie mit Diphtherie Heilserum. Deutsche Med Wochenschr 19: 543–544

Bell R, Sheil AGR, McDonald JA, McCaughan GW (1989) The role of CMV immune prophylaxis in patients at risk of primary CMV infection following orthotopic liver transplantation. Transplant Proc 21: 3781–3782

Blacklock HA, Griffiths P, Stirk P, Prentice HG (1985) Successful treatment of cytomegalovirus pneumonitis after allogeneic bone marrow transplantation using high titre CMV immunoglobulin. Exp Hematol 13: 76

Bowden RA, Sayers M, Flourney N et al. (1986) Cytomegalovirus immune globulin and seronegative infection after marrow transplantation. N Engl J Med 314: 1006–1010

Brunkhorst U, Stürner M, Willers H, Deicher H, Schedel I (1990) Efficacy of intravenous immunoglobulins in patients with advanced HIV-1 infection. A randomised clinical study. Infection 18(2): 86–91

Callandra T, Glauser MP, Schellekens J, Verhoef J, Swiss–Dutch J5 Immunoglobulin Study Group (1988) Treatment of Gram-negative septic shock with human IgG antibody to *Escherichia coli* J5: A prospective, double-blind randomised study. J Infect Dis 158: 312–319

Centers for Disease Control Morbidity and Mortality Weekly Report (1984) MMWR 33: 393–408

Chirico G, Rondini G, Plebani A, Chiara A, Massa M, Ugazio AG (1987) Intravenous gammaglobulin therapy for prophylaxis of infection in high-risk neonates. J Pediatr 110: 437–442

Choo QL, Kuo G, Weiner AJ, Overby LR, Bradley DW, Houghton M (1989) Isolation of a cDNA clone derived from a blood-borne non-A, non-B hepatitis genome. Science 244: 359–361

Cohn EJ (1945) Blood proteins and their therapeutic value. Science 101: 51–56

Cohn EJ, Strong LE, Hughes LE et al. (1946) Preparation and properties of serum and plasma

proteins. IV. A system for the separation into fractions of the proteins and lipoprotein components of biological tissues and fluids. J Am Chem Soc 68: 459–475
Cometta A, Baumgartner JD, Lee M, Glauser MP (1990) Prophylaxis of infection in high risk surgical patients with standard IVIG or with antibody to core glycolipid. Abstract 476, 30th Interscience Conference on Antimicrobial Agents and Chemotherapy, Atlanta, USA
Condie RM, O'Reilly R (1984) Prevention of cytomegalovirus infection by prophylaxis with an intravenous, hyperimmune, native, unmodified cytomegalovirus globulin. Am J Med 76: 134–141
Conway SP, Ng PC, Howel D, MacLain B, Gooi HC (1990) Prophylactic intravenous immunoglobulin in preterm infants: A controlled trial. Vox Sang 59: 6–11
Cooperative Group for the Study of Immunoglobulin in Chronic Lymphocytic Leukemia (1988) Intravenous immunoglobulin for the prevention of infection in chronic lymphocytic leukemia. N Engl J Med 319: 902–907
Cross AS (1992) The use of IVIG for bacterial infections. In: Yap PL (ed) Intravenous immunoglobulin therapy. Churchill Livingstone, Edinburgh, pp 139–166
Dominioni L (1991) Clinical results of high dose immunoglobulin administration in severely septic surgical patients, 2nd International Congress on the Immuno Consequences of Trauma, Shock and Sepsis Mechanisms and Therapeutic Approaches. Abstract SY80
Duswald KH, Muller K, Seifert J, Ring J (1980) Wirksamkeit von i.v. Gammaglobulin gegen bakterielle Infektionen chirurgischer Patienten. Ergebnisse einer kontrolierten, randomisierten klinischen Studie. Munchener Med Wochenschr 122: 832–836
Ehrlich KS, Dix RD, Mills J (1987) Prevention and treatment of experimental herpes simplex virus encephalitis with human immune serum globulin. Antimicrob Agents Chemother 31: 1006–1009
Felton LD (1930) Concentration of antipneumococcus serum. JAMA 94: 319–320
Finland M (1930) The serum therapy of lobar pneumonia. N Engl J Med 202: 1244–1247
Frickhofen N, Abkowitz JL, Safford M et al. (1990) Persistent B19 parvovirus infection in patients infected with human immunodeficiency virus type 1 (HIV-1): A treatable cause of anemia in AIDS. Ann Intern Med 113: 926–933
Glinz W, Grob PJ, Nydegger UE et al. (1985) Polyvalent immunoglobulin for prophylaxis of bacterial infections in patients following multiple trauma. A randomised, placebo-controlled study. Intensive Care Med 11: 288–294
Greenman M, Schein RMN, Martin MA et al. (1991) A controlled clinical trial of E5 murine monoclonal IgM antibody to endotoxin in the treatment of gram-negative sepsis. JAMA 266: 1097–1102
Gregor B, Kurth J, Schareck WD, Muller GH, Hopt UT, Bockhorn H (1985) CMV-prophylaxis after kidney transplantation. Immunol Infect 5: 215–219
Griffiths H, Brennan V, Lea J, Bunch C, Lee M, Chapel H (1989) Crossover study of immunoglobulin replacement therapy in patients with low-grade B-cell tumors. Blood 73: 366–368
Hague RA, Yap PL, Mok JYQ et al. (1989) Intravenous immunoglobulin in HIV infection: Evidence for the efficacy of treatment. Arch Dis Child 64: 1146–1150
Haque KN, Zaidi MH, Haque SK, Bahakim H, el-Hazmi M, el-Swailam M (1986) Intravenous immunoglobulin for prevention of sepsis in preterm and low birth weight infants. Pediatr Infect Dis J 5: 622–625
Harper TE, Christensen RD, Rothstein G, Hill HR (1986) Effect of intravenous immunoglobulin G on neutrophil kinetics during experimental Group B streptococcal infection in neonatal rats. Rev Infect Dis 8: S401–S408
Hemming VG, Prince GA, Horswood RL et al. (1985) Passive immunotherapy of respiratory syncytial virus respiratory tract infections: Studies in a primate model. J Infect Dis 152: 1083–1087
Hemming VG, Rodriguez W, Kim HW (1987) Intravenous immunoglobulin treatment of respiratory syncytial virus infections in infants and young children. Antimicrob Agents Chemother 31: 1882–1886
Jacobson MA, O'Donnell JJ, Rousell R, Dionian B, Mills J (1990) Failure of adjunctive cytomegalovirus intravenous immune globulin to improve efficacy of ganciclovir in patients with acquired immunodeficiency syndrome and cytomegalovirus retinitis: A phase 1 study. Antimicrob Agents Chemother 34: 176–178
Janeway CA (1970) The development of clinical uses of immunoglobulins – a review. In: Merler E (ed) Immunoglobulins, biologic aspects and clinical uses. National Academy of Sciences, Washington DC, pp 3–14

Joint Committee on Vaccination and Immunisation (1990) Immunisation against infectious disease. HMSO, London.

Just HM, Vogel W, Metzger M, Pelka RD, Daschner FD (1986) Treatment of intensive care unit patients with severe nosocomial infections. In: Morell A, Nydegger UE (eds) Clinical use of immunoglobulins. Academic Press, London, pp 345–353

Kurtzman G, Frichofen N, Kimball J, Jenkins DW, Nienhuis AW, Young NS (1989) Pure red cell aplasia of 10 years' duration due to persistent parvovirus B19 infection and its cure with immunoglobulin therapy. N Engl J Med 321: 519–523

Leen CLS, Yap PL, McClelland DBL (1986) Increase of serum immunoglobulin level into the normal range in primary hypogammaglobulinaemia by dosage individualisation of intravenous immunoglobulin. Vox Sang 51: 278–286

McClelland DBL, Yap PL (1984) Clinical use of immunoglobulins. Clin Haematol 13: 39–74

Mease PJ, Ochs HD, Wedgwood RJ (1981) Successful treatment of echovirus meningoencephalitis and myositis-fasciitis with intravenous immune globulin therapy in a patient with X-linked agammaglobulinemia. N Engl J Med 304: 1278–1281

Meyers JD, Leszczynski J, Zaia JA et al. (1983) Prevention of cytomegalovirus infection by cytomegalovirus immune globulin after marrow transplantation. Ann Intern Med 98: 442–446

Mitchell SA, Welch JM, Weston-Smith S et al. (1990) Parvovirus infection and anaemia in a patient with AIDS: A case report. Genitourin Med 66: 95–96

Murray R, Ratner F (1953) Safety of immune serum globulin with respect to homologous serum hepatitis. Proc Soc Exp Biol Med 83: 544–555

National Institute of Child Health and Human Development Intravenous Immunoglobulin Study Group (1991) Intravenous immune globulin for the prevention of bacterial infections in children with symptomatic human immunodeficiency virus infection. N Engl J Med 325: 73–80

Piazza M (1990) Periodic gammaglobulin to prevent hepatitis C in at-risk sexual partners. Lancet 336: 823

Polsky B, Gold JWM, Whimbey E et al. (1986) Bacterial pneumonia in patients with the acquired immunodeficiency syndrome. Ann Intern Med 104: 38–41

Preiksaitis JK, Rosno S, Rasmussen L, Merigan TC (1982) Cytomegalovirus infection in heart transplant recipients: Preliminary results of a controlled trial of intravenous gammaglobulin. J Clin Immunol 2: 365–415

Prince GA, Hemming VG, Horswood RL, Chanock RL (1985) Immunoprophylaxis and immunotherapy of respiratory syncytial virus infection in the cotton rat. Virus Res 3: 193–206

Ringden O, Pihlstedt P, Volin L et al. (1987) Failure to prevent cytomegalovirus infection by cytomegalovirus hyperimmune plasma: A randomised trial by the Nordic Bone Marrow Transplantation Group. Bone Marrow Transplant 2: 299–305

Saliba F, Arulnaden JL, Gugenheim J et al. (1989) CMV hyperimmune globulin prophylaxis after liver transplantation: A prospective randomised controlled study. Transplant Proc 21: 2260–2262

Salmon SE, Samal BA, Hayes DM, Hosley H, Miller SP, Schilling A (1967) Role of gammaglobulin for immunoprophylaxis in multiple myeloma. N Engl J Med 227: 1336–1340

Samuel S, Bismuth A, Mathieu D et al. (1991) Passive immunoprophylaxis after liver transplantation in HBsAg-positive patients. Lancet 337: 813–815

Schaad UB, Gianella-Borradori A, Perret B, Imbach P, Morell A (1988) Intravenous immune globulin in symptomatic pediatric human immunodeficiency infection. Eur J Pediatr 147: 300–303

Schafers HJ, Haverich A, Wahlers T, Milbradt H, Flik J, Fieguth HG (1987) Cytomegalovirus prophylaxis after heart transplantation using specific hyperimmunoglobulin. Transplant Proc 19: 4061–4062

Schedel I (1986) Application of immunoglobulin preparations in multiple myeloma. In: Morell A, Nydegger UE (eds) Clinical use of intravenous immunoglobulins. Academic Press, New York, pp 123–132

Schmidt RE, Hartlapp JH, Niese D, Illiger HJ, Stroehmann I (1984) Reduction of infection frequency by intravenous gammaglobulins during intensive induction therapy for small cell carcinoma of the lung. Infection 12: 167–170

Schrappe-Bächer M, Rasokat H, Bauer P et al. (1990) High-dose intravenous immunoglobulins in HIV-1-infected adults with AIDS-related complex and Walter-Reed 5. Vox Sang 59 (suppl 1): 3–14

Seeff CB, Hoofnagle JH (1979) Immunoprophylaxis of viral hepatitis. Gastroenterology 77: 161–182
Selwyn PA, Feingold AR, Hartel D et al. (1988) Increased risk of bacterial pneumonia in HIV-infected intravenous drug users without AIDS. AIDS 2: 267–272
Shenep JL, Mogan KA (1984) Kinetics of endotoxin release during antibiotic therapy for experimental gram-negative bacterial sepsis. J Infect Dis 150: 380–388
Snydman DR, Werner BG, Heinze-Lacey B et al. (1987) Use of cytomegalovirus immune globulin to prevent cytomegalovirus disease in renal transplant recipients. N Engl J Med 317: 1049–1054
Snydman DR, Werner BG, Meissner HC, Schwab J, Zaleski A, Neonatal CMVIG Study Group (1990) Use of cytomegalovirus immune globulin (CMVIG) in multiply transfused, premature neonates. Abstract 208, 31st ICAAC, Atlanta, Georgia
Steinmuller DR, Graneto D, Swift C et al. (1989) Use of intravenous immunoglobulin prophylaxis for primary cytomegalovirus infection post living-related-donor renal transplantation. Transplant Proc 21: 2069–2071
Sullivan KM, Kopecky KJ, Jocom J et al. (1990) Immunomodulatory and antimicrobial efficacy of intravenous immunoglobulin in bone marrow transplantation. N Engl J Med 323: 705–712
Takahashi M, Koike T, Moriyama Y, Shibata A (1991) Neutralizing activity of immunoglobulin preparation against erythropoietic suppression of human parvovirus. Am J Hematol 37: 68
Twomey JJ (1973) Infections, complications, multiple myeloma and chronic lymphocytic leukaemia. Arch Intern Med 132: 562–565
Waymack JP, Jenkins ME, Alexander JW et al. (1989) A prospective trial of prophylactic intravenous immune globulin for the prevention of infections in severely burned patients. Burns 15: 71–76
Weidermann G, Ambrosch F, Kollaritsch H et al. (1990) Safety and immunogenicity of an activated hepatitis A candidate vaccine in healthy adult volunteers. Vaccine 8: 581–584
Wenzel R, Bone R, Fein A et al. (1991) Results of a second double-blind randomised controlled trial of antiendotoxin antibody E5 in gram-negative sepsis. Abstract 1170, 31st Interscience Conference on Antimicrobial Agents and Chemotherapy, Chicago, USA
WHO Expert Committee on Rabies Sixth Report (1983) Technical report, Series No. 523: 50–51
Williams PE, Scott FM, Russell L, Yap PL (1991a) Benefit of intravenous IgG therapy in reducing infections in chronic lymphocytic leukaemia. EOS J Immunol Immunopharmacol 11: 10–11
Williams PE, Thompson C, Yap PL, Brettle RP (1991b) Controlled study of IV IgG therapy for HIV-infected adults with recurrent bacterial infections. Vox Sang 60: 126–127
Williams PE, Todd AAM, Yap PL (1992) IVIG therapy in primary and secondary immunodeficiency. In: Yap PL (ed) Intravenous immunoglobulin therapy. Churchill Livingstone, Edinburgh, pp 63–92
Williams PE, Yap PL, McClelland DBL (1987) Dose of intravenous IgG in primary hypogammaglobulinaemia. Lancet i: 1435–1436
Winston DJ, Ho WG, Lin C-H et al. (1987) Intravenous immune globulin for prevention of cytomegalovirus infection and interstitial pneumonia after bone marrow transplantation. Ann Intern Med 106: 12–18
Winston DJ, Pollard RB, Ho WG et al. (1982) Cytomegalovirus immune plasma in bone marrow transplant recipients. Ann Intern Med 97: 11–18
Yap PL (1990) Intravenous immunoglobulin for secondary immunodeficiency. Blut 60: 8–14
Yap PL (ed) (1992) Intravenous immunoglobulin therapy. Churchill Livingstone, Edinburgh
Yap PL, Todd AAM, Williams PE et al. (1991) Use of intravenous immunoglobulin in AIDS. Cancer (suppl) 68: 1440–1450
Ziegler EJ, Fisher CJ, Sprung CL et al. (1991) Treatment of gram-negative bacteremia and septic shock with HA-1A human monoclonal antibody against endotoxin: A randomized, double-blind, placebo-controlled trial. N Engl J Med 324: 429–436
Ziegler EJ, McCutchan JA, Fierer J et al. (1982) Treatment of Gram-negative bacteremia and shock with human antiserum to a mutant *Escherichia coli*. N Engl J Med 307: 1225–1230

9 Immunological Therapy of Endotoxaemia: Anti-endotoxin Antibodies

A.P. Wheeler and G.R. Bernard

Introduction

Sepsis syndrome is a constellation of clinical findings that includes altered temperature, tachycardia and an increased minute ventilation together with a major organ system failure (renal, hepatic, circulatory, haematological or neurological). More than 400 000 cases of sepsis syndrome occur in the USA alone each year, resulting in the expenditure of 5–10 billion dollars annually (1). The case fatality rate for sepsis syndrome ranges from 20% to 60% (2,3). Interestingly, up to one-half of patients who develop sepsis syndrome have no demonstrable infection (4) and several non-infectious disorders mimic the physiological and biochemical changes of sepsis syndrome. These two facts have prompted some investigators to rename "sepsis syndrome" the "systemic inflammatory response syndrome" (SIRS), emphasizing that not all patients have infection as the cause and that the host response is the critical determinant of severity. Although SIRS may result from non-infectious causes or viral, fungal or Gram-positive infections, Gram-negative bacteria constitute the single most frequent group of organisms, accounting for approximately one-third of all SIRS cases (1,4–6).

Despite the development of sophisticated support technologies including critical care units, broad-spectrum antibiotics, bedside haemodynamic monitors, mechanical ventilators, haemodialysis and intravenous nutrition, it is not clear that the mortality rate of Gram-negative bacteraemia has been substantially reduced in the last century. Likewise, investigational use of corticosteroids and opiate antagonists has failed to improve mortality, making innovation in therapy imperative (4,7–10).

The Role of Endotoxin in Sepsis

In Gram-negative sepsis, the important factor is the release of toxins contained within organisms that stimulate a systemic host response. The bacteria themselves are less important. Killed bacteria, extracted endotoxin and synthetic lipid A (the major active component of endotoxin) are all comparably toxic in animal models (11). Endotoxin, an integral Gram-negative cell wall lipopolysaccharide (LPS), is the principal toxin responsible for triggering host reactions during Gram-negative sepsis. Most of the physiological changes of sepsis are not directly attributable to endotoxin, but instead result from the rapid production of endogenous mediators such as tumour necrosis factor (TNF) and interleukin-1 (IL-1).

In some forms of Gram-negative sepsis the level of circulating LPS correlates well with mortality (12–15), but endotoxin concentrations do not tell the whole story. For example, LPS levels in volunteers receiving endotoxin approach those of septic patients (16). However, only 30%–40% of patients with septic shock have endotoxaemia (17–19). Failure to detect circulating LPS in patients may be explained by the results of human experiments in which LPS injection results in only transient appearance of endotoxaemia (20). LPS rapidly induces inflammation. In vitro, LPS causes irreversible cellular injury with exposures as short as 5 min and in animals significant physiological changes occur within approximately 1 h (21–23). These findings indicate that while endotoxaemia is often brief, such exposures are sufficient to provoke the inflammatory cascade.

Patients at risk of developing SIRS have a high risk of endotoxaemia. Haemorrhagic shock (19,24,25), bowel ischaemia (26,27), profound hypoxaemia (28), ionizing radiation (29), graft-versus-host disease (30), hyperthermia (31,32), burns (33,34), multiple trauma (35), gastroenteritis (36,37), excessive use of vasoconstrictive agents (38) and decompression sickness (39) are all associated with endotoxaemia. As the diverse nature of these conditions suggests, endotoxaemia can and does occur in the absence of bacteraemia. Free endotoxin may be shed into the circulation by growing bacteria; LPS from faecal material may leak directly across the bowel wall (18,37); and LPS may be precipitously released by treatment of bacteraemia with bactericidal antibiotics (24,25,40). The correlation between bacteraemia and endotoxaemia varies widely (41–45). Interestingly, some patients with documented Gram-negative bacteraemia do not have detectable circulating endotoxin (18).

It is the occurrence of non-bacteraemic endotoxaemia and the failure of antibiotics to neutralize endotoxin that explains why antibiotics are not a panacea for SIRS. Unfortunately, a high rate of false positive and false negative test results prevents clinical use of current assays for endotoxaemia and precludes early identification of patients who might benefit from anti-endotoxins (46–48).

Endotoxin: Relationship of Structure to Function

Producing an anti-endotoxin is not a simple matter of manufacturing one antibody that will promptly bind and neutralize every LPS molecule. The fact that attempts have been made for more than a century to produce just such a compound attests to the complexity of the problem. To understand the capability and limitations of immunotherapy, it is important to understand the structure of LPS. Endotoxin includes three major regions. The highly variable outermost "O antigen" region is composed of oligosaccharide polymers of varying length that impart a "smooth" appearance to bacterial colonies. The O region is the most variable portion of the LPS molecule, differing both among species and strains of the same species and within a single strain depending on bacterial growth rate (49–51). In addition, the stereochemistry of LPS in vitro may be substantially different from that of naturally released LPS or endotoxin in intact bacterial cell walls (52,53). The O region is the most antigenic portion of the LPS molecule, hence when oligosaccharide-containing bacteria or endotoxin are used as immunogens, the vast majority of antibody produced is specific for the O region. Although the addition of oligosaccharides to the lipid A core structure prolongs the circulating half-life of LPS somewhat, it does not substantially enhance the toxicity of LPS (52,54).

The discovery of oligosaccharide-deficient bacterial mutants having a common exposed core and hence a "rough" appearance in culture raised hopes that a cross-reactive core-directed antibody could be engineered. Rough mutants lack vital enzymes that catalyze either the polymerization or attachment of oligosaccharides to the core region. Except for minor differences, the core region is constant among most Gram-negative bacteria (51,55–58) and links the O antigen region to the toxic innermost lipid A portion of LPS (51). Lipid A alone can reproduce the effects of the entire LPS molecule (51,59) and preservation of the structure of lipid A is critical to its toxicity. Cleavage of even a single bond linking the components of lipid A can transform it into a non-toxic compound, "lipid X" (60–62). Both purified naturally occurring and synthetically produced lipid A are highly toxic.

Choice of the proper immunogen is critical in producing a neutralizing, cross-reactive antibody. Although lipid A antibodies exhibit nearly universal cross-reactivity with a variety of endotoxins, they do not uniformly prevent the physiological effects of LPS (51,59,63–67). Even incubation of such antibodies directly with lipid A prior to animal administration has minimal protective effects (67). Conversely, it is easy to produce high-titre, high-affinity, neutralizing antibodies to the O antigens of smooth LPS. Unfortunately, such antibodies only reliably protect against challenge with homologous LPS or bacteria (63,64, 68–76): as expected, there is poor cross-reactivity of O antigen-directed antibodies. Because of the limitations of oligosaccharide and lipid A-directed antibodies, some investigators turned their efforts to active immunization strategies, some to non-immunological methods of LPS antagonism and others to producing antibodies to the common LPS core region.

Approaches to Endotoxin Antagonism

Research into the antagonism of endotoxin has fallen into two basic areas, passive anti-endotoxin therapy (77–84) and all other methods. Passive anti-endotoxin therapy is currently the subject of intensive clinical investigation and will be discussed in detail below. Other research groups have tested the possibility of active immunization and non-immunological methods of LPS antagonism. A recent report suggests that absorption of LPS from plasma using immobilized polymyxin B may be possible (85). Partially hydrolysed, non-toxic forms of LPS have also been developed. One of these compounds, lipid X, is an inactive structural LPS analogue that blocks the effect of endotoxin in sheep and other animals (60–62). While further testing of such approaches is warranted, their use in humans remains speculative.

Despite its effectiveness in experimental animals, active immunization of humans is not practical because even low doses of LPS are extremely toxic, there is significant delay in producing antibodies following immunization, and without repeated injections the antibody titre rapidly wanes.

Mechanism of Anti-endotoxin Antibody Action

As early as 1896 Pfeiffer and Kolle recognized that transfer of convalescent sera from humans surviving typhoid fever could prevent death in guinea-pigs challenged with *Salmonella typhi* (86). More than 60 years later, Abernathy and Spink showed that human serum could neutralize a specific bacterial endotoxin (87). Within a few years it was shown that antiserum could provide protection both against homologous and heterologous bacterial strains and that antibodies were the protective component of antiserum (88–92).

Even these early studies demonstrated a protective effect of antibodies against homologous and heterologous endotoxins, but the protective mechanism remains obscure. LPS neutralization and enhanced clearance of LPS or bacteria are possibilities, but there is little in vitro evidence for a direct neutralizing effect of antibody. Likewise, while some studies suggest that homologous LPS is more rapidly cleared in the presence of antibody, the same is not true for heterologous bacteria or endotoxin (54,68,93). Enhancement of complement-mediated bacterial lysis, toxin opsonization and non-specific immune stimulation are also possible mechanisms. There is little evidence to support the role of antibody-enhanced complement-mediated bacterial lysis (54,94,95). In addition, opsonization does not seem to be a viable explanation for the anti-LPS action of core-directed antibodies because of great differences in the effectiveness of anti-core and anti-oligosaccharide antibodies. O-directed antibodies are up to 100-fold more effective than anti-core antibodies in enhancing opsonic activity (11,63,68,70,82,94,96,97). Although "non-specific" immune stimulation has been postulated as a mechanism of action, there are few, if any, data to support this postulate.

The Use of Anti-core Antibodies

The concept of cross-protection by anti-core antibodies is supported by four lines of evidence:

1. In vitro, anti-core antibodies bind to both smooth and rough mutant LPS.
2. Active and passive immunization with anti-core antibodies can prevent the effects of bacteraemia in experimental sepsis (11,54,63,64,93,94,97–102). However, several investigators have been unable to demonstrate protective

effects against heterologous LPS or bacteria (76,103,104). Passive transfer of anti-core antibody can also offer protection in animal models of endotoxaemia (68,76,105–108). Passive immunization has been claimed to provide "tolerance" to heterologous and homologous LPS-induced fever in animals (109,110). Unfortunately, original data supporting these claims have not been published. Active immunization with rough mutants to induce production of anti-core antibody has also been attempted as a protective mechanism against Gram-negative pneumonias. Although the results are complex, parenteral administration of rough mutant vaccine does not seem to protect against heterologous Gram-negative pneumonias (64,70,111–113). Protection against the local and generalized Shwartzman reaction has also been demonstrated (93,95,108,109).

3. Analysis of plasma from patients with Gram-negative bacteraemia shows that those with high titres of anti-core antibodies at the onset of sepsis have improved survival rates (78,96).

4. Clinical studies using human polyclonal antisera suggest that survival is increased by antisera to rough mutants (79,83).

Unfortunately, many contradictory results have been reported and there are several situations in which anti-core/lipid A antibodies have failed to prevent the effects of endotoxaemia (22,114–116).

Antibodies to rough mutant LPS or bacteria are able to bind to the core region of a wide variety of Gram-negative bacteria and hence a single antibody can protect animals from a large number of endotoxins. *Escherichia coli 0111:B4 J5* and *Salmonella minnesota Re 595* rough mutants have been the most widely used immunogens. Hyperimmune anti-core sera from animals vaccinated with rough-mutant organisms reduce the mortality and morbidity of septic and haemorrhagic shock induced by both homologous and heterologous LPS in animals and are accepted therapy and prophylaxis in veterinary medicine (54,65,66,93,97–99,117,118). These studies imply that anti-core antibodies can circumvent the potential steric interference of the O region of heterologous LPS and bind to core regions of both smooth and rough bacterial mutants (54). While having wide cross-reactivity, the magnitude of the protection offered by anti-core antibodies is less than that offered by homologous O antigen antibodies (96). Morbidity and mortality rates are improved by anti-core antibodies in clinical (79,83) and laboratory studies (24,26–29,36,37,67,94,100,119,120), and anti-core antibodies can occasionally have dramatic effects on the haemodynamic abnormalities of sepsis (36,121,122).

Impact of Anti-core Antibody Class and Titre on Efficacy

The relative importance of the origin of antibodies and of antibody isotypes in endotoxaemia is not clear. In general, however, monoclonal antibodies have been found to be significantly less effective than polyclonal antibodies in combating endotoxaemia (52,107,123,124). In animal models, Kim and Watson (107) have shown that the 19S fraction (predominantly IgM) antibodies reduce mortality. McCabe has also demonstrated that greater protection was afforded to mice challenged with bacteria or endotoxin when IgM class anti-core antibodies were administered than when IgG class anti-core antibodies were used (125). In contrast, rabbit studies by Greisman et al. (115) demonstrated that the antipyretic effects of antisera were contained in both the IgG and IgM fractions to core glycolipid and oligosaccharides. Early studies in this area by Braude and colleagues also confirmed the effectiveness of the IgG fractions (93,95).

Studies by McCabe, Pollack, Zinner and Baumgartner have contributed to our understanding of the role of naturally occurring LPS antibodies in humans. Using a haemagglutination assay, McCabe found that high titres of naturally occurring human antibodies to the core regions of *S. minnesota Re* mutants present at the onset of Gram-negative bacteraemia correlated positively with survival (96). Survival did not correlate with the titre of anti-O region antibodies. Zinner and McCabe (126) later re-examined the same anti-sera using immunofluorescence techniques and concluded that survival correlated best with titres of IgG O-specific antibodies directed against the infecting organism. There was no correlation between oligosaccharide-specific IgM antibody levels and outcome. These investigators also reconfirmed that high titres of anti-core antibodies, regardless of isotype, correlated with survival. Using ELISA technology in patients with *Pseudomonas aeruginosa* bacteraemia, Pollack found that high titres of both IgG and IgM antibodies to core glycolipid were associated with improved survival. Multivariate analysis suggested that high titres of strain-specific antibodies were the best predictor of outcome, followed by IgM then IgG anti-core antibodies (78). Interestingly, Young and colleagues (11,99,118) have shown that the majority of the anti-LPS antibody produced in humans convalescing from Gram-negative sepsis is of the IgG class.

The controversy over the relative importance of antibody classes was further fuelled by the studies of Callandra et al. (6) and Baumgartner et al. (127) who showed that there were no differences between the levels of IgG and IgM antibodies to *E. coli J5* or *S. minnesota Re* LPS, nor IgG class antibodies to lipid A, among surviving and fatal cases of human Gram-negative bacteraemia with shock. The only significant difference was that the titre of IgM antibodies to lipid A was higher in non-survivors.

The conflicting results of these studies show that no single antibody class is exclusively responsible for protection against endotoxaemia. Animal data showing that both polyclonal IgG and IgM antibodies are capable of combating endotoxaemia (79,93,95,107) and that even partially digested (Fab) fragments can protect against lethal sepsis (97,128) bring into serious question the critical role of IgM isotype antibodies.

Prospective Studies of Human Polyclonal Core Antiserum

In a small study in 1978 Ziegler et al. (80) demonstrated that administration of human J5 antiserum halved the mortality rate in 136 patients with Gram-negative bacteraemia (26% in controls versus 14% in J5 recipients).

In patients with Gram-negative bacteraemia and shock, the mortality rate was reduced from 89% in controls to 29% in J5 recipients. These early results prompted a larger formal study of J5 antisera in humans with sepsis.

In a study in 1982 Ziegler et al. (79) administered human sera rich in core-directed antibodies or control serum to 304 patients with sepsis syndrome in a randomized, double-blind study. Antisera were produced by injection of human volunteers with a killed *E. coli J5* rough mutant. A total of 212 patients comprised 191 with Gram-negative bacteraemia and 21 patients with a Gram-negative site of infection and sterile blood cultures but who had received antibiotics before blood cultures were obtained. Of these patients, 109 received control serum and 103 J5 antisera. A mortality rate of 39% (42/109) in controls and 22% (23/103) in bacteraemic recipients of J5 antisera suggested a treatment effect ($p<0.05$). Even more impressive were the mortality figures in the subgroup of 80 patients with refractory hypotension. Patients in shock had a reduction in mortality from 77% (30/39) in controls to 44% (18/41) in antisera-treated patients ($p<0.05$). Because of the very high incidence of Gram-negative bacteraemia observed in this study, many have questioned the applicability of the results to more heterogeneous groups of patients with sepsis syndrome. Other practical problems in this study include the omission of a defined endpoint for observation of mortality, and exclusion of deaths occurring as the result of multiple organ system failure weeks after an episode of sepsis. The study would not detect the possibility that J5 antiserum prolonged the dying process without any ultimate effect on mortality, or that J5 may have contributed to late multiple organ system failure deaths.

The study of Ziegler et al. (79) spurred two prophylactic trials of antisera in patients at high risk of Gram-negative infections. McCutchan et al. (81) studied a group of neutropenic patients receiving intensive chemotherapy. Patients received either control sera or that from *E. coli J5* immunized humans before the onset of neutropenia. Treatment did not reduce the risk of acquiring new infections during neutropenia: 8/59 infections in controls and 8/52 in treated patients. Likewise, there was no reduction in the risk of bacteraemia: 12% in controls versus 15% in the treated group. In addition, there was no impact on mortality: 3% (2/59 deaths) in controls and 8% (4/52 deaths) in treated patients. There was a significant but clinically unimportant reduction in the incidence of fever in a single subgroup of patients. There are several possible explanations for failure of this intervention. First, the sample size was small and the incidence of infection was low. Furthermore, because only a single dose of antisera was given at the initiation of chemotherapy, it is unlikely that significant amounts of transfused antisera remained to provide protection by the time neutropenia developed (approximately 1 week).

Baumgartner et al. (83) undertook a prophylactic trial of human J5 antibodies in surgical patients at high risk for sepsis. The study of Ziegler et al. (79) failed to show a protective effect in patients with Gram-negative intra-abdominal infections. Antibodies obtained by plasmapheresis were used to provide large quantities of material. Patients developed sepsis despite prophylactic plasma administered every 5 days. Patients were also given additional units of immune plasma if signs of sepsis developed. Plasma from *E. coli J5*-immunized donors did not prevent new Gram-negative infections, but did reduce the risk of developing Gram-negative septic shock: 11% (15/136) in placebo-treated patients versus 5% (6/126) in J5 plasma recipients ($p < 0.05$). J5 immune plasma also reduced the risk of death from 7% (9/136) in controls to 2% (2/126) in treated patients ($p<0.05$). As might be expected, treatment had no impact on the outcome of patients with Gram-positive or fungal sepsis. The findings of this study have been questioned because of the low incidence of Gram-negative bacteraemia and because effects were limited to the subgroup of patients who underwent abdominal surgery. In that subgroup, mortality was reduced from 16% (13/83) in controls to 3% (2/71) in patients ($p < 0.05$). Little patient detail was provided and it is difficult to compare the two groups with respect to severity of illness. Wolff et al. (129) also demonstrated a reduction in the incidence of fever in a subgroup of neutropenic patients receiving prophylactic administration of J5 antiserum.

In neither the Baumgartner et al. (83) nor Ziegler et al. (79) studies did the titre of anti-core antibodies correlate with survival. Recently, Girardin et al. (84) conducted a randomized, double-blind, placebo-controlled study of J5 immune plasma in 70 children with meningococcaemia. The immune plasma used in this study was produced using methods similar to those employed in the above (79,83). Failure to observe beneficial effects at interim analysis resulted in early termination of the study.

Many workers have studied the effects of purified intravenous human globulin preparations. Callandra et al. (6) tested an intravenous human IgG preparation against *E. coli J5* (J5 IVIG) in patients with Gram-negative septic shock. Treatment with 200 mg/kg of J5-rich IgG did not reduce 2-week mortality in the treated group (15/30 deaths (50% mortality) versus 20/41 deaths (49% mortality) in the group treated with control IgG). J5 IVIG also did not reduce the incidence of organ system failures resulting from shock. The most likely explanation for this failure was the low titre of specific anti-J5 in the J5 IVIG preparation. There was only a 2.2-fold difference in ELISA titre between J5 IVIG and control IgG. Alternative explanations include the possibility that patients with fully developed septic shock cannot benefit from an anti-endotoxin antibody or that IgG isotype antibodies are ineffective. Neither explanation is satisfactory. However, in the 1982 study of Ziegler et al. (79), patients with established septic shock had the greatest proportional reduction in mortality. Furthermore, there are multiple models in which IgG class antibodies provide protection against Gram-negative bacteraemia and endotoxaemia and there is little apparent relationship between antibody isotype titre and clinical outcome.

Four other studies by Duswald et al. (130), Glinz et al. (131), Rommelshein (132) and Class and Schorer (133) have described the use of intravenous immunoglobulin preparations in humans. These studies used either polyspecific IgG, IgM-enriched IgG or IgG enriched with high levels of IgM antibodies to *P. aeruginosa*. Patient populations varied, but consistently included patients at high risk of nosocomial infection and Gram-negative sepsis. Each study showed some benefit in terms of fever duration, antibiotic usage, shortened intensive care unit (ICU) time, decreased risk of nosocomial pneumonia and a decreased need for respiratory therapy treatments. However, none of these studies showed an improvement in mortality and all had methodological limitations.

The most recent trial of a polyclonal human intravenous immunoglobulin preparation was conducted by Schedel et al. (134) in 55 patients with septic shock. The results were very striking. Mortality rates in patients with septic shock were reduced from 32% (9/28) in patients receiving placebo to 4% (1/27) in patients given intravenous immunoglobulin daily for 3 days. Both groups in this study were well matched for entry criteria. Immunological and physiological data were provided to complement the survival data. Improvements in the APACHE II scores of treated patients were rapidly apparent after immunoglobulin administration and reached statistical significance in the treated group after 5 days.

Taken together, this large group of trials offers only inconsistent evidence to suggest that human antisera/plasma or purified immunoglobulin preparations can benefit patients with Gram-negative sepsis.

Studies with Anti-core/Lipid A Monoclonal Antibodies

Two unrelated developments have substantially shaped the course of anti-endotoxin development. The first was the emergence of monoclonal antibody technology (135,136). The prospects of developing a constant, pure, specific anti-endotoxin antibody in unlimited quantities in vitro were inviting. At least eight different monoclonal antibodies to various determinants on endotoxin were produced (137–141). Two of these compounds, XOMEN E5 and HA1A, have been tested in large-scale clinical trials (135,136). The second development was recognition of the human acquired immunodeficiency syndrome (AIDS). The association of blood products and AIDS transmission had a stifling effect on research into the use of polyclonal human antisera. The advent of AIDS, the evolution of monoclonal antibody technology and data from McCabe suggesting that IgM class antibodies were superior to IgG antibodies in large part explains the design of XOMEN E5 and HA1A.

XOMEN E5

Animal Studies

There is a dearth of evidence to support the efficacy of monoclonal anti-endotoxins in vivo. XOMEN E5, a monoclonal IgM antibody derived from *E. coli J5*-immunized mice, was initially reported to be effective in combination with antibiotic therapy in bacteraemic animals (136). This study conflicts with subsequent studies of endotoxaemic animals using XOMEN E5 in chronically instrumented sheep (22). In conscious sheep with chronic lung lymph fistulas, and extensive haemodynamic and airway monitoring, multiple physiological measurements were made before and after infusion of endotoxin in the presence or absence of XOMEN E5. Animals in this study received an infusion of XOMEN E5 (2 mg/kg) 4 h before LPS (0.75 μg/kg) challenge or were given a mixture of LPS (0.75 μg/kg) and XOMEN E5 that had been incubated in vitro at 37°C for 30 min before infusion. A control group given only 2 mg/kg of antibody showed no change in any measured parameter, while animals receiving LPS alone exhibited a typical endotoxin response. In all animals receiving endotoxin, lung compliance declined by approximately 50% within 30–60 min and was accompanied by a six-fold increase in resistance to airflow. There was also pulmonary hypertension, leukopenia, and widening of the A-aDO_2 (alveolar–arterial oxygen difference). Pretreatment with XOMEN E5 or infusion of an in vitro antibody–LPS mixture modestly blunted the early pulmonary artery (PA) pressure rise when compared with LPS controls; however, no other variable was significantly improved (22). Similar results were seen in pilot studies when lower doses of LPS (0.075, 0.05 and 0.005 μg/kg) were infused 1 h after antibody (2 mg/kg) administration (unpublished observations). In vitro, incubation of LPS with XOMEN E5 in molar ratios from 1:10^3 to 1:10^6 for 30 min at 37°C did not reduce LPS-induced limulus activation under serum-free or serum-containing conditions. These studies suggest that XOMEN E5 does not effectively neutralize the *E. coli* endotoxins used in these studies, in spite of the fact that E5 was made specifically against one of these (*E. coli 0111, J5*).

In two human studies (142,143) using XOMEN E5, conflicting results have been reported. In the pivotal (phase III) trial of XOMEN E5, a widely accepted clinical definition for sepsis syndrome was used. Patients were required to have at least two of the following manifestations of sepsis: fever or hypothermia, leukocytosis or leukopenia, a blood culture growing a Gram-negative organism within the 48 h preceding study entry or a suspected focus of Gram-negative infection. In addition, at least one of the following manifestations of a failing organ system due to sepsis was required: tachypnoea (or evidence of pulmonary dysfunction), hypotension (or decreased systemic vascular resistance), acidosis, renal dysfunction, central nervous system dysfunction or coagulopathy.

After enrolment, patients received two doses of XOMEN E5 (2 mg/kg) 24 h apart or two doses of an equal volume of 5% dextrose in isotonic saline. No other aspect of patient care was controlled during this 30-day study. Of 486 enrolled patients, 468 were considered to be appropriate. Gram-negative infection was seen in 316 of 468 patients (68%) and Gram-negative bacteraemia in 171 of 468 (37%). Shock occurred in 56% (262/468) of the total group and in 57% of the patients with Gram-negative infection (179/316). Of the total study population, patients who received the monoclonal antibody had a mortality rate of 31% (75/242) compared with 37% (83/226 deaths) in placebo-treated patients, but this was not statistically significant. Similarly, there was no significant difference in mortality in all patients with Gram-negative bacteraemia: 33% (31/94) in antibody-treated patients compared with 42% (32/77) in those given placebo. Even when the group of patients with Gram-negative bacteraemia was subdivided into patients with or without shock, no treatment effect could be observed. For patients with Gram-negative bacteraemia without shock, mortality rates were 9% (4/44) in treated patients and 19% (5/27) in placebo recipients. Of the patients without Gram-negative bacteraemia, there was also no difference in mortality: 30% (44/148) in E5 recipients versus 34% (51/149) in placebo-treated patients.

In this study the only subgroup appearing to benefit from XOMEN E5 were patients who had evidence of Gram-negative infection without bacteraemia and who were not in shock. Adding to the complexity of the analysis, the beneficial effects of E5 were only seen at 30 days follow-up but not at 14 days. No physiologic data were presented to suggest an early effect of treatment.

The mortality was 33% (24/72) in treated patients and 43% (28/65) in placebo patients ($p < 0.05$) after p value adjustment for covariates. The resolution rate of organ system failures in the E5 study was also reported. A total of 66 organ failure reversals was seen in the 137 patients without shock. In treated patients, 19 of 53 organ failures (36%) resolved compared with eight of 31 (26%) in the placebo group ($p<0.05$ by chi-square).

Much criticism has been levelled at the E5 study because of reported low APACHE scores in the 40% of patients in whom these scores were reported. Despite the low APACHE scores in this subset of patients, the population enrolled in the E5 trial was undoubtedly quite ill with a 50% incidence of shock and a high prevalence of multiple organ failure. The mortality rate and incidence of organ failures in the E5 study support the contention that the population was significantly more ill than the APACHE scores suggest. The prevalence of organ failures in the study and placebo groups at the time of study entry was well balanced. Others have criticized the study for its choice of placebo. The most appropriate placebo in both this and in the HA1A studies would have been irrelevant monoclonal IgM class antibodies.

E5 appears to be safe. The incidence of allergic reactions was only 1.6% and all allergic reactions resolved spontaneously. Although not associated with clinical illness, almost half of E5 recipients developed human anti-mouse antibodies (HAMA) as determined by a highly sensitive assay. The authors concluded that E5 was safe and effective in Gram-negative sepsis, a conclusion not widely accepted. E5 benefited only a small subset of patients and there is no clear and compelling rationale as to why the treatment effect should be limited to this subgroup. Even this benefit is of limited clinical significance because the subgroup cannot be identified prospectively.

A second phase III study of E5 was undertaken in patients with suspected Gram-negative infection without shock. The results of the second phase III trial were presented at the 1991 ICCAAC conference and reproduced in the lay press (144,145). Of 811 enrolled patients, 530 (65%) were found to have Gram-negative infection and 139 of these had organ system failures (52 cases of adult respiratory distress syndrome, 73 cases of acute renal failure and 40 cases of disseminated intravascular coagulation). There was no benefit of treatment in patients with Gram-negative infection. Thirty-day survival was 70% in the treated group and 74% in the placebo group. Among the subgroup of 139 patients with organ system failures, survival was 59% in E5 recipients and 53% in patients receiving placebo. None of these differences was significant. More episodes of organ failure were reversed in the treated group (48%) than in the placebo-treated group (25%). However, this effect failed to reach statistical significance. In the subgroup of patients with Gram-negative infection and acute renal failure, 63% had reversal of renal failure if treated and 29% recovered renal function if given placebo ($p<0.05$).

In the second trial E5 was again relatively safe with only a 2.6% incidence of adverse reactions (four cases of anaphylaxis, five episodes of rash). Although deemed to be clinically unimportant, 48% of treated patients developed a HAMA response as compared with 12% of placebo-treated patients. As in the first phase III trial, there was no clear benefit of XOMEN E5 treatment. Furthermore, in the second study the group that seemed to have benefited in the first study did not benefit. Given current data, XOMEN E5 does not have a substantial biological effect in the population studied.

HA1A

Animal Studies

Like XOMEN E5, there are few published animal data on the effectiveness of HA1A, a chimeric human–mouse monoclonal IgM class antibody directed against *E. coli J5*. Teng et al. (135) showed that HA1A in hybridoma fluid from the peritoneum of mice prevented the dermal Shwartzman reaction in rabbits and reduced the mortality of lethal Gram-negative bacteraemia in a mouse model (135). Because this peritoneal fluid probably contains substances other than HA1A, these data are inconclusive. Later studies reported contradictory results. For example, Baumgartner et al. have reported that purified HA1A does not block Gram-negative bacteraemia and LPS-induced death in mice, and also fails to prevent the Schwartzman reaction in rabbits (114). Similar to the findings of Wheeler et al. (22) with XOMEN E5, studies in sheep using HA1A have failed to show protective effects. No effect was seen on haemodynamic alterations and there was only minor attenuation of fever. Failure to block LPS-induced physiological alterations in these studies does not appear to be an aberration of the sheep model: there are LPS-directed antibodies that offer protection to the chronically instrumented endotoxaemic sheep (Zapol, personal communication). In vitro, HA1A failed to prevent LPS-induced generation of cytokines (114). Furthermore, a recent study from Quezado et al. failed to establish efficacy of HA1A in a canine septic shock model (146). Indeed, the mortality in HA1A-treated dogs was 85% (11/13) compared with a mortality of only 43% (6/14) in the placebo group ($p < 0.05$). Thus, the specificity of the binding of HA1A to endotoxin and the mechanism of LPS inactivation, if this occurs, is unknown.

A clinical trial of HA1A in patients with sepsis syndrome has been completed. The entry criteria for this trial differed slightly from the E5 study. Patients were required to have fever or hypothermia, tachycardia and tachypnoea and hypotension in the presence of an adequate fluid challenge or at least two of six signs of organ failure: acidosis, hypoxaemia, acute renal failure, coagulopathy, altered mental status or increased cardiac index with a decreased systemic vascular resistance. After enrolment, patients received 100 mg of HA1A or human serum albumin. Patients were followed until death, 28 days or study withdrawal.

Of a total of 543 patients, 262 were given HA1A and 281 were given albumin. Overall 58% of patients (317/543) had Gram-negative infection and 37% (200/543) had Gram-negative bacteraemia. There was no significant difference in mortality at 28 days between the HA1A treated (39%) and albumin (43%) groups. In the patients with Gram-negative bacteraemia, mortality was 49% in the placebo group and 30% in the HA1A group ($p < 0.05$ after adjustment for covariates). The p value prior to adjustment was not given. These benefits extended to the smaller subgroup of bacteraemic patients with shock. In this group, mortality was 57% in the placebo group and 33% in treated patients. Published data also divided the bacteraemic patients into two groups. Bacteraemic patients with APACHE scores greater than 25 and less than 25 both seemed to benefit from HA1A administration.

Two out of 291 patients had adverse reactions to HA1A, but both reactions were transient. Only 116 of the treated patients underwent testing for anti-chimeric antibody formation; no antibodies were found. The methods to assess the HAMA response were not described. The true incidence of antibody formation is unknown, as is the biological significance of such antibody formation.

Much criticism has been levelled at this study (147). Many have suggested that the most appropriate placebo would be an identical quantity of an irrelevant monoclonal antibody of the same species and isotype. The two groups in the HA1A study were not statistically different with respect to any single entry characteristic, yet the two populations have clear differences. The APACHE score was 2.1 points higher in the placebo group. This seemingly small increase in APACHE score reflects a higher average incidence of failing organ systems. Even small increases in APACHE score can have significant effects on mortality. In addition, organ system failure was more prevalent in the placebo group: the incidence of ARDS, acute renal failure and hepatic failure were all lower in the HA1A-treated group. There was a strikingly higher incidence of *Pseudomonas* bacteraemia, known to be associated with an exceptionally bad prognosis, in the placebo group. Division of patients into groups of high and low APACHE scores is an artificial and relatively unhelpful comparison. Because of imbalance in the incidence of organ failure and *Pseudomonas* bacteraemia, the results of this study are open to question. It is not clear from the published data whether the authors of this study performed appropriate corrections for imbalances between treatment groups at entry.

In addition, attempts have been made to compare this study with the 1982 study of Ziegler et al. (79). Despite obvious problems in comparing mortality statistics for groups with different entry characteristics treated 10 years apart, the analysis is interesting and perhaps worth pursuing because of the parallels drawn by the authors. The mortality rates in the antibody-treated groups were similar in both studies, but the same is not true for the placebo groups. For patients with Gram-negative bacteraemia, the 1991 study has a significantly higher mortality rate in the placebo group than in any other group in either study. Furthermore, while the percentage improvement in mortality rates was similar between the two studies, the patient populations clearly were not. The 1982 study had a ten-fold higher incidence of neutropenia and higher rates of *Pseudomonas* bacteraemia, neoplasia and liver disease. Critical examination of the 1982 data also reveals imbalances between the treated and placebo groups at entry. Overall, the 1991 trial studied a less-ill group of patients and found similar mortality rates. Even ignoring the above concerns, there remains the problem of prospectively identifying the subgroups for which therapy could be potentially useful.

Impact of Anti-endotoxins on Cytokine Generation in Human Sepsis

The cytokines appear to be critical in the development of SIRS. If anti-endotoxins are to be effective, one potential mechanism would be the inhibition of the generation of cytokines such as TNFα and IL-1. At least three groups have now examined the role of anti-endotoxins in cytokine generation and have produced conflicting data. DeGroote et al. (148) and Baumgartner et al. (114) have shown that use of XOMEN E5 and HA1A fails to inhibit cytokine generation in vitro and in vivo. In contrast, Wortel (149) reported a reduction in TNFα and IL-6 levels in endotoxaemic patients treated with HA1A.

Advantages and Limitations of Anti-endotoxin Antibodies

Anti-LPS antibodies have several potential advantages over other pharmacological agents in sepsis. First, they may directly antagonize LPS, a potent trigger of the inflammatory cascade. Second, unlike antibiotics, anti-endotoxins may be useful in non-bacteraemic endotoxaemia. Third, anti-endotoxins could be used prophylactically in high-risk patients. Finally, polyclonal anti-endotoxins have been shown to be safe and effective in animals.

Despite the advantages over antibiotics, there are many disadvantages of anti-endotoxins. Only 30%–40% of patients with SIRS have endotoxaemia or Gram-negative bacteraemia. Thus anti-endotoxins will fail to offer benefit to roughly two-thirds of patients with SIRS. Furthermore, because of the structural diversity of endotoxin, even anti-LPS antibodies recognizing the core region will bind to endotoxins with different affinities and, in some cases, not at all.

The mechanisms by which anti-endotoxin antibodies afford protection are not clear. They probably include bacterial opsonization, complement-mediated bacterial lysis, non-specific immune stimulation and direct LPS neutralization. Although direct binding and neutralization of endotoxin or enhanced circulatory clearance of LPS are the most likely explanations, there is little evidence to support this mechanism for the currently studied anti-endotoxins. HA1A and E5 bind not only to endotoxin, but also to Gram-positive bacteria, some fungi and to some serum proteins.

The critical site within the organism for the action of anti-endotoxins is unknown. Because of their high molecular weight, IgM antibodies are confined to the circulation. Lower molecular weight antibodies or antibody fragments capable of gaining access to a larger volume of distribution should prove more effective in neutralizing LPS closer to its source.

Even if LPS–antibody binding is complete, avid and irreversible, it is possible that the antibodies will not sequester the toxic portion of LPS sufficiently to prevent inflammation. This appears to be the case with HA1A and E5. LPS–antibody complexes may themselves be toxic. Because of the speed with which LPS may initiate an inflammatory cascade, therapy after the onset of SIRS is likely to be less successful than pretreatment. The appropriate time window for anti-endotoxin has also yet to be defined: it may be that antibodies cannot be administered rapidly enough to protect against the effects of isolated episodes of endotoxaemia. On the other hand, in the setting of continuous or repeated LPS release, it is reasonable to believe some patients might benefit from the late administration of an anti-endotoxin.

Antibodies are large and complex molecules. The presence of the Fc portion allows antibodies to activate complement and bind to the surface of mononuclear cells. These two actions can stimulate immediate allergic and long-term immunological reactions raising the possibility of allergic reactions on re-challenge.

Finally, the cost of monoclonal therapy is immense. With a condition as common as SIRS, financial limitations may prove to be the limiting factor preventing their widespread use.

Summary

The production of high-affinity, widely cross-reactive antibodies to endotoxin is a difficult undertaking, but represents the first step in the development of immunological therapy for septic shock. There is no doubt that crude antisera and polyclonal anti-endotoxins can bind and neutralize endotoxin in vitro. This neutralization can afford in vivo protection to animals challenged with endotoxin or Gram-negative bacteria. Using human polyclonal antisera, Ziegler et al. (79) and Baumgartner et al. (83) have performed the only studies that demonstrate a convincing survival advantage. However, because of the potential risks of transfusion of human blood products in the age of AIDS it is unlikely that a human polyclonal anti-endotoxin will be developed.

Unlike polyclonal antisera, there are few data to support the efficacy of monoclonal anti-endotoxins in vivo and the available data are sometimes contradictory. Similarly, very few animal data demonstrating the efficacy of either XOMEN E5 or HA1A have been published. Evidence of improved survival rates from three large clinical trials of monoclonal anti-endotoxins in humans with sepsis syndrome is subject to different interpretations. Furthermore, the apparent benefits of XOMEN E5 demonstrated in an initial randomized, double-blind, phase III trial have not been reproduced in a second study.

Though administration of HA1A confers a survival benefit in the subgroup of patients with Gram-negative bacteraemia, the practical value of this therapy is much less clear. Even taking account of methodological factors in the structure of the study, the data indicate that two-thirds of patients will not benefit from treatment with HA1A. Because patients who might benefit cannot be prospectively identified, most patients would receive the drug unnecessarily, with the further problems of untoward reactions and substantial financial liability. The potential of anti-endotoxin therapy is undoubtedly attractive. However, the problems of the human clinical trials and the contradictory animal data indicate that much further work is needed before the use of anti-endotoxins becomes standard practice.

References

1. Centers for Disease Control (1990) MMWR 39: 31–34
2. Balk RA, Bone RC (1989) The septic syndrome. Definition and clinical implications. Crit Care Clin 5: 1–8

3. Bone RC, Fisher CJ, Clemmer TP, Slotman GJ, Metz CA, Balk RA (1989) Sepsis syndrome: A valid clinical entity. Crit Care Med 17: 389–393
4. Bone RC, Fisher CJ, Clemmer TP et al. (1987) A controlled clinical trial of high-dose methyl-prednisolone in the treatment of severe sepsis and septic shock. N Engl J Med 317: 653–658
5. Ispahani P, Perason NJ, Greenwood D (1987) An analysis of community and hospital acquired bacteremia in a large teaching hospital in the United Kingdom. Q J Med 241: 427–440
6. Callandra T, Glauser MP, Schellekens J, Verhoef J, Swiss–Dutch J5 Immunoglobulin Study Group (1988) Treatment of Gram-negative septic shock with human IgG antibody to *Escherichia coli J5*: A prospective, double blind, randomized trial. J Infect Dis 158: 312–319
7. Bone RC, Fisher CJ, Clemmer TP et al. (1987) Early methylprednisolone treatment for septic syndrome and adult respiratory distress syndrome. Chest 932: 1032–1036
8. Neugebauer E, Schirren J, Lorenz W (1988) High dose steroids and sepsis. N Engl J Med 318: 514
9. Veterans Administration Systemic Sepsis Cooperative Study Group (1987) Effect of high dose glucocorticoid therapy on mortality in patients with signs of systemic sepsis. N Engl J Med 317: 659–665
10. DeMaria A, Craven DE, Heffernan JJ, McIntosh TK, Grindlinger GA, McCabe WR (1985) Naloxone versus placebo in the treatment of septic shock. Lancet 1: 1363–1365
11. Young LS, Stevens P, Ingram J (1975) Functional role of antibody against "core" glycolipid of Enterobacteriaceae. J Clin Invest 56: 850–861
12. Brandtzag P, Kieruli P, Gaustad P et al. (1989) Plasma endotoxin as a predictor of multiple organ failure and death in systemic meningococcal disease. J Infect Dis 159: 195–204
13. Brandtzag P, Mollnes TE, Kierrulf P (1989) Complement activation and endotoxin levels in systemic meningococcal disease. J Infect Dis 160: 58–65
14. Brandtzag P, Sandset PM, Joo GB, Ovstebo R, Abildgaard U, Kieruli P (1989) The quantitative association of plasma endotoxin, anti-thrombin, protein C, extrinsic pathway inhibitor and fibrinopeptide A in systemic meningococcal disease. Thromb Res 55: 459–470
15. Brandtzag P, Ovstebo RM, Bruscetto B, Kierulf P (1990) Plasminogen activator inhibitor 1 and 2, alpha 2 anti-plasmin, plasminogen and endotoxin levels in systemic meningococcal disease. Thromb Res 57: 271–278
16. van Deventer SJH, Pauw W, ten Cate JW, Janssen ME, Buller HR, Sturk A (1987) Clinical evaluation in febrile patients of an optimized endotoxin assay in blood. Prog Clin Biol Res 231: 489–499
17. Danner RL, Elin RJ, Hosseini JM, Wesley RA, Reilly JM, Parillo JE (1991) Endotoxemia in human septic shock. Chest 99: 169–175
18. Dofferhoff ASM, Bom VJJ, van Ingen J et al. (1991) Patterns of cytokines, plasma endotoxin, and acute phase proteins during the treatment of severe sepsis in humans. In: Sturk A, van Deventer SJH, Wouter ten Cate J, Büller HR, Thijs LG, Levin J (eds) Bacterial endotoxins: Cytokine mediators and new therapies of severe sepsis in humans. Wiley Liss, New York, pp 43–54
19. Schlag G, Redl H, Dinges HP, Davies J (1991) Sources of endotoxin in the posttraumatic setting. In: Sturk A, van Deventer SJH, Wouter ten Cate J, Büller HR, Thijs LG, Levin J (eds) Bacterial endotoxins: Cytokine mediators and new therapies of severe sepsis in humans. Wiley Liss, New York, pp 121–134
20. van Deventer SJH, Hack CE, Wolbink CE et al. (1991) Endotoxin-induced neutrophil activation – the role of complement revisited. In: Sturk A, van Deventer SJH, Wouter ten Cate J, Büller HR, Thijs LG, Levin J (eds) Bacterial endotoxins: Cytokine mediators and new therapies of severe sepsis in humans. Wiley Liss, New York, pp 101–109
21. Meyrick B, Hoover R, Jones M, Berry LC, Brigham KL (1989) In vitro effects of endotoxin on bovine and sheep lung microvascular and pulmonary artery endothelial cells. J Cell Physiol 138: 165–174
22. Wheeler AP, Hardie WD, Bernard G (1990) Studies of an anti-endotoxin antibody in preventing the physiologic changes of endotoxemia in awake sheep. Am Rev Resp Dis 142: 775–781
23. Michie HR, Manogue KR, Spriggs DR et al. (1988) Detection of circulating tumor necrosis factor after endotoxin administration. N Engl J Med 318: 1481–1486
24. Gaffin SL, Grinberg Z, Abraham C, Birkhan J, Shechter (1981) Protection against

hemorrhagic shock in the cat by human plasma containing endotoxin-specific antibodies. J Surg Res 31: 18–21
25. Papa M, Halperin Z, Rubinstein E (1983) The effect of ischemia of the dogs's colon on transmural migration of bacteria and endotoxin. J Surg Res 35: 264
26. Gathiram P, Gaffin SL, Wells MT, Brock Utne JG (1986) Superior mesenteric artery occlusion shock in cats: Modification of the endotoxemia by anti-lipopolysaccharide antibodies (anti-LPS). Circ Shock 19: 231–237
27. Zanotti AM, Gaffin SL (1985) Prophylaxis of superior mesenteric artery occlusion shock in rabbits by anti-lipopolysaccharide (anti-LPS antibodies). J Surg Res 38: 113–115
28. Gaffin SL, Brock-Utne JG, Zanotti AM (1986) Hypoxia-induced endotoxemia in primates: Role of the reticulo-endothelial system function and anti-lipopolysaccharide plasma. Aviat Space Environ Med 57: 1044
29. Gaffin SL, Wells M, Jordan JP (1985) Anti-lipopolysaccharide toxin therapy for whole body X-irradiation overdose. Br J Radiol 58: 881–884
30. Walker RI, Ledney G, Galley G (1975) Septic endotoxemia in radiation injury and graft-versus-host disease. Radiat Res 62: 242–249
31. Graber C, Reinhold R, Bremen J, Harley R (1971) Fatal heatstroke. JAMA 216: 1195–1196
32. Neuman F, Gaffin S, Epstein Y, Magazanik, Shapiro Y (1978) Changes in membrane permeability to endotoxin in heat stroke. Isr Soc Int Med Proc Herzliya 6: 38–42
33. Hammer-Hodges D, Woodruff P, Cuevas P (1974) Role of intraintestinal Gram-negative bacterial flora on response to major burn. Surg Gynecol Obstet 138: 599
34. Cuevas P, Ishiyama N, Koizumi S, Woodruff P, Kaufmann A, Fine J (1974) Role of endotoxemia of intestinal origin in early death from large burns. Surg Gynecol Obstet 138: 725–731
35. Michaeli D (1979) Medicine on the battlefield. J R Soc Med 72: 370–373
36. Gaffin SL, Baker B, DuPreez J, Katzwinkel R, Fleming J, Brock Utne JG (1982) Prophylaxis and therapy with anti-endotoxin hyperimmune serum against gastroenteritis and endotoxemia in horses. Proc Congr Am Assoc Eq Pract 28: 335–340
37. Wessels BC, Gafffin SL, Wells MT (1987) Circulating plasma endotoxin (LPS) concentration in healthy and hemorrhagic enteric dogs: Anti-endotoxin immunotherapy in hemorrhagic enteric endotoxemia. J Am Anim Hosp Assoc 23: 291
38. Cuvas P, Fine J (1973) Production of fatal endotoxin shock by vasoactive substances. Gastroenterology 64: 285–291
39. Daily O, Uddin S, Walker RI, Spaur W (1978) Endotoxemia during hyperbaric stress. Undersea Biomed Res 5 (suppl): 37–38
40. Shenep JL, Morgan K (1984) Kinetics of endotoxin release during antibiotic therapy for experimental Gram-negative bacterial sepsis. J Infect Dis 150: 380
41. Buller HR, ten Cate JW, Sturk A, Thomas LL (1985) Validity of the endotoxin assay in post-surgical patients. In: ten Cate JW, Buller HR, Sturk A, Levin J (eds) Bacterial endotoxins: Biomedical significance and detection with the limulus amebocyte lysate test. Alan R Liss, New York, p 405
42. Dolan SA, Riegle L, Berzofsky R, Cooperstock M (1987) Clinical evaluation of the plasma chromogenic limulus assay. In: Watson SW, Levin J, Novitsky TJ (eds) Detection of bacterial endotoxins with the limulus amebocyte lysate test. Alan R Liss, New York, p 405
43. Pearson FC, Dubczak J, Weary M, Bruszer G, Donohue G (1987) Detection of endotoxemia in plasma of patients with Gram-negative bacterial sepsis by the limulus amebocyte lysate assay. J Clin Microbiol 21: 865
44. McCartney AC, Piotrowicz BI, Edlin SE, Ledingham I McA (1987) Evaluation of the chromogenic LAL assay in septic shock. In: Watson SW, Levin J, Novitsky TJ (eds) Detection of bacterial endotoxins with the limulus amebocyte lysate test. Alan R Liss, New York, p 459
45. Cooperstock MS, Tucker RP, Baublio JV (1975) Possible pathogenic role of endotoxin in Reye's syndrome. Lancet 1: 1272
46. van Deventer SJH (1988) Endotoxaemia: An early predictor of septicaemia in febrile patients. Lancet 1: 605–608
47. Sturk A, Janssen ME, Muylaert FR, Thomas JK, ten Cate JW (1987) Endotoxin testing in blood. In: Watson SW, Levin J, Novitsky TJ (eds) Detection of bacterial endotoxins with the limulus amebocyte lysate test. Alan R Liss, New York, pp 371–385
48. van Deventer SJH, Buller HR, ten Cate JW, Aarden LA, Hack E, Sturk A (1994)

Experimental endotoxemia in humans. Analysis of cytokine release and coagulation, fibrinolytic and complement pathways. Blood (in press)
49. Goldman RC, Leive L (1980) Heterogeneity of antigenic-side-chain length in lipopolysaccharide from *Escherichia coli 0111* and *Salmonella typhimurium LT2*. Eur J Biochem 107: 145–153
50. Munford RS, Hall CL, Rick PD (1980) Size heterogeneity of *Salmonella typhimurium* lipopolysaccharides in outer membranes and culture supernatant membrane fragments. J Bacteriol 144: 630–640
51. Luderitz O, Galanos C, Lehmann V et al. (1973) Lipid A: Chemical structure and biological activity. J Infect Dis 128: S17–29
52. Gigliotti E, Shenep JL (1985) Failure of monoclonal antibodies to core glycolipid to bind intact smooth strains of *Escherichia coli*. J Infect Dis 151: 1005–1011
53. Johns MA, Bruins SC, McCabe WR (1977) Immunizations with R mutants of *Salmonella minnesota*. II. Serological response to lipid A and the lipopolysaccharide of Re mutant. Infect Immun 17: 9–15
54. Chedid L, Parant M, Parant F, Boyer F (1968) A proposed mechanism for natural immunity of enterobacterial pathogens. J Immunol 100: 292–301
55. Pollack M, Chia JKS, Koles NL, Miller M, Guelde G (1989) Specificity and cross-reactivity of monoclonal antibodies reactive with the core and lipid A regions of bacterial lipopolysaccharide. J Infect Dis 159: 168–188
56. Fuller NA, Wv M, Wilkinson RG, Heath EC (1973) The biosynthesis of cell wall lipopolysaccharide in *Escherichia coli*. J Biol Chem 248: 7938–7950
57. Jansson P, Lindberg A, Wollin R (1981) Structural studies on the hexose region of the core in lipopolysaccharides from Enterobacteriaceae. Eur J Biochem 115: 571
58. Retschel ET, Wollenweber HW, Russa R, Brade H, Zahringer U (1984) Concepts of the chemical structure of lipid A. Rev Infect Dis 6: 432–438
59. Galanos C, Luderitz O, Westphal O (1971) Preparation and properties of antisera against the lipid A component of bacterial lipolpolysaccharides. Eur J Biochem 24: 116–122
60. Golenbock DT, Will JA, Raetz CR, Proctor RA (1987) Lipid X ameliorates pulmonary hypertension and protects sheep from death due to endotoxin. Infect Immun 55: 2471–2476
61. Golenbock DT, Ebert S, Will JA, Proctor RA (1988) Elimination and tissue distribution of the monosaccharide lipid A precursor, lipid X in mice and sheep. Antimicrob Agents Chemother 32: 37–41
62. Golenbock DT, Leggett JE, Rasmussen P, Craig WA, Raetz CR, Proctor RA (1988) Lipid X protects mice against fatal *Escherichia coli* infection. Infect Immun 56: 779–784
63. Bruins SC, Stumacher R, Johns MA, McCabe WR (1977) Immunization with R mutants of *Salmonella minnesota*. III. Comparison of the protective effect of immunization with lipid A and the Re mutant. Infect Immun 17: 16–20
64. McCabe WR, Bruins SC, Craven DE, Johns M (1977) Cross reactive antigens: Their potential for immunization-induced immunity to Gram-negative bacteria. J Infect Dis 136: S161–S166
65. Hodgin L, Drevis J (1976) Effect of active immunizations with lipid A and *Salmonella minnesota* Re 595 on Gram-negative infections in mice. Infection 4: 5–13
66. Mullan WA, Newsome PM, Cunnington PG, Palmer GH, Wilson ME (1974) Protection against Gram-negative infections with anti-serum to lipid A from *Salmonella minnesota* R595. Infect Immun 10: 1195–1201
67. Reitschel ETh, Galanos C (1977) Lipid A antiserum-mediated protection against lipopolysaccharide and lipid A-induced fever and skin necrosis. Infect Immun 15: 34–49
68. Tate WJ, Douglas H, Braude AE (1966) Protection against lethality of *E. coli* endotoxin with "O" antiserum. Ann NY Acad Sci 133: 746–762
69. McCabe WR, Greeley A (1972) Immunization with R mutants of *S. minnesota*. I. Protection against challenge with heterologous Gram-negative bacilli. J Immunol 108: 601–610
70. Pennington JE, Menkes E (1981) Type-specific vs. cross-protective vaccination for Gram-negative bacterial pneumonia. J Infect Dis 144: 599–603
71. Pennington JE, Hickey WF, Blackwood LL, Arnaut MA (1981) Active immunization with lipopolysaccharide *Pseudomonas* antigen for chronic *Pseudomonas* bronchopneumonia in guinea pigs. J Clin Invest 68: 1140–1148
72. Wolberg G, Dewitt CW (1969) Mouse virulence of K(L) antigen containing strains of *Escherichia coli*. J Bacteriol 100: 730–737

73. Markley K, Smallman E (1968) Protection by vaccination against *Pseudomonas* infection after thermal injury. J Bacteriol 96: 867–874
74. McCabe WR, DeMaria A, Berberich H, Johns MA (1988) Immunization with rough mutants of *Salmonella minnesota*: Protective activity of IgM and IgG antibody to the R595 (Re chemotype) mutant. J Infect Dis 158: 291–300
75. Davis D, Brown K, Douglas H, Take W, Braude AI (1969) Prevention of death from endotoxin with antiserum. J Immunol 102: 563–567
76. Ng A, Chen CLH, Chang CM, Nowotny A (1976) Relationship of structure to function in bacterial endotoxins: Serologically cross-reactive components and their effect on protection of mice against some Gram-negative organisms. J Gen Microbiol 94: 107–116
77. Lachman E, Pitsoe SB, Gaffin SL (1984) Anti-lipopolysaccharide immunotherapy in management of septic shock of obstetric and gynaecological origin. Lancet 1: 981–983
78. Pollack M, Huang AI, Prescott RK et al. (1983) Enhanced survival in *Pseudomonas aeruginosa* septicemia associated with high levels of circulating antibody to *Escherichia coli* endotoxin core. J Clin Invest 72: 1874–1881
79. Ziegler EJ, McCutchan JA, Fierer J et al. (1982) Treatment of Gram-negative bacteremia and shock with human antiserum to a mutant *Escherichia coli*. N Engl J Med 307: 1225–1230
80. Ziegler EJ, McCutchan JA, Braude AI (1978) Clinical trial of core glycolipid antibody in Gram-negative bacteremia. Trans Assoc Am Phys 91: 253–258
81. McCutchan JA, Wolf JL, Ziegler EJ, Braude AI (1983) Ineffectiveness of single dose human anti-serum to core glycolipid (*E. coli J5*) for prophylaxis of bacteremic Gram-negative infections in patients with prolonged neutropenia. Schweiz Med Wschr 113 (suppl 14): 40–45
82. Ziegler EJ, McCutchan JA, Douglas H, Braude AI (1975) Prevention of lethal *Pseudomonas* bacteremia with epimerase deficient *E. coli* antiserum. Trans Assoc Am Phys 88: 101–108
83. Baumgartner JD, Glauser MP, McCutchan JA et al. (1985) Prevention of Gram-negative shock and death in surgical patients by antibody to endotoxin core glycolipid. Lancet 2: 59–63
84. Girardin E, Grau G, Dayer J, Roux-Lombard P, J5 Study Group, Lambert PH (1988) Tumor necrosis factor and interleukin 1 in serum of children with severe infectious purpura. N Engl J Med 319: 397–400
85. Bysani GK, Shenep JL, Hildner WK et al. (1990) Detoxification of plasma containing lipopolysaccharide by adsorption. Crit Care Med 18: 67–71
86. Pfeiffer R, Kolle W (1986) Uber die speccifiscle Immunitatsreactin der Typhus-bacillii. Z Hyg Infektionskr 21: 203–214
87. Abnernathy RS, Spink WW (1958) Studies with *Brucella* endotoxin in humans, the significance of susceptibility to endotoxin in the pathogenesis of brucellosis. J Clin Invest 37: 219–231
88. Morgan HR (1941) Immunological properties of an antigenic material isolated from *Eberthella typhosa*. J Immunol 41: 161–180
89. Creech HJ, Hamilton MA, Nishimura ET, Hankwitz RF Jr (1948) The influence of antibody containing fractions on the lethal and tumor necrotizing actions of poylysaccharides from *Serratia marscesnus (Bacillus prodigiosus)*. Cancer Res 8: 330–338
90. Watson DW, Kim YB (1963) Modification of host responses to bacterial endotoxins. I. Specificity of pyrogenic tolerance and role of hypersensitivity in pyrogenicity, lethality and skin reactivity. J Exp Med 118: 425–446
91. McCabe WR, Greely A (1973) Common enterobacterial antigen. II. Effect of immunization on challenge with heterologous bacilli. Infect Immun 7: 386–392
92. McCabe WR, Johns M, DiGenio T (1973) Common enterobacterial antigen. III. Initial titer and antibody response in bacteremia caused by Gram-negative bacilli. Infect Immun 7: 393–397
93. Braude AI, Douglas H (1972) Passive immunization against the local Schwartzman reaction. J Immunol 108: 505–512
94. Ziegler EJ, Douglas H, Sherman JE, Davis CE, Braude AI (1973) Treatment of *E. coli* and *Klebsiella* bacteremia in agranulocytic animals with antiserum to a UDP-GAL-epimerase-deficient mutant. J Immunol 111: 433–438
95. Braude AI, Douglas H, Davis CE (1973) Treatment and prevention of intravascular coagulation with antiserum to endotoxin. J Infect Dis 128: S157–S164

96. McCabe WR, Kreger BE, Johns M (1972) Type specific and cross-reactive antibodies in Gram-negative bacteremia. N Engl J Med 287: 261–267
97. Dunn D, Furgeson R (1982) Immunotherapy of Gram-negative bacterial sepsis: Enhanced survival in a guinea pig model by use of rabbit antiserum to *Escherichia coli J5*. Surgery 92: 212–219
98. McCabe WR (1972) Immunization with R mutants of *S. minnesota*. I. Protection against challenge with heterologous Gram-negative bacilli. J Immunol 108: 601–610
99. Young LS, Stevens PR (1977) Cross-protective immunity to Gram negative bacilli: Studies with core glycolipid of *Salmonella minnesota* and antigens of *Streptococcus pneumoniae*. J Infect Dis 136 (suppl): S174–S180
100. Marks MI, Ziegler EJ, Douglas H, Corbeil LB, Braude AI (1982) Induction of immunity against lethal *Haemophilus influenza* type b infection by *Escherichia coli* core lipopolysaccharide. J Clin Invest 69: 742–749
101. Braude AI, Ziegler EJ, Douglas H, McCutchan JA (1977) Antibody to cell wall glycolipid of Gram-negative bacteria: Induction of immunity to bacteria and endotoxin. J Infect Dis 136: S167–S173
102. McCabe WR, Greely A, DiGenio T, Johns MA (1973) Humoral immunity to type-specific and cross-reactive antigens of Gram-negative bacilli. J Infect Dis 128: S284–289
103. Greisman SE, Dubut JB, Woodward CL (1978) Experimental Gram-negative bacterial sepsis: Re-evaluation of the ability of rough mutant antisera to protect mice. Proc Soc Exp Biol Med 158: 482–490
104. van Dijk WC, Verbrugh HA, Van Erne-Van der Tol ME, Peters R, Verhoef J (1981) *Escherichia coli* antibodies in opsonization and protection against infection. J Med Microbiol 14: 381–389
105. Brown KR, Douglas H, Braude AI (1971) Prevention of death from endotoxin with antiserum. II. Elimination of risk of anaphylaxis to endotoxin. J Immunol 106: 324–333
106. Freedman H (1959) Passive transfer of protection against lethality of homologous and heterologous endotoxins. Proc Soc Exp Biol Med 102: 504–506
107. Kim YB, Watson DW (1965) Modification of host responses to bacterial endotoxins. II. Passive transfer of immunity to containing 19S antibodies. J Exp Med 121: 751–759
108. Ziegler EJ, Douglas H, Braude A (1973) Human antiserum for prevention of the local Shwartzman reaction and death from bacterial lipopolysaccharide. J Clin Invest 52: 3236–3238
109. Braude AE (1980) Endotoxic immunity. Adv Intern Med 26: 427–445
110. Greisman S, Hornick R (1973) Mechanism of endotoxin tolerance with special reference to man. J Infect Dis 128: S265–S276
111. Pennington JE, Menkes E (1981) Type specific vs. cross-protection vaccination for Gram-negative bacterial pneumonia. J Infect Dis 144: 599–603
112. Pennington JE (1979) Lipopolysaccharide *Pseudomonas* vaccine: Efficacy against pulmonary infection with *Pseudomonas aeruginosa*. J Infect Dis 140: 73–80
113. Pennington JE (1980) Mechanism for pulmonary protection by lipopolysaccharide *Pseudomonas* vaccine. J Infect Dis 142: 191–198
114. Baumgartner JD, Heuman D, Weinbreck P, Grau GE, Glauser MP (1990) Association between protective efficacy of anti-lipopolysaccharide (LPS) antibodies and suppression of PS-induced tumor necrosis factor α and interleukin-6. J Exp Med 171: 889–896
115. Greisman SE, Young EJ, Dubut B (1973) Mechanisms of endotoxin tolerance. VIII. Specificity of serum transfer. J Immunol 111: 1349–1360
116. Baumgartner JD, Glauser MP (1990) Immunotherapy of Gram-negative septic shock. In: Vincent JL (ed) Update in intensive care and emergency medicine. Springer-Verlag, New York, 109–120
117. Mutharia LM, Crockford G, Bogard WC, Hancock RE (1984) Monoclonal antibodies specific for *E. coli J5* lipopolysaccharide: cross-reaction with other Gram-negative bacterial species. Infect Immun 45: 631–636
118. Young LS, Hoffman KR, Stevens P (1975) "Core" glycolipid of Enterobacteriaceae. Immunofluorescent detection of antigen and antibody. Proc Soc Exp Biol Med 149: 389–396
119. Lachman E, Samkar D, Pitsoe SB et al. (1985) Septic abortion in rats: Protection by human lipopolysaccharide-specific globulin. S Afr J Sci 81: 525–526
120. Wessels BC, Gaffin SL (1986) Anti-endotoxin immunotherapy for canine parvovirus endotoxemia. J Small Anim Pract 27: 609

121. Lachman E, Pitsoe SB, Gaffin SL (1984) Anti-lipopolysaccharide immunotherapy in management of septic shock of obstetric and gynaecological origin. Lancet 1: 981–983
122. Gaffin SL, Lachman E (1984) The use of anti-lipopolysaccharide (anti-LPS antibodies) in the management of septic shock. S Afr Med J 65: 158–161
123. Dunn DL, Bogard WC, Cerra FB (1985) Efficacy of type specific and cross-reactive murine monoclonal antibodies directed against endotoxin during experimental sepsis. Surgery 98: 283–290
124. Gorelick KJ, Harkonen S, Rosendorf LR, Wilson K, Greenberg RN (1988) Clinical investigation of anti-lipid A monoclonal antibody XOMEN-E5 in patients with Gram-negative sepsis (abstr). Critical Care Med 16: 166–167
125. McCabe WR, De Maria A, Berberich H, Johns MA (1988) Immunization with rough mutants of *Salmonella minnesota*: Protective activity of IgM and IgG antibody to the 595 (Re chemotype) mutant. J Infect Dis 158: 291
126. Zinner S, McCabe WR (1976) Effects of IgM and IgG antibody in patients with bacteremia due to Gram-negative bacilli. J Infect Dis 133: 37
127. Baumgartner JD, Heumann D, Callandra T, Glauser MP (1989) Antibodies to core LPS in patients with Gram-negative septic shock: Absence of correlation with outcome. In: Proceedings of the Interscience Am Soc Congress. Microbiol, Washington DC
128. Dunn DL, Mach PA, Condie RM, Cerra FB (1984) Anticore endotoxin Fab_2 equine immunoglobulin fragments protect against lethal effects of Gram-negative bacterial sepsis. Surgery 96: 440–446
129. Wolff JL, McCutchan JA, Ziegler EJ, Braude Al (1975) Prophylactic antibody to core lipopolysaccharide in neutropenia. In: Nelson JD, Grossi C (eds) Proceedings of the 17th Interscience Congress on Antimicrobial Agents and Chemotherapy. American Society for Microbiology, Washington DC, pp 439–441
130. Duswald KH, Muller K, Seifert J, Ring J, Wirksamkeit von IV (1980) Gammaglobulin gegen bakterielle Infektionen chirurgisher Patienten. Munch Med Wschr 122: 832–836
131. Glinz W, Grob PJ, Nydegger UE (1985) Polyvalent immunoglobulins for prophylaxis of bacterial infections in patients following multiple trauma. Int Care Med 11: 288–294
132. Rommelshein K (1989) Prophylaktische Einsatz von Pentaglobin in der Traumapatienten. Anasth Intensivther Notfallmed 24: 162–166
133. Class I, Schorer R (1989) Adjuvante Therapie mit Pseudomonas Immunoglobulin. Anasth Intensivther Notfallmed 24: 167–171
134. Schedel I, Dreikhausen U, Nentwig B et al. (1991) Treatment of Gram-negative septic shock with an immunoglobulin preparation: A prospective, randomized clinical trial. Crit Care Med 19: 1104–1113
135. Teng NNH, Kaplan HS, Hebert JM et al. (1985) Protection against Gram-negative bacteremia in endotoxemia with human monoclonal IgM antibodies. Proc Natl Acad Sci USA 82: 1790–1794
136. Young LS (1984) Functional activity of monoclonal antibodies against lipopolysaccharide (LPS) antigens of Gram-negative bacilli. Clin Res 32: 518A
137. Appelmelk BJ, Verweij-von vught AMJJ, Maaskant JJ, Schouten WF, Thijs LG, Maclaren DM (1987) Monoclonal antibodies detecting novel structures in the core region of *Salmonella minnesota* lipopolysaccharide. FEMS Microbiol Lett 40: 71–74
138. Pollack M, Chia JK, Koles NL, Guelde G (1988) Monoclonal antibodies that recognize epitopes in the core and lipid A region of lipopolysaccharides. Prog Clin Biol Res 272: 327–328
139. Young LS, Gascon R, Alam S, Bermeudez LE (1989) Monoclonal antibodies for treatment of Gram-negative infections. Rev Infect Dis 11 (suppl S7): 1564–1571
140. Kirkland TN, Colwell DE, Michalek SM, McGhee JR, Ziegler EJ (1986) Analysis of the fine specificity and cross-reactivity of monoclonal anti-lipid A antibodies. J Immunol 137: 3614–3619
141. Miner KM, Manyak CL, Williams E (1986) Characterization of murine monoclonal antibodies to *Escherichia coli J5*. Infect Immun 52: 56–62
142. Gorelick K, Jacobs R, Chmel H, Trenholme G, Greenman R, XOMA Sepsis Study Group (1990) Efficacy results of a randomized multi-center trial of E5 anti-endotoxin antibody in patients with Gram-negative sepsis. In: 29th International Conference on Antimicrobial Agents and Chemotherapy. Am Soc Microbiol, Washington DC 101 (abstr 2)
143. Gorelick K, Scannon PJ, Hannigan J, Wedel N, Ackerman SK (1990) Randomized placebo controlled study of E5 monoclonal anti-endotoxin antibody. In: Larrick J, Borrebaeck C (eds) Therapeutic monoclonal antibodies. Stratton, New York, pp 253–264

144. SCRIP World Pharmaceutical Newsletter (1991) PJB Publications, UK, vol 1659, October 11, p 22
145. Swarz JR (1991) Goldman Sachs Investment Research, Centocor Inc., November 11
146. Quezado ZMN, Natanson C, Banks SM et al. (1992) A human IgM monoclonal antibody (MAb) against endotoxin (HA-1A) decreased survival in a canine model of Gram-negative bacterial septic shock. Clin Res 40(2): 286A (abstr)
147. Letters (1991) N Engl J Med 325: 279–283
148. deGroote MA, Martin MA, Densen P, Pfaller MA, Wenzel RP (1989) Plasma tumor necrosis factor levels in patients with presumed sepsis: results in those treated with anti-lipid A antibody versus placebo. JAMA 262: 249–251
149. Wortel CH, Sprung CL, Van Deventer SJH, Lubbers MJ, ten Cate JW (1990) Anti-endotoxin treatment with HA1A: Possible mechanism of beneficial effects in patients with Gram-negative septicemia. In: Proceedings of the Interscience Congress for Infectious Diseases and Antimicrobial Agents and Chemotherapy, Montreal Am Soc Microbiol, Washington DC, p 206

10 Cytokine Antibodies and Antagonists in the Treatment of Sepsis

A.P. Wheeler and K.L. Brigham

Introduction

Sepsis syndrome is a constellation of clinical findings that includes three major features: a site of inflammation; presence of abnormal vital signs (altered temperature, tachycardia and an increased minute ventilation); and at least one organ system failure (renal, hepatic, circulatory, haematological or neurological). More than 400 000 cases of sepsis syndrome occur in the USA alone each year, resulting in the expenditure of 5–10 billion dollars annually (1). The case fatality rate ranges from 20% to 60% (2,3). Importantly, one-half of afflicted patients have no demonstrable infection (4) and numerous non-infectious disorders mimic sepsis syndrome. These two facts have prompted investigators to propose renaming "sepsis syndrome" the "systemic inflammatory response syndrome" (SIRS), emphasizing that infection is not essential and that the host response is the critical determinant of severity. Although SIRS may result from non-infectious causes or viral, fungal or Gram-positive infections, Gram-negative bacteria constitute the single largest group of microbiological isolates, accounting for about one-third of all cases (1,4–6).

Despite the development of critical care units, antibiotics, haemodynamic monitoring, mechanical ventilators, haemodialysis and intravenous nutrition, the mortality rate of SIRS remains high. The use of agents such as corticosteroids and opiate antagonists has failed to improve mortality, making innovative immunological therapies attractive (4,7–10).

Toxin Initiation of Sepsis

To initiate SIRS, it is less important that live microorganisms are present in the host than it is that toxins from these agents stimulate host cells. Dead microorganisms, exotoxins, endotoxins and lipid A (the active component of endotoxin) are all highly toxic. Endotoxin, a Gram-negative bacterial cell wall lipopolysaccharide (LPS), is the principal toxin triggering inflammation during Gram-negative sepsis and as such, has attracted the most attention as a target for immunological intervention.

Despite some valuable properties, there are substantial limitations to LPS antagonists. First, only 30%–40% of patients with sepsis syndrome have demonstrable endotoxaemia (11) suggesting that LPS antagonists will consistently fail to offer benefit to roughly two-thirds of treated patients. Secondly, because of the structural heterogeneity of endotoxins, even antibodies designed to be cross-reactive will bind some LPS poorly and fail to bind others. Even complete, avid and irreversible LPS–antibody binding does not guarantee LPS inactivation. Thirdly, because of the usually brief duration of endotoxaemia and the rapidity with which LPS initiates inflammation, therapy after the onset of sepsis will be less than uniformly successful. As a practical matter, endotoxin antagonists may not be administered rapidly enough to protect against LPS in the clinical setting.

Most physiological changes of SIRS are not directly caused by microbiological toxins but instead result from the endogenous mediators tumour necrosis factor alpha (TNFα), interleukin-1 (IL-1) and interleukin-6 (IL-6). Hence, an understanding of the actions of these proteins, collectively known as cytokines, is essential. Cytokines exhibit autocrine, paracrine and endocrine effects mediated by binding to specific receptors on target cells. These cytokines are in general inflammatory, causing the production of acute-phase reactants and leukocyte adhesion molecules while suppressing production of constitutive proteins such as albumin, cytochrome P450 enzymes and lipoprotein lipase. Cytokines are critical intermediaries in the production of prostaglandins (12–15), platelet activating factor (16,17), coagulant proteins (18,19) and other cytokines. The attenuated production of TNF after repeated endotoxin challenge is at least a partial explanation for the tolerance to LPS observed in vivo (20).

Properties of TNF, IL-1, IL-6 and their Receptors

Tumour Necrosis Factor

Tumour necrosis factor alpha (TNFα), also known as cachectin, is a highly conserved 233 amino acid, 17.4 kDa protein (21–24). While it is likely that TNFα can be produced by all nucleated cells, it is thought to be predominantly a blood monocyte and tissue macrophage product (25). The active form of TNFα is a trimer of the basic protein (26–28). A similar lymphocyte product, TNFβ, also known as lymphotoxin, circulates in low concentrations and probably plays a minor role in SIRS (29). In man, the TNFα and TNFβ genes are closely linked on chromosome 6 near the major histocompatibility complex region.

Within minutes of stimulation, TNFα messenger RNA can be recovered from cultured cells and mature protein can be found in cell supernatants and the circulation of animals (30–34). After a discrete intravenous challenge in vivo, TNFα levels typically peak within 1–3 h and wane within 4–6 h; however, lower levels of TNFα production and prolonged TNFα elaboration have been described in some models. Two receptors (type I and type II) specific for TNF have been cloned (35–43), both of which bind TNFα and TNFβ (44). With the exception of red blood cells, all cells studied have either type I, II or both TNFα receptors.

The effects of TNFα mimic the sepsis syndrome. These effects include altered haemodynamics, lung mechanics, oxygenation, fever and cachexia, as well as leukocyte and coagulation activation, and the production of acute-phase reactants (21,22,45–50). Neutrophils accentuate the degree of injury caused by TNFα, but even profound reduction in neutrophil counts does not preclude the development of acute lung injury (46). The effects of TNFα depend both on the TNF level and on the site of production (51–53). TNF is distinguished from most other cytokines by its ability to lyse some transformed cells. Bioactive TNF can be detected by measuring mouse L929 fibroblast or WEHI cell lysis (54,55). Immunoreactive TNF can be measured using radioimmunoassay and enzyme-linked immunoassay. Measurement of bioactivity and immunological reactivity are complementary because allosteric alterations can alter bioactivity without changing immunoreactivity, and binding to soluble receptors and antibodies may negate biological activity while immunoreactivity is preserved.

Interleukin-1

In almost all aspects studied, IL-1 mimics the biological effects of TNFα (15,56,57). Unlike TNF, IL-1 also causes T-cell proliferation through the induction of IL-2 but does not cause cytolysis. Alone and together, TNFα and IL-1 have potent effects on endothelial cell–neutrophil adhesion and activation (58,59). Although endothelial production of IL-1 is likely to be important, blood monocytes and tissue macrophages are the predominant cell sources. In vivo IL-1 tends to be produced more slowly and for longer periods than TNF.

Two structurally diverse forms of IL-1 (IL-1α and IL-1β) have been identified. Both produce identical actions by binding to a common receptor (60–63). Two different IL-1 receptors have been isolated and their presence has been demonstrated on the surface of most mammalian cells (64). The gene for the murine IL-1β receptor (IL-1βR) has been cloned and codes for an 80 kDa plasma membrane glycoprotein (62,65). Both forms of IL-1 result from processing a larger precursor into mature 17 kDa proteins (60,61). The carboxy terminus of IL-1 is the critical portion of the molecule for biological activity (61). IL-1β represents more than 90% of both the IL-1 mRNA and active protein secreted in vitro by human monocytes following LPS challenge and is the predominant form of IL-1 circulating in septic animals. Biological assay is based on the ability of IL-1β to potentiate mitogen effects on thymocytes (66). Radioimmunoassay and ELISAs for human and murine IL-1β and IL-1α are also available.

Interleukin-6

IL-6, originally named interferon β2 (IFN-β2), is a 21 kDa 184 amino acid glycoprotein (67) having a specific 80 kDa receptor (68,69). IL-6 is produced by many cells including endothelial cells, activated T cells, lung fibroblasts and monocytes. IL-6 production may be induced by TNF or IL-1 (70). Multiple biological activities have been attributed to IL-6, but the role in sepsis is unknown (71,72). IL-6 causes hepatic production of acute-phase reactants and reduces albumin synthesis (73,74) while simultaneously stimulating B lymphocytes to augment immunoglobulin production (75). IL-6 is a pyrogen (76), promotes expression of IL-2 and IL-2 receptors (77) and cytolytic T cell differentiation (78) and stimulates thrombopoiesis (79–81). A human 80 kDa IL-6 glycoprotein receptor for IL-6 has been isolated. This receptor is unique in that it does not require the cytoplasmic domain for signal transduction. A 50 kDa soluble form of the receptor produced by proteolytic cleavage of the extracellular domain from cell surfaces has also been detected (82). Detection of IL-6 by bioassay uses an IL-6 dependent cell line in a similar fashion to that described for IL-1 (66). Unlike TNF, the structure of IL-6 is not highly conserved. Murine and human amino acid sequences are only 41% homologous making it surprising that in most cases IL-6 is not species specific. Like TNF and IL-1, IL-6 expression is not exclusively due to sepsis (83–87).

Cytokine Interactions in Inflammation

The actions of cytokines are complex. On occasions a single agent may have contrasting actions on different target cells. For example, TNFα is cytolytic for some cell lines (54,55), inhibitory for others (88), but acts as a growth factor for still others (89–92). The actions of cytokines also commonly overlap as is the case with TNFα and IL-1β (93).

Because cytokine functions may be redundant and because one cytokine may stimulate or inhibit the production of another, it is often difficult to distinguish the compound responsible for a given action (76,94). For example, in vivo and in vitro, TNFα administration results in its own production (94), as well as that of IL-1 (95–97) and IL-6 (98–102). IL-1 also induces itself, TNFα and IL-6 (103,104). In contrast, IL-6 does not cause TNFα or IL-1 production. IL-2 may also induce TNFα (94,105,106), and IL-6 (101,107) production. Cytokines also act synergistically: this is the case with TNFα and IL-1β induced septic shock (108–110); with IL-1β and IL-6 induced thymocyte stimulation (111) and immunoglobulin production (93,112–114); and with the inflammatory effects of TNFα and interferon gamma (114–116).

Recognition of the synergistic and autoamplifying interactions of cytokines is important because it suggests that inhibition of one cytokine could interrupt the inflammatory cascade. This suspicion has been borne out in vivo where TNFα antibodies dramatically reduce IL-1 and IL-6 production (117,118). TNF may also directly synergize with endotoxin in causing injury in vivo (119). The actions of one cytokine may also be inhibited by another as when IL-6, IL-1 or TGFβ down-regulate TNFα or IL-1 production (120–123), or when IL-1 exposure blunts the action of TNFα, LPS or other inflammatory stimuli (123). Interestingly, low doses of TNFα or IL-1 given several hours in advance prevent death from an otherwise lethal TNFα challenge (124).

Cytokines are normally tightly regulated by unique mechanisms. For example, when used prophylactically, LPS-induced TNFα production is inhibited by corticosteroids (125), prostaglandin E_2 (126) and pentoxifylline (127), while these same compounds usually have no effect on IL-1 or IL-6 production (57,127–131). Timing of application is also a critical issue with these inhibitors. Corticosteroids and pentoxifylline are potent inhibitors of TNFα production when applied before LPS stimulation, but have no effect when applied afterwards (127,132–135). Cytokines are also regulated by arachidonic acid products and treatment with cyclooxygenase inhibitors before septic stimulation may even augment TNF production (136).

Cytokines are not entirely detrimental and some are necessary for normal immune function. For example, the removal of TNFα dramatically reduces the ability to control infection (123–125,137–141) and pretreatment with IL-1 or TNF may augment bacterial defenses (123,124). However, at high local concentrations or when released into the circulation, cytokines are deleterious. Knowledge of the beneficial effects of cytokines dictates that therapy designed to interrupt cytokine action during sepsis must be specific and brief.

Evidence that Cytokines are Involved in Sepsis

TNFα Deficiency Prevents the Effects of Endotoxin

C3HeJ mice are resistant to the effects of endotoxin, a property conferred by their inability to produce TNFα (125). Sensitivity to LPS can be restored by marrow transplantation using endotoxin-sensitive donors. Although a genetic deficiency of TNFα has not been described in humans, this experiment of nature suggests that TNFα plays a pivotal role in SIRS. While resistant to LPS, the C3HeJ mouse remains sensitive to live bacteria suggesting a beneficial role for TNFα in vivo.

Cytokines Circulate Following Toxin Challenge

The appearance of cytokines in the circulation following toxin challenge has now been measured in numerous animal and human studies despite technical problems complicating these measurements (142). Most studies demonstrate that limited intravenous infusions of bacteria or their toxins cause a sequential rise in TNFα, IL-1β and IL-6 (128). Following a discrete stimulus, TNFα elevations are brief (24,31–34,128,143–145) and sometimes negligible (31). However in some experimental models (33) and in septic humans, especially those in shock, TNFα levels may remain elevated for days (146–150).

Zaneti et al. (33) and Bagby et al. (151) have provided enlightening data in this area. Following intravenous (IV) challenge of mice with lethal doses of endotoxin or bacteria, rapid transient increases in plasma TNFα levels are followed by increases in IL-1 and IL-6. A dose–response relationship exists between LPS or bacterial dose and cytokine response. Bacterial clearance in this model is neither impeded nor enhanced by TNFα antibody. In IV-challenged animals, TNFα returns to baseline prior to death, while IL-1 and IL-6 levels remain elevated until death. Similar results have been seen in bacteraemic baboons (117). However, striking differences in peak cytokine levels and duration occur when the challenge is an intraperitoneal infected clot. Although a dose–response relationship between inoculum and TNFα level is maintained, peak levels occur more slowly and reach only 1%–2% of those seen after IV challenge. Substantially lower levels of plasma TNFα after peritoneal challenge have been reported by Bagby et al. (151). Zaneti et al. (33) also found that plasma TNFα levels after peritoneal challenge usually remain elevated until death. IL-1 levels are very low or undetectable in surviving animals, while IL-6 levels are strongly correlated with mortality.

Michie et al. (152) infused 4 ng/m^2 of *Escherichia coli* endotoxin into 13 healthy men, then measured serum TNFα and IL-1β. TNFα levels rose from a baseline of 35 pg/ml to peak at 240 pg/ml 1 h later, but IL-1β levels did not increase. TNFα rose concurrently with the onset of fever, tachycardia and increases in adrenocorticotrophic hormone (ACTH) and epinephrine concentrations. Suffredini et al. (153) also found brief elevations in plasma TNFα in nine of 12 volunteers given 4 ng/m^2 of LPS. Specific organ production of TNFα has also been demonstrated during experimental human endotoxaemia (154,155). Cannon et al. (156) reported that both plasma TNFα and IL-1β increased in LPS-challenged humans, but also noted that TNFα elevations were of greater magnitude and occurred faster (peak levels at 90 min) than IL-1β, where peak concentrations occurred at 180 min. Similar timing in peak TNFα (90 min) and IL-1β (120 min) levels were seen in four humans and four baboons injected with LPS by Hesse et al. (31). Not only do TNFα and IL-1 levels increase after LPS, but IL-6 and G-CSF levels also rise with peak concentrations observed 2–4 h after challenge (157,158).

Cytokines Circulate in Inflammatory States

The presence of cytokines cannot be regarded exclusively as a marker of infection (31, 159). For example, elevation of TNFα has been reported in parasitic infestation (160), renal allograft rejection (161,162), heart failure (163) and neoplasia (164). TNFα, IL-1 and IL-6 have also been recovered from localized sites of inflammation such as bronchoalveolar lavage fluid from patients with adult respiratory distress syndrome (ARDS) (165–168) and animals given intraperitoneal LPS (151); in the blood and joint fluid of patients with rheumatoid arthritis (169–174); and the cerebrospinal fluid of patients with bacterial meningitis and head trauma (175–184). Local and systemic increases in cytokines have also been observed in patients with thermal burns (147), surgery (86), psoriasis (84) and renal allograft rejection (161,162).

TNFα, IL-1β and IL-6 circulate in humans with sepsis syndrome and there is a relationship between cytokine concentration and host reaction. Debets et al. (159) detected TNFα in 25% of 43 patients with sepsis syndrome. Marks et al. (146) found TNFα at a similar frequency (33%) in serial plasma samples from 25 patients with Gram-negative septic shock compared with only 10%

in a non-septic control population. Waage et al. (175,176) reported that ten of 11 patients who died from meningococcal disease had elevated TNFα levels while only eight of 68 survivors had similar elevations. All five patients with TNFα levels exceeding 100 pg/ml died (175,176). Casey et al. (185,186) found that TNFα, IL-1 and LPS were frequently elevated in septic (Gram-positive and Gram-negative) shock patients; there was no clear prognostic value of LPS or cytokine levels, although persistent elevation of TNFα and IL-1 and high TNFα levels were associated with greater likelihood of developing shock. Regression analysis suggested that endotoxaemia occurring in the absence of detectable IL-1 was a lethal combination. Dofferhoff et al. (187) measured TNFα and IL-6 in 20 bacteraemic patients. Ninety-four per cent had detectable TNFα and all had detectable IL-6, by contrast to low or absent levels in non-septic intensive care unit (ICU) patients. Non-survivors had higher TNFα and IL-6 levels at entry (187). Although Gram-positive and Gram-negative sepsis causes cytokine release (146,159,185,186), some microorganisms are more likely to cause profound TNFα elevations. For example, Girardin et al. (188) and Waage et al. (175,176) have described elevated plasma TNFα as a nearly universal feature of severe meningococcaemia.

Among burned patients, a relationship exists between TNFα levels and sepsis. Eleven of 16 (69%) patients with clinical episodes of sepsis had detectable TNFα levels, whereas only nine of 27 (33%) without sepsis had detectable TNFα (146). TNF elevations in these patients were brief but repetitive and the mortality in patients with detectable TNFα exceeded 70% compared with only 33% in patients without detectable TNFα.

The relationship between IL-1 level and mortality is less certain. It has been reported that IL-1β is increased in up to 21% of patients with Gram-negative sepsis (188), but neither the absolute IL-1 level nor its duration has been associated with increased mortality (185,186,189). Plasma IL-6 concentrations are elevated in 90% of patients with sepsis syndrome and correlate with elevated plasma lactate levels, tachycardia, hypotension and thrombocytopenia (176,190,191). Hack et al. (192) reported that over 85% of culture-positive septic patients had detectable levels of IL-6. Neither the type of bacteria nor the site of infection had a significant impact on IL-6 levels. Plasma IL-6 concentrations in septic shock were sometimes 100-fold greater than those of normotensive septic patients (192).

Magnitude and Duration of Cytokine Responses Correlate with Illness Severity

Several studies have examined the relationship between cytokine levels, severity of sepsis and mortality. Taken together, the findings indicate that persistent or profound elevations of TNFα, IL-1β and IL-6 are associated with a higher mortality.

In sepsis, TNFα levels correlate with the severity of pulmonary dysfunction (146), illness scores (146,175,176,189), level of plasma fibrinogen (188) and mortality rate (146,159,188). Damas et al. (189) found a positive correlation between plasma TNFα concentration and sepsis severity score; the highest scores were seen in patients with fatal bacteraemia (189). In this study, a

92% (12/13) mortality rate was observed in patients with TNFα levels greater than 200 pg/ml, but only 36% (5/14) of patients died when TNF levels were below 200 pg/ml. Debets et al. (159) reported a similar relationship between TNFα level and mortality, where death was roughly twice as common in 43 ICU patients with detectable TNFα than in patients with undetectable TNFα levels: 73% (8/11) versus 34% (11/32). Because of the small numbers, no correlation could be drawn between TNFα level and outcome. Baud et al. (149) have also reported TNFα levels in a small group of patients with septic shock. All patients had elevated TNFα levels on admission. The patients could be divided into two groups, those with persistent TNF elevations who always died, and those with declining levels who had a lower mortality rate (20%) (149).

In contrast to Damas et al. (189), studies by Callandra et al. (193,194) and Dofferhoff et al. (187) indicate that the duration of cytokine elevation is more critical than absolute level. Dofferhoff et al. found that substantial elevations of cytokines at the onset of sepsis may be associated with death, but that the duration of cytokine circulation is more important (187). Occasionally TNFα and IL-1 circulate for days after the onset of septic shock (193,194). Persistent cytokine elevation in humans is a poor prognostic sign and agrees with experimental models in which TNFα levels are more likely to remain elevated in non-survivors (33). Pinsky et al (150) found that TNFα levels were elevated in 52 septic shock patients when compared with a hypotensive control group. A mortality rate of 33% was seen in patients with elevated TNFα levels; however, no consistent pattern of cytokine elevation was observed. Although TNFα and IL-6 levels were higher in the septic group, there was no correlation between initial or peak TNFα or IL-6 level and outcome. However, in patients with a plasma TNF greater than 150 pg/ml 24 h after study entry, the mortality rate was 50%.

Waage et al. (175,176) also reported an association between IL-1β and IL-6 levels and a fatal outcome, and suggested that TNFα alone may not be sufficient to cause death. In this study, high levels of IL-6 combined with elevated TNFα levels were associated with a fatal outcome. Elevations of IL-1β occurred exclusively in patients with high levels of IL-6 and TNFα and a rapidly fatal outcome. Callandra et al. have reported that IL-6 levels are detectable in most patients at an early stage of Gram-negative septic shock, but these levels rapidly decline. In contrast to the findings of Dofferhoff et al. (187), the poor predictive value of IL-6 levels in these patients rendered IL-6 levels clinically useless (194). In 40 patients with *Plasmodium falciparum* infection, Kern et al. (190) found a correlation between serum concentrations of TNFα and IL-6 and the density of parasitaemia. Grau et al. (191) have also reported a correlation between TNFα plasma level and mortality in children with malaria. Dofferhoff et al. (187) found a correlation between IL-6 level and outcome. Callandra et al. (193) noted that the initial serum levels of TNFα were elevated and remained elevated for 10 days in 13 non-survivors compared with lower and decreasing levels in 34 survivors of Gram-negative sepsis. Marano et al. (147) reported similar findings in 43 burn victims in whom the presence of detectable TNFα in the peripheral circulation predicted mortality. Data from Hack et al. (192) indicated that IL-6 levels are elevated in both survivors and non-survivors of sepsis, but there was a correlation between admission IL-6 level and mortality in both shock and non-shock patients.

Administration of Purified Cytokines Mimics Sepsis

In animals and man the infusion of recombinant TNFα, IL-1β and IL-2 results in physiological alterations identical to those seen in SIRS (153,195–197). It is likely that IL-2-induced hypotension is caused by production of IL-1 and TNFα (107). In rodents, recombinant TNFα (rTNFα) causes neutrophilia, haemoconcentration and hypovolaemic shock by increasing vascular permeability (198,199). Similar organ damage and circulatory collapse are seen during TNFα infusions in dogs (200,201) and rabbits (202). Studies in sheep and pigs have also shown that TNFα has comparable effects on haemodynamics and extravascular lung water as LPS, although TNFα acts more rapidly (203). Johnson et al. (204) infused rTNFα into chronically instrumented conscious sheep and found that it caused pulmonary hypertension, hypoxaemia, leukopenia and the generation of prostanoid mediators. Increases in protein-rich lymph flow suggested an increased pulmonary microvascular permeability. Changes in vascular permeability have also been shown by Stephens et al. (205) and Goldblum et al. (206,207). Administration of TNFα to chronically instrumented sheep has demonstrated intense pulmonary sequestration of granulocytes and perivascular oedema (208). In sheep, Wheeler et al. (209) confirmed the haemodynamic results and demonstrated a decline in lung compliance and increases in airway resistance and airway reactivity after TNFα. TNF-induced enhanced airway reactivity has been confirmed in rodents (210). Similar changes in sheep given TNF have also been shown by Redl et al. (211) and Kreil et al. (212). Kettelhut, Evans, Wheeler and others have demonstrated that many of the effects of TNFα are attenuated by cyclooxygenase inhibitors (12,14,213).

In man and animals, TNFα causes rapid leukopenia followed by leukocytosis and lymphopenia, fever, increased serum cortisol and C-reactive protein levels, a decrease in serum zinc levels, and alterations in amino acid metabolism (108,214). However, TNFα is unique in that it is the only cytokine that can produce shock and death on its own (199). While synergy with IL-1 (108,118,215) or interferon gamma (216) may accelerate death in these models, IL-1 and interferon gamma cannot cause death by themselves (199,200).

In rabbits, large intravenous doses of either TNFα or IL-1β increase cardiac output, reduce systemic vascular resistance and cause hypotension (108,109,217). Doses of IL-1β and TNFα that on their own cannot alter haemodynamics, result in a profound shock state when given in combination (108). Like TNFα the effects of IL-1 can be altered by cyclooxygenase inhibitors (108).

The investigations leading to the discovery of TNFα focused not on the induction of sepsis or shock but rather on the cachexia producing properties of TNF. The metabolic effects of TNFα and other cytokines have been reviewed by Tracey et al. (218) and Grimble (219). Acute inflammation is usually associated with an alteration in the profile of circulating proteins referred to as the acute-phase reaction. The acute-phase reaction includes increases in the concentration of fibrinogen, C-reactive protein, α-1 protease inhibitor, ceruloplasmin, haptoglobin and complement factor C3, and decreases in the serum albumin concentration. In vitro studies with IL-1β, TNFα, and IL-6 suggest that cytokines are central to the alteration of protein metabolism (220). Mortensen et al. (221) reported that recombinant IL-1β and recombinant TNFα synergistically increased the appearance of acute-phase reactants and serum amyloid P-component. TNFα and IL-1β decreased albumin synthesis and enhanced the production of acute-phase proteins in cultured hepatoma cells (73,222). Gauldie et al. (73) and Morrone et al. (220) showed that IL-6 is a major inducer of acute-phase protein stimulation in vivo. Clinical studies showing a relationship between IL-6 and the acute-phase reaction are emerging. For example, Nijsten et al. (223) reported a relationship between IL-6 activity in serum and C-reactive protein levels in 21 burn patients. There is a sequential relationship between endotoxin treatment, a rise in IL-6 levels and the appearance of C-reactive protein in the circulation of man (223). TNFα also has potent effects on the clotting system including stimulation of plasminogen activator inhibitor (187,224).

Watters et al. (225) injected seven volunteers three times daily for 4 days with etiocholanolone, which is thought to induce in vivo production of IL-1β. This caused fever, leukocytosis and increased serum C-reactive protein production. IL-1 has also been infused into humans in an attempt to treat refractory malignancies; however the dose is limited by hypotension (226). The effects of IL-1 are in part ameliorated by cyclooxygenase inhibitor treatment. The hypotension caused by IL-1 is not entirely due to prostaglandin production because nitric oxide also plays a role (227). Intravenous administration of IL-1 in humans produces toxicity at doses less than 1μg/kg thus limiting human use (228).

Several studies have reported the pharmacodynamics of rTNFα treatment in man (214,228–233). Chapman et al. (231) infused rTNFα in 26 patients with advanced cancer. In these patients, initial serum concentrations of TNFα ranged from 2.5 ng/ml to 80 ng/ml following IV administration of 35 $\mu g/m^2$ and 200 $\mu g/m^2$, respectively, with a half-life of 20 min. The short half-life of exogenous TNFα in humans has been confirmed by Blick et al. (214). Starnes et al. (230) infused TNFα in humans with similar results. Demetri et al. (234) also infused TNFα into humans with cancers with or without interferon gamma. Chills, rigors and fever were universal. Nausea and vomiting were common and doses in excess of 91 $\mu g/m^2$ always caused hypotension. The hypotension observed with TNF infusion was exacerbated by the administration of interferon gamma, an effect similar to that seen in animals (202). The uncontrolled use of indomethacin reportedly resulted in attenuation of symptoms due to TNF and interferon. Administration of TNFα to cancer patients increased IL-6 levels within minutes, peaking 2–3 h later (235).

Therapeutic Strategies

Two recent studies claim that antibodies to LPS improve survival of Gram-negative bacteraemia in humans, (236,237) but conflicting data exist (238–240) and the biological effectiveness of these antibodies is not striking. Endotoxin antagonists are reviewed in detail elsewhere in this volume. Some evidence suggests that anti-endotoxins blunt cytokine production (131); however, direct antagonism of cytokines offers an independent opportunity for intervention with cytokine antibodies, soluble inhibitors and receptor antagonists.

Anti-cytokine Antibodies

Beutler et al. were the first to report that pretreatment with a polyclonal rabbit antiserum to murine TNFα prevented LPS-induced death. However, these studies indicated only a narrow therapeutic window (241). In mice, Grau et al. (242) have suggested that post-treatment with anti-TNFα antibodies may have limited effectiveness. Similar results were obtained by Mathison et al. (202) using polyclonal anti-TNFα prophylactically in rabbits. Hypotension, fibrin deposition and death were prevented by antisera given before LPS challenge (202). Silva et al. (243) have reported beneficial effects with TNFα monoclonal antibodies in bacteraemic mice. Antibodies given before or up to 30 min after the LD_{90} of *E. coli: 0111* improved 72 h survival rates to near 80%. However, the physical appearance of the mice was not improved, suggesting that non-TNFα pathways are also active. Delay in antibody treatment of 2.5 h reduced survival to only 25%. A 50% improvement in survival at 72 h was observed using anti-TNF antibodies before giving *Pseudomonas aeruginosa*, but there was no improvement in survival when cyclophosphamide-conditioned mice were challenged with *Klebsiella pneumoniae*. Regardless of the type of septic challenge, administration of TNF antibody reduced serum TNFα levels but did not impair or enhance clearance of bacteria from blood or tissue. Interestingly, serum TNFα levels were highest in *E. coli*-challenged animals and were ten-fold greater than those previously reported in LPS-challenged mice (244), rabbits (202) or baboons (215). Similar improvements in survival with anti-TNF antibodies have also been demonstrated in rats with *Pseudomonas* bacteraemia (245,246).

However, there are conflicting data. Peritonitis models have not demonstrated any benefit of anti-TNFα treatment despite effectiveness in intravenous models of endotoxaemia (151,247,248). Using a murine model of sepsis, Zaneti et al. (33) have shown that the site of inflammation affects the profile of cytokines generated and hence the effectiveness of TNFα antibodies. Mice challenged with lethal doses of intravenous *E. coli* LPS had brief but profound TNFα elevations and were highly protected by anti-TNF antibody. In contrast, following mucin-clot peritonitis, anti-TNFα was ineffective in reducing cytokine generation or improving survival (33); furthermore, the profile of cytokine release was dramatically different. Bagby et al. (151) reported low plasma levels of TNFα in rats with peritonitis; anti-TNFα antibodies were not protective. By contrast, intravenously challenged rats had substantial protection by TNF antibody therapy. In addition to blocking the acute effects of TNFα administration, TNF antibodies may prevent the chronic wasting effects of TNFα (249)

In baboons, Tracey et al. (215) administered TNFα monoclonal $F(ab')_2$

antibody fragments prior to lethal *E. coli* challenge. $F(ab')_2$ given 2 h before bacteraemia prevented shock and organ failure, but treatment 1 h before *E. coli* challenge was not beneficial. Fong et al. (117) later reported that the $F(ab')_2$ antibody abolished detectable serum TNF and attenuated IL-1β and the IL-6 production by more than 95%. Zaneti et al. (33) have confirmed the quenching effect of TNFα antibodies on IL-1 and IL-6 production in mice. Further studies by Hinshaw et al. (34) investigated the usefulness of anti-TNFα after the onset of sepsis. Anaesthetized baboons were given a lethal intravenous dose of *E. coli*, then were treated with TNF antibody or placebo 30 min later. All six treated baboons survived for 7 days without evidence of organ failure. By contrast, all baboons receiving placebo died within 34 h. TNFα antibody had no effect on leukopenia, thrombocytopenia or hypofibrinogaemia. Tachycardia, tachypnoea and decreases in blood pressure were observed in both groups but were more marked in the placebo group. Cortisol levels increased in antibody-treated animals but not in controls. Anti-TNF treatment did not affect bacterial clearance. Both groups also had elevated lactate and creatinine concentrations, but these abnormalities were more marked in the placebo group. The histological damage to the lungs, adrenals, spleen and liver was attenuated by TNF antibody. In contrast to other models of sepsis, the baboons had no evidence of bowel, stomach, gallbladder or pancreatic damage.

After demonstrating beneficial effects in primates (250), Exley et al. reported preliminary observations of a phase I study of a murine monoclonal antibody (CB0006) to TNFα in 14 patients with septic shock (251). Administration of the antibody was free of immediate toxicity and was associated with a rise in mean arterial pressure. Unfortunately, mortality remained high and lack of a control group prevents interpretation of either the physiological or survival data. Anomalous findings in this study included a 100% incidence of endotoxaemia and only a 14% incidence of detectable TNFα in plasma. Using the same TNFα antibody in ten patients, Vincent et al. (252) reported disappointing results. Minimal reductions in heart rate and increases in left ventricular stroke work index were seen in treated patients, together with transient improvements in gas exchange. Despite achieving statistical improvements in two cardiovascular parameters, the changes are of questionable biological significance. Again the lack of a control group precludes interpretation except to confirm there is no major immediate toxicity associated with the antibody.

Grau et al. (254) have demonstrated that TNFα antibodies block lethal brain damage in murine models of malaria. Concerns that removal of TNFα might hamper the host clearance of bacteria from the circulation are unfounded (33,34,215,243). However, there are data to suggest that use of anti-TNFα antibodies may worsen the outcome (141,255,256).

Circulating Cytokine Inhibitors and Receptor Antagonists

Soluble inhibitors have been described for IL-1 (257–267), IL-2 (264), IL-6 (82) and TNFα (103,266). These proteins are structurally similar to either the cytokine itself or the extracellular domain of the cytokine receptor.

The largest amount of data has been generated using a 20–25 kDa IL-1 receptor antagonist (IL-1ra) originally named the IL-1 inhibitor. Prieur et al. (260) originally reported an IL-1 inhibitor in serum and urine of children with juvenile arthritis. Seckinger et al. then purified an 18–25 kDa IL-1α inhibitor from human urine (257,258). This protein binds to the IL-1 receptor; it blocks access by IL-1 but does not activate the receptor (257,258,263) or block the effects of TNFα or IL-2 (257–259). The IL-1 inhibitor also blocks synovial cell PGE_2 production, thymocyte proliferation and insulin release from pancreatic tissue. Human IL-1ra has been shown to be produced by monocytes and alveolar macrophages (267). Eisenberg et al. (261) isolated the cDNA for the IL-1 receptor inhibitor and found a structure similar to IL-1β. The IL-1 inhibitor/receptor antagonist has now been cloned (261,262).

IL-1ra prevents death in endotoxaemic rabbits (217) and in those given lethal *E. coli* bacteraemia (266) or IL-1 injections. An initial reduction in systemic vascular resistance results in hypotension in both treated and untreated animals, but hypotension occurs to a lesser degree in IL-1ra treated animals and reverses more quickly. IL-1ra blunts the decline in peripheral leukocyte count and pulmonary accumulation of neutrophils, but has no effect on thrombocytopenia. TNFα and IL-1 levels were not reduced by IL-1ra treatment (217,266). IL-1ra can also prevent lethal *Klebsiella* sepsis in newborn rats (268) and *E. coli* sepsis in baboons. It also has the attractive potential of being effective after the onset of sepsis, working 2 h after lethal *E. coli* bacteraemia in rabbits (217). IL-1ra has also delayed death and blunted the occurrence of hypotension in bacteraemic baboons. A recent open-label trial of IL-1ra in septic humans reported a dose-dependent reduction in mortality from 44% in placebo recipients to 16% in patients treated with 133 mg/h of IL-1ra (269). Even though substantial reductions in mortality have been reported, data from a non-blind trial must remain suspect until a full-scale randomized double-blind placebo-controlled trial of the drug is completed.

IL-1ra has potent anti-inflammatory effects in non-sepsis models. For example, IL-1ra reduces inflammation in models of immune complex colitis (270,271), meningitis (272) and adjuvant-induced arthritis. It also blocks the soporific, febrile and neutrophil chemoattractant effects of IL-1 (273). In vitro IL-1ra blocks IL-1-induced production of IL-1, TNF and IL-6 from human peripheral blood monocytes. One potential problem in using IL-1ra clinically may be the dose requirements for the drug. In vitro and in vivo 50–500-fold molar excesses of IL-1ra have been required to confer protection (217,265,266) and the effects of the drug are very dose dependent (217,269). Such huge doses of drug may preclude economical clinical use.

The IL-1 inhibitors described above differ from the soluble IL-1 inhibitor reported by Giri et al. (274), which has characteristics of the extracellular binding domain of the IL-1 receptor. Antibodies to the murine IL-1 receptor have also been produced and are reported to reduce the severity of IL-1-induced and radiation-induced injury and death (275–277).

Two soluble receptors (27 and 30 kDa) for TNFα have been isolated from human urine (82,278). The human TNFα receptor represents a shed portion of the cell surface receptor (279). Seckinger et al. (280) and Engelmann et al. (281) described a 27 kDa and 33 kDa inhibitor that blocked TNFα binding to the TNFα receptor. This has been further characterized by Heller et al. (40).

Administration of the soluble TNFα receptor can prevent death in mice from LPS-induced shock.

Novick et al. (282) have reported a soluble extracellular fragment of the IL-6 receptor that functions as a soluble IL-6 inhibitor. To date there are no data to support a significant role of the IL-6 inhibitor in sepsis.

Summary

The discovery of the cytokines and their role in inflammation has provided an exciting and potentially useful type of therapy for SIRS. Unfortunately, there are still few human data showing that cytokine antagonists can effectively curtail established sepsis. In animals, the type of inflammatory challenge (endotoxin versus bacteria) and the location (intravenous versus peritoneal) are critical determinants of the effectiveness of cytokine antagonists. As with endotoxin antagonists, logistical problems in administration, uncertain efficacy and high cost may prove problematic.

Furthermore, cytokines have beneficial effects in appropriate local concentrations: abolition of their actions may therefore prove to be dangerous. Although bacterial clearance has not been hindered by anti-cytokine antibodies, the local immune response may be impaired. To maximize the cost–benefit ratio, safety and efficacy, it is desirable to have inexpensive, avidly binding and neutralizing, low molecular weight compounds with large volumes of distribution and short half-lives. The production of antagonists specific to human cytokines will preclude adequate preclinical study of the safety and efficacy of such compounds. For each cytokine antagonist, large, multi-centre, randomized double-blind, placebo-controlled trials in septic humans will be required to demonstrate safety and efficacy. Because of the complexity of cytokine interactions a single cytokine antagonist may fail to treat human sepsis syndrome, and an approach to SIRS not unlike that of combined chemotherapy for cancer may be required.

References

1. Centers for Disease Control (1990) MMWR 39: 31–34
2. Balk RA, Bone RC (1989) The septic syndrome: Definition and clinical implications. Crit Care Clin 5: 1–8
3. Bone RC, Fisher CJ, Clemmer TP et al. (1989) Sepsis syndrome: A valid clinical entity. Crit Care Med 17: 389–393
4. Bone RC, Fisher CJ, Clemmer TP et al. (1987) A controlled clinical trial of high-dose methyl-prednisolone in the treatment of severe sepsis and septic shock. N Engl J Med 317: 653–658
5. Ispahani P, Perason NJ, Greenwood D (1987) An analysis of community and hospital acquired bacteremia in a large teaching hospital in the United Kingdom. Q J Med 241: 427–440

6. Callandra T, Glauser MP, Schellekens J, Verhoef J, Swiss-Dutch J5 Immunoglobulin Study Group (1988) Treatment of Gram-negative septic shock with human IgG antibody to *Escherichia coli J5*: A prospective, double blind, randomized trial. J Infect Dis 158: 312–319
7. Bone RC, Fisher CJ, Clemmer TP et al. (1987) Early methylprednisolone treatment for septic syndrome and adult respiratory distress syndrome. Chest 932: 1032–1036
8. Neugebauer E, Schirren J, Lorenz W (1988) High dose steroids and sepsis. N Engl J Med 318: 514
9. Veterans Administration Systemic Sepsis Cooperative Study Group (1987) Effect of high dose glucocorticoid therapy on mortality in patients with signs of systemic sepsis. N Engl J Med 317: 659–665
10. DeMaria A, Craven DE, Heffernan JJ et al. (1985) Naloxone versus placebo in the treatment of septic shock. Lancet 1: 1363–1365
11. Danner RL, Elin RJ, Hosseini JM, Wesley RA, Reilly JM, Parillo JE (1991) Endotoxemia in human septic shock. Chest 99: 169–175
12. Wheeler AP, Hardie W, Bernard GR (1992) The role of cyclooxygenase products in lung injury induced by tumor necrosis factor. Am Rev Resp Dis 145: 632–639
13. Cifone MG, Alesse E, Reale M, Bologna M, Angeletti PU, Conti P (1986) Stimulating effects of hr tumor necrosis factor on TxB2 release by polymorphonuclears and macrophages. Agents and Actions 19: 349–350
14. Kettelhut IC, Fiers W, Goldberg AL (1987) The toxic effects of tumor necrosis factor in vivo and their prevention by cyclooxygenase inhibitors. Proc Natl Acad Sci USA 84: 4273–4277
15. Bernehim HA (1986) Is prostaglandin E_2 involved in the pathogenesis of fever? Effects of interleukin-1 on the release of prostaglandins. Yale J Biol Med 59: 151
16. Bonavida B (1989) The involvement of platelet activating factor (PAF)-induced monocyte activation and tumor necrosis factor (TNF) production in shock. In: Schlag G, Redl H (eds) Progress in Clinical Biological Research, vol 308: Second Vienna Shock Forum. Alan R Liss, New York, pp 485–490
17. Horvath CJ, Kaplan JE, Malik AB (1991) Role of platelet-activating factor in mediating tumor necrosis factor-induced pulmonary vasoconstriction and plasma-lymph protein transport. Am Rev Resp Dis 144: 1337–1341
18. Nawroth PP, Stern DM (1986) Modulation of endothelial cell hemostatic properties by tumor necrosis factor. J Exp Med 163: 740–745
19. Bevilacqua MP, Pober JS, Majeau GR et al. (1986) Recombinant tumor necrosis factor induces procoagulant activity in cultured human vascular endothelium: Characterization and comparison with the actions of interleukin 1. Proc Natl Acad Sci USA 831: 4533–4537
20. Mathison JC, Virca GD, Wolfson E, Tobias PA, Glaser K, Ulevitch RJ (1990) Adaptation to bacterial lipopolysaccharide controls lipopolysaccharide induced tumor necrosis factor production in rabbit macrophages. J Clin Invest 85: 1108–1118
21. Beutler B, Greenwald D, Hulmes JD et al. (1986) Identity of tumor necrosis factor and the macrophage-secreted factor cachectin. Nature 316: 552–554
22. Beutler B, Cerami A (1986) Cachectin: More than a tumor necrosis factor. N Engl J Med 316: 379–385
23. Sherry B, Cerami A (1988) Cachectin/tumor necrosis factor exerts endocrine, paracrine, and autocrine control of inflammatory responses. J Cell Biol 107: 1269–1277
24. Beutler BA, Milsark IW, Cerami A (1985) Cachectin/tumor necrosis factor, production, distribution and metabolic fate in vivo. J Immunol 135: 3972–3977
25. Wang AM, Creasey AA, Ladner MB et al. (1985) Molecular cloning of the complementary DNA for human tumor necrosis factor. Science 228: 149
26. Jones EY, Stuart DI, Walker NPC (1989) Structure of tumor necrosis factor. Nature 338: 225–228
27. Eck MJ, Sprang SR (1989) The structure of tumor necrosis factor at 2.6 A resolution. J Biol Chem 264: 17595–17605
28. Tavernier J, van Ostade, Hauuquier G et al. (1989) Conserved residues of tumor necrosis factor and lymphotoxin structure constitute the framework of the trimeric structure. FEBS Lett 257: 315–318
29. Caput D, Beutler B, Hartog K, Thayer R, Brown-Shimer S, Cerami A (1986) Identification of a common nucleotide sequence in the 3′ untranslated region of mRNA molecules specifies inflammatory molecules. Proc Natl Acad Sci USA 83: 1670–1674

30. Ulich TR, Guo K, del Castillo J (1989) Endotoxin-induced cytokine gene expression in vivo. I. Expression of tumor necrosis factor mRNA in visceral organs under physiologic conditions and during endotoxemia. Am J Pathol 134: 11–14
31. Hesse DG, Tracey KJ, Fong Y et al. (1988) Cytokine appearance in human endotoxemia and primate bacteremia. Surg Gynecol Obstet 166: 147
32. Kelly N, Cross A (1990) Non-lethal and lethal production of cytokines (TNF and IL-6) in response to bacterial LPS. In: Dinarello CA, Kluger MJ, Powanda MC, Oppenheim JJ. The physiological and pathological effects of cytokines (eds), Wiley-Liss, New York, pp 147–152
33. Zaneti G, Heumann D, Gerain J et al. (1992) Cytokine production after intravenous or peritoneal Gram-negative bacterial challenge in mice. J Immunol 148: 1890–1897
34. Hinshaw LB, Tekamp-Olson P, Chang ACK et al. (1990) Survival of primates in LD100 septic shock following therapy with antibody to tumor necrosis factor (TNFα). Circ Shock 30: 279–292
35. Schall TJ, Lewis M, Koller KJ et al. (1990) Molecular cloning and expression of a receptor for human tumor necrosis factor. Cell 61: 361–370
36. Loetscher H, Pan YCE, Lahm HW et al. (1990) Molecular cloning and expression of the human 55 kD tumor necrosis factor receptor. Cell 61: 351–359
37. Smith CA, Davis T, Anderson D et al. (1990) A receptor for tumor necrosis factor defines an unusual family of cellular and viral proteins. Science 248: 1019–1023
38. Heller RA, Song K, Onasch MA, Fischer W, Chang D, Ringold GM (1990) Complementary cloning of a receptor for tumor necrosis factor and demonstration of a shed form of the receptor. Proc Natl Acad Sci USA 87: 6151–6155
39. Shepard VL, Abdolrasulnia R (1989) Isolation of a receptor for tumor necrosis factor from human lung tissue. Cytokine 1: 96
40. Heller RA, Song K, Onasch MA, Fischer WH, Chang D, Ringold GM (1990) Complementary DNA cloning of a receptor for tumor necrosis factor and demonstration of a shed form of the receptor. Proc Natl Acad Sci USA 87: 6151–6155
41. Gray P, Barrett K, Chantry D, Turner M, Feldman M (1990) Cloning of human tumor necrosis factor (TNF) receptor cDNA and expression of recombinant soluble TNF-binding protein. Proc Natl Acad Sci USA 87: 7380–7384
42. Nophar Y, Kemper O, Brakebush C (1990) Soluble forms of tumor necrosis factor receptors (TNF-s). The cDNA for the type I TNF-R, cloned using amino acid sequence data of its soluble form, encodes both the cell surface and a soluble form of the receptor. EMBO J 9: 3269–3278
43. Kohno T, Brewer MT, Baker SL (1990) A second tumor necrosis factor receptor gene product can shed a naturally occuring tumor necrosis factor inhibitor. Proc Natl Acad Sci USA 87: 8331–8335
44. Aggarwal BB, Eessalu TE, Hass PE (1985) Characterization of receptors for human tumor necrosis factor and their regulation by gamma interferon. Nature 318: 655–667
45. Ziegler EJ (1988) Tumor necrosis factor in humans. N Engl J Med 318: 1533–1535
46. Stephens KE, Ishizaka A, Wu Z, Larrick JW, Raffin TA (1988) Granulocyte depletion prevents tumor necrosis factor-mediated acute lung injury in guinea-pigs. Am Rev Resp Dis 138: 1300–1307
47. Ferrari-Baliviera E, Mealy K, Smith RJ, Wilmore DW (1989) Tumor necrosis factor induces adult respiratory distress syndrome in rats. Arch Surg 124: 1400–1405
48. Kuei JH, Tashkin DP, Figlin RA (1989) Pulmonary toxicity of recombinant human tumor necrosis factor. Chest 96: 334–338
49. Aderka D (1991) Role of tumor necrosis factor in the pathogenesis of intravascular coagulopathy of sepsis: Potential new therapeutic implications. Israel J Med Sci 27: 52–60
50. Gamble JR, Harlan JM, Klebanoff SJ, Vadas MA (1985) Stimulation of the adherence of neutrophils to umbilical vein endothelium by human recombinant tumor necrosis factor. Proc Natl Acad Sci USA 82: 8667–8671
51. Oliff A, Defeo-Jones D, Boyer M et al. (1987) Tumors secreting human TNF/cachectin induce cachexia in mice. Cell 50: 555–563
52. Tracey KJ, Morgello S, Koplin B et al. (1990) Metabolic effects of cachectin/tumor necrosis factor are modified by site of production. Cachectin/tumor necrosis factor-secreting tumor in skeletal muscle induces chronic cachexia, while implantation in brain induces predominantly acute anorexia. J Clin Invest 86: 2014–2024

53. Martinet Y, Yamauchi K, Crystal RG (1988) Differential expression of the tumor necrosis factor/cachectin gene by blood and lung mononuclear phagocytes. Am Rev Resp Dis 138: 659–665
54. Flick DA, Gifford GE (1984) Comparison of in vivo cell cytotoxic assays for tumor necrosis factor. J Immunol Meth 68: 167–175
55. Hay H, Cohen J (1989) Studies on the specificity of the L929 cell bioassay for the measurement of tumor necrosis factor. J Clin Lab Immunol 29: 151–155
56. Dinarello CA (1988) New concepts on the pathogenesis of fever. Rev Infect Dis 10: 168
57. Dinarello CA (1991) The proinflammatory cytokines interleukin-1 and tumour necrosis factor and treatment of the septic shock syndrome. J Infect Dis 163: 1177–1184
58. Pohlman TH, Stanness KA, Beatty PG, Ochs HD, Harlan JM (1986) An endothelial cell surface factor(s) induced in vitro by lipopolysaccharide, interleukin 1 and tumor necrosis factor increases neutrophil adherence by a CDW18 dependent mechanism. J Immunol 136: 4548–4553
59. Bevilacqua MP, Pober JS, Wheeler ME, Cotran RS, Gimbrone MA (1985) Interleukin 1 acts on cultured human vascular endothelium to increase the adhesion of polymorphonuclear leukocytes, monocytes and related leukocyte cell lines. J Clin Invest 76: 2003–2011
60. March CJ, Mosley B, Larsen A et al. (1985) Cloning, sequence and expression of two distinct human interleukin-1 complementary DNAs. Nature 315: 641
61. Auron PE, Webb AC, Rosenwasser LJ et al. (1984) Nucleotide sequence of human monocyte interleukin-1 precursor cDNA. Proc Natl Acad Sci USA 81: 7907
62. Sims JE, March C, Cosman D et al. (1988) cDNA expression cloning of the IL-1β receptor, a member of the immunoglobulin superfamily. Science 243: 585–589
63. Matsushima KT, Akahoshi T, Yamada M, Furutani Y, Oppenheim JJ (1986) Properties of a specific interleukin-1 receptor on human Epstein-Barr virus transformed B lymphocytes: Identity of the receptor for IL-1α and IL-1β. J Immunol 136: 4496–4502
64. Dower SK, Sims JE (1990) Structure and function of murine and human IL-1 receptors. In: Cochrane CG, Gimbrone MA (eds) Cellular and molecular mechanisms of inflammation: Receptors of inflammatory cells: Structure and function relationships. Academic Press, San Diego, pp 137–172
65. Bomsztyk K, Sims JE, Stanton TH (1989) Evidence for different interleukin 1 receptors in murine B- and T-cell lines. Proc Natl Acad Sci USA 86: 8034–8038
66. Helle M, Boeije L, Aarden LA (1988) Functional discrimination between interleukin 1 and interleukin 6. Eur J Immunol 18: 1535–1539
67. Zilberstein A, Ruggieri R, Korn JH, Revel M (1988) Structure and expression of the interferon β_2/B cell differentiation factor BSF-2/hepatocyte stimulating factor gene in human fibroblasts by other cytokines. J Immunol 140: 974–977
68. Munck-Peterson C, Davidson O, Moestrup SK, Sonne O, Nykjaer A, Moller BK (1990) Cellular targets and receptors for interleukin 6. II. Characterization of the IL-6 binding and receptors in peripheral blood cells and macrophages. Eur J Clin Invest 20: 377–384
69. Yamasaki K, Taga T, Hiratas Y et al. (1988) Cloning and expression of the human interleukin-6 receptor. Science 243: 825–828
70. Van Snick J (1990) Interleukin 6 an overview. Ann Rev Immunol 8: 253–278
71. Wong GG, Clark SC (1988) Multiple actions of interleukin-6 within a cytokine network. Immunol Today 8: 137–139
72. Le J, Vilcek J (1989) Interleukin 6: A multifunctional cytokine regulating immune reactions and the acute phase protein response. Lab Invest 61: 588–602
73. Gauldie J, Richards C, Harnish M (1988) Interferon β_2/BSF-2 shares identity with monocyte derived hepatocyte stimulating factor and regulates the major acute phase response in liver cells. Proc Natl Acad Sci USA 9: 7252–7255
74. Geiger T, Andus T, Klapproth J, Hirano T, Kishimoto T, Heinrich PC (1988) Induction of rat acute phase proteins by interleukin 6 in vivo. Eur J Immunol 18: 717–722
75. Sehgal PB, May LT, Tamm I, Vilcek J (1987) Human β_2 interferon and B-cell differentiation factor BSF-2 are identical. Science 235: 731–732
76. Helle M, Brakenhoff JPJ, DeGroot ER, Aarden LA (1988) Interleukin 6 is involved in interleukin 1 induced activities. Eur J Immunol 18: 957–959

77. Hirano T, Taga T, Nakano N et al. (1985) Purification to homogeneity and characterization of human B-cell differentiation factor (BCDF, BSF p-2). Proc Natl Acad Sci USA 82: 5490–5494
78. Okada M, Kitahara M, Kishimoto S, Matsuda T, Hirano T, Kishimoto T (1988) IL-6/BSF2 functions as a killer helper factor in the in vitro induction of cytotoxic T-cells. J Immunol 141: 1543–1549
79. Ishibashi T, Kimura H, Shikama Y et al. (1989) Interleukin 6 is a potent thrombopoetic factor in vivo in mice. Blood 74: 1241–1244
80. Asano S, Okano A, Ozawa K et al. (1990) In vivo effects of recombinant human interleukin-6 in primates stimulated production of platelets. Blood 75: 1602–1605
81. Hill RJ, Warren MK, Levin J (1990) Stimulation of thrombopoiesis in mice by human recombinant interleukin 6. J Clin Invest 85: 1242–1247
82. Novick D, Engelmann H, Wallach D, Rubenstein M (1989) Soluble cytokine receptors are present in normal human urine. J Exp Med 170: 1409–1414
83. Maury CPJ, Teppo AM (1987) Raised serum levels of cachectin/tumor necrosis factor alpha in renal allograft rejection. J Exp Med 166: 1132–1137
84. Grossman RM, Kreuger J, Yourish D et al. (1988) Interleukin 6 is expressed in high levels in psoriatic skin and stimulates proliferation of cultured human keratinocytes. Proc Natl Acad Sci USA 86: 6367–6371
85. Houssiau FA, Bukasa K, Sindic CJM, Van Damme J, Van Snick J (1988) Elevated levels of the 26K human hybridoma growth factor (interleukin 6) in cerebrospinal fluid of patients with acute infection of the central nervous system. Clin Exp Immunol 71: 320
86. Shenkin A, Fraser WD, Series J et al. (1989) The serum interleukin 6 response to elective surgery. Lymphokine Res 8: 123–127
87. McClain CJ, Cohen D, Phillips R, Miller B, Talwalkar R, Young B (1990) Increased plasma interleukin 6 levels in head injury patients. In: Dinarello CA, Kluger MJ, Powanda MC, Oppenheim JJ (eds) The physiological and pathological effects of cytokines. Wiley-Liss, New York, pp 61–67
88. Elias JA (1988) Tumor necrosis factor interacts with interleukin 1 and interferons to inhibit fibroblast proliferation via fibroblast prostaglandin-dependent and independent mechanisms. Am Rev Resp Dis 138: 652–658
89. Sugarman BJ, Aggarwal BB, Hass PE, Figari IS, Palladino MA, Shepard HM (1985) Recombinant tumor necrosis factor α: Effects on proliferation of normal and transformed cells in vitro. Science 230: 943–945
90. Vilcek J, Palombella VJ, Henriksen-DeStefano D et al. (1986) Fibroblast growth enhancing activity of tumor necrosis factor and its relationship to other polypeptide growth factors. J Exp Med 163: 632
91. Sugarman BJ, Lewis GD, Eessalu TE, Aggarwal BB, Shepard M (1987) Effects of growth factors on the antiproliferative activity of tumor necrosis factor. Cancer Res 47: 780–786
92. Sato N, Goto T, Haranaka K et al. (1986) Actions of tumor necrosis factor on cultured vascular endothelial cells: Morphologic modulation, growth inhibition and cytotoxicity. JNCI 76: 1113–1121
93. Dinarelo CA (1989) Interleukin 1 and its biologically related cytokines. Adv Immunol 44: 153–205
94. Oppenheim JJ, Matsushima K, Yoshimura T, Leonard EJ, Neta R (1989) Relationship between interleukin-1, tumor necrosis factor and a neutrophil attracting peptide. Agents and Actions 26: 134–140
95. Le J, Vilcek J (1987) Tumor necrosis factor and interleukin 1: Cytokines with multiple overlapping biological actions. Lab Invest 56: 234–248
96. Dinarello CA, Cannon JG, Wolff SM et al. (1986) Tumor necrosis factor (cachectin) is an endogenous pyrogen and induces production of interleukin-1. J Exp Med 163: 1433–1450
97. Nawroth PP, Bank I, Handley D, Cassimeris J, Chess L, Stern D (1986) Tumor necrosis factor/cachectin interacts with endothelial cell receptors to induce release of interleukin-1. J Exp Med 163: 1363–1375
98. Van Damme J, Opdenakker G, Simpson RJ et al. (1987) Identification of the human 26 kD protein interferon β2 (IFN β2) as a growth factor induced by interleukin 1 and tumor necrosis factor. J Exp Med 165: 914
99. McIntosh JK, Jablons DM, Mule JJ et al. (1989) In vivo induction of IL-6 by administration of exogenous cytokines and detection of de novo serum levels of IL-6 in tumor bearing mice. J Immunol 143: 162–167

100. Kohase MD, Henriksen-DeStefano, May LT, Vilcek J, Sehgal P (1986) Induction of β-2-interferon by tumor necrosis factor: A homeostatic mechanism in the control of cell proliferation. Cell 45: 659
101. Jablons DM, Mule JJ, McIntosh JK et al. (1989) IL-6/IFN-β-2 as a circulating hormone: Induction by cytokine administration in humans. J Immunol 142: 1542–1547
102. Brouckaert P, Sprigggs DR, Demetri G, Kufe DW, Fiers W (1989) Circulating IL-6 during a continuous infusion of tumor necrosis factor and interferon gamma. J Exp Med 169: 2257–2262
103. Warner SJC, Auger KR, Libby P (1987) Interleukin-1 induces interleukin-1: Recombinant human interleukin-1 induces interleukin-1 production by adult human vascular endothelial cells. J Immunol 139: 1911–1917
104. Dinarello CA, Ikejima T, Warner SJC et al. (1987) Interleukin-1 induces interleukin-1: Induction of circulating interleukin-1 in rabbits in vivo and in human mononuclear cells in vitro. J Immunol 139: 1902–1910
105. Strieter RM, Remick DG, Lynch JP, Spengler RN, Kunkel RL (1989) Interleukin-2-induced tumor necrosis factor-α gene expression in human alveolar macrophages and blood monocytes. Am Rev Resp Dis 139: 335–342
106. Steuer MR, Moser RP, Blacklock B, Crump W, Grimm EA (1990) Cytokines in the cerebrospinal fluid following intraventricular injection of interleukin 2 in patients with leptomeningeal carcinomatosis. In: Dinarello CA, Kluger MJ, Powanda MC, Oppenheim JJ (eds) The physiological and pathological effects of cytokines. Wiley-Liss, New York, pp 49–54
107. Mier JW, Vachino G, Van der Meer JWM et al. (1988) Induction of circulating tumor necrosis factor (TNFα) as a mediator for the febrile response to interleukin 2 (IL 2) in cancer patients. J Clin Immunol 8: 426–436
108. Okusawa S, Gelfand JA, Ikejima T, Connolly RJ, Dinarello CA (1988) Interleukin-1 induces a shock-like state in rabbits. J Clin Invest 81: 1162–1172
109. Weinberg JR, Wright DJM, Guz A (1988) Interleukin-1 and tumor necrosis factor cause hypotension in the conscious rabbit. Clin Sci 75: 251–255
110. Waage A, Espevik T (1988) Interleukin-1 potentiates the lethal effect of tumor necrosis factor a/cachectin in mice. J Exp Med 167: 1987–1992
111. Elias JA, Trinchieri G, Beck JM et al. (1989) A synergistic interaction of IL-6 and IL-1 mediates the thymocyte stimulating activity produced by recombinant IL-1 stimulated fibroblasts. J Immunol 142: 509–514
112. Kunimoto DY, Nordan RP, Striber W (1989) IL-6 is a potent cofactor of IL-1 in IgM synthesis and of IL-5 in IgA synthesis. J Immunol 143: 2230–2235
113. Elias JA, Lentz V (1990) Interleukin 1 and tumor necrosis factor synergistically stimulate fibroblast IL-6 production and stabilize IL-6 mRNA. J Immunol 145: 161–166
114. Heremans H, van Damme J, Dillen C, Dijkmans R, Billiau A (1990) Interferon gamma, a mediator of lethal lipopolysaccharide-induced Shwartzman-like shock reactions in mice. J Exp Med 171: 1853–1869
115. Heinzel FP (1990) The role of IFN gamma in experimental endotoxemia. J Immunol 145: 2920–2924
116. Kiner PA, Marek F, Rodges G, Lin PF, Warr G, Desiderio J (1988) Induction of tumor necrosis factor, IFN gamma and acute lethality in mice by toxic and non-toxic forms of lipid A. J Immunol 141: 870–874
117. Fong Y, Tracey KJ, Moldawer LL et al. (1989) Antibodies to cachectin/tumor necrosis factor reduce interleukin-1 β and interleukin-6 appearance during lethal bacteremia. J Exp Med 270: 1627
118. Brennan FM, Jackson A, Chantry D, Maini R, Feldman M (1989) Inhibitory effect of TNFα antibodies on synovial cell interleukin-1 production in rheumatoid arthritis. Lancet 2(8657): 244–247
119. Rothstein JL, Schreiber H (1988) Synergy between tumor necrosis factor and bacterial products causes hemorrhagic necrosis and lethal shock in normal mice. Proc Natl Acad Sci USA 85: 607–611
120. Schindler RJ, Mancilla J, Endres S, Ghorbani R, Clark SC, Dinarello CA (1990) Correlations and interactions in the production of interleukin-6, IL-1β, and tumor necrosis factor in human blood mononuclear cells: IL-6 suppresses IL-1β and TNFα. Blood 75 (suppl 1): 40
121. Moriarity JL, Starnes HF (1990) Transforming growth factor β reduces lethal effects of *E.*

coli infection. In: Dinarello CA, Kluger MJ, Powanda MC, Oppenheim JJ (eds) The physiological and pathological effects of cytokines. Wiley-Liss, New York, pp 153–158
122. Espevik T, Figari IS, Shalaby MR et al. (1987) Inhibition of cytokine production by cyclosporin A and transforming growth factor β. J Exp Med 166: 571–576
123. Cross AS, Sadoff JC, Kelly N, Bernton E, Gemski F (1989) Pretreatment with recombinant murine tumor necrosis factor α/cachectin and murine interleukin 1α protects mice from lethal bacterial infection. J Exp Med 169: 2021–2027
124. Sheppard BC, Norton JA (1991) Tumor necrosis factor and interleukin-1 protection against the lethal effects of tumor necrosis factor. Surgery 109: 698–705
125. Beutler B, Krochinin N, Milsdark IN, Leedke C, Cerami A (1986) Control of cachectin (tumor necrosis factor) synthesis: Mechanisms of endotoxin resistance. Science 232: 977–980
126. Strieter RM, Remick DG, Lynch JP, Raiford GC, Spengler R, Kunkel SL (1989) Differential regulation of tumor necrosis factor-alpha in human alveolar macrophages and peripheral blood monocytes: A cellular and molecular analysis. Am J Resp Cell Mol Biol 1: 57–63
127. Zabel P, Kreiker C, Schonharting MM, Schade UF (1990) Endotoxin-induced tumor necrosis factor α formation in man and its reversal by pentoxifylline. In: Dinarello CA, Kluger MJ, Powanda MC, Oppenheim JJ (eds) The physiological and pathological effects of cytokines Wiley-Liss, New York, pp 43–48
128. Waage A (1987) Production and clearance of tumor necrosis factor in rats exposed to endotoxin and dexamethasone. Clin Immunol Immunopathol 45: 348–355
129. Waage A, Bakke O (1988) Glucocorticoids suppress the production of tumor necrosis factor by lipopolysaccharide-stimulated human monocytes. Immunology 63: 299–302
130. Badgar AM, Olivera D, Talmadge JE, Hanna N (1989) Protective effect of SK&F 86002, a novel dual inhibitor of arachadonic acid metabolism in murine models of endotoxic shock. Circ Shock 27: 51–61
131. Baumgartner JD, Heumann D, Gerain J, Weinbreck P, Grau GE, Glauser MP (1990) Association between protective efficacy of anti-lipopolysaccharide (LPS) antibodies and suppression of LPS-induced tumor necrosis factor α, and interleukin 6: Comparison of O side-chain-specific antibodies with core LPS antibodies. J Exp Med 171: 889
132. Strieter RM, Remick DG, Ward PA et al. (1988) Cellular and molecular regulation of tumor necrosis factor-alpha production by pentoxifylline. Biochem Biophys Res Comm 155: 1230–1236
133. Schade UF (1989) The role of prostacyclin in the protective effects of pentoxifylline and other xanthine derivatives in endotoxin action in mice. Eicosanoids 2: 183–188
134. Welsh CH, Lien D, Worthen GS, Weil JV (1988) Pentoxifylline decreases endotoxin-induced pulmonary polymorphonuclear sequestration and extravascular protein accumulation in the dog. Am Rev Resp Dis 138: 1106–1114
135. Bertini R, Bianchi M, Ghezzi P (1988) Adrenalectomy sensitizes mice to the lethal effects of interleukin 1 and tumor necrosis factor. J Exp Med 167: 1708–1712
136. Spinas GA, Bloesch D, Keller U, Zimmerli W, Cammisuli S (1991) Pretreatment with ibuprofen augments circulating tumor necrosis factor α, interleukin 6 and elastase during acute endotoxemia. J Infect Dis 163: 89–95
137. Nelson S, Bagby GJ, Bainton BG, Wilson LA, Thompson JJ, Summer WR (1989) Compartmentalization of intra-alveolar and systemic lipopolysaccharide-induced tumor necrosis factor and the pulmonary inflammatory response. J Infect Dis 159: 189–194
138. Nelson S (1990) LPS induced inhibition of lung TNF. In: Dinarello CA, Kluger MJ, Powanda MC, Oppenheim JJ (eds) The physiological and pathological effects of cytokines. Wiley-Liss, New York, pp 141–146
139. Kindler V, Sappino AP, Grau GE, Piquet PF, Vassal P (1989) The inducing role of tumor necrosis factor in the development of bactericidal granulomas during BCG infection. Cell 56: 731–740
140. Titus RG, Sherry B, Cerami A (1989) Tumor necrosis factor plays a protective role in experimental murine cutaneous leishmaniasis. J Exp Med 170: 2097–2104
141. Nakane A, Minagawa T, Kato K (1988) Endogenous tumor necrosis factor (cachectin) is essential to host resistance against *Listeria monocytogenes* infection. Infect Immun 56: 2563–2569
142. Engelberts I, Moller A, Schoen GJM, Van der Linden CJ, Buurman WA (1991) Evaluation of measurement of human TNF in plasma by ELISA. Lymphokine Cytokine Res 10: 69–76

143. Gibson RL, Redding GJ, Henderson WR, Truog WE (1991) Group B *Streptococcus* induces tumor necrosis factor in neonatal piglets. Am Rev Resp Dis 143: 598–604
144. Zuckerman SH, Bendele AM (1989) Regulation of serum tumor necrosis factor in glucocorticoid senstive and resistant rodent endotoxin models. Infect Immun 57: 3009–3013
145. Hinshaw L, Olson P, Kuo G (1989) Efficacy of post-treatment with anti-TNF monoclonal antibody in preventing the pathophysiology and lethality of sepsis in the baboon (abstr). Circ Shock 27: 362
146. Marks JD, Marks CB, Luce JM, Montgomery AB, Turner J, Murray JF (1990) Plasma tumor necrosis factor in patients with septic shock: Mortality rate, incidence of adult respiratory distress syndrome. Am Rev Resp Dis 141: 94–97
147. Marano MA, Fong Y, Maldawer LL et al. (1990) Serum cachectin/tumor necrosis factor in critically ill patients with burns correlates with infection and mortality. Surg Gynecol Obstet 170: 32–38
148. Swiss-Dutch J5 Immunoglobulin Study Group (1990) Prognostic values of tumor necrosis factor/cachectin, interleukin-1, interferon-α, and interferon-gamma in the serum of patients with septic shock. J Infect Dis 161: 982–987
149. Baud L, Cadranel J, Offenstadt G et al. (1990) Tumor necrosis factor and septic shock (letter). Crit Care Med 18: 349–350
150. Pinsky MR, Vincent JL, Kahn RJ, Schandene L, Dupont E, Content J (1990) Inflammatory mediators of septic shock in man. Am Rev Resp Dis 141: A512
151. Bagby GJ, Plessala KJ, Wilson LA, Thompson JJ, Nelson S (1991) Divergent efficacy of antibody to tumor necrosis factor α in intravascular and peritonitis models of sepsis. J Infect Dis 163: 83
152. Michie HR, Manogue KR, Spriggs DR et al. (1988) Detection of circulating tumor necrosis factor after endotoxin administration. N Engl J Med 318: 1481
153. Suffredini AF, Fromm RE, Parker MM et al. (1989) The cardiovascular response of normal humans to the administration of endotoxin. N Engl J Med 321: 280–287
154. Fong Y, Marano MA, Moldawer LL et al. (1988) Splanchnic monokine and metabolic response to endotoxin in man. Surgery Forum 39: 21–23
155. Fong Y, Marano MA, Moldawer LL, Wei H, Calvano SE, Kennedy JS (1990) The acute splanchnic and peripheral tissue metabolic response to endotoxin in humans. J Clin Invest 85: 1896–1904
156. Cannon JG, Tompkins RG, Gelfand JA et al. (1990) Circulating interleukin-1 and tumor necrosis factor in septic shock and experimental endotoxin fever. J Infect Dis 161: 79–84
157. Fong Y, Moldawer LL, Marano M et al. (1989) Endotoxemia elicits increased circulating β2 IFN/IL-6 in man. J Immunol 142: 2321–2324
158. Mackensen A, Galanos C, Englehardt R (1991) Treatment of cancer patients with endotoxin induces release of endogenous cytokines. Pathobiology 59: 264–267
159. Debets JM, Kampmeijer R, van der Linden MP, Buurman WA, van der Linden CJ (1989) Plasma tumor necrosis factor and mortality in critically ill septic patients. Crit Care Med 17: 489–494
160. Scuderi P, Lam KS, Ryan EJ et al. (1986) Raised serum levels of tumour necrosis factor in parasitic infections. Lancet 2: 1364–1365
161. Maury CPJ, Teppo AM (1987) Raised serum levels of cachectin/tumor necrosis factor α in renal allograft rejection. J Exp Med 166: 1132–1137
162. Imagawa DK, Millis JM, Olthoff KM, Busuttil RW et al. (1990) The role of tumor necrosis factor in allograft rejection. Transplantation 50: 219–225
163. Levine B, Kalman J, Mayer L, Fillit HM, Packer M (1990) Elevated circulating levels of tumor necrosis factor in severe chronic heart failure. N Engl J Med 323: 236–241
164. Balkwell F, Burke R, Talbot D et al. (1987) Evidence for tumor necrosis factor/cachectin production in cancer. Lancet 2: 1229–1232
165. Millar AB, Singer M, Meager A, Foley NM, Johnson NM, Rook GAW (1989) Tumor necrosis factor in bronchopulmonary secretions of patients with adult respiratory distress syndrome. Lancet 2: 712–714
166. Hyers TM, Tricomi SM, Dettenmeier PA, Fowler AA (1991) Tumor necrosis factor levels in serum and bronchoalveolar lavage fluid in patients with the adult respiratory distress syndrome. Am Rev Resp Dis 144: 268–271
167. Suter PM, Suter S, Girardin E, Roux-Lombard P, Grau GE, Dayer JM (1992) High bronchoalveolar levels of tumor necrosis factor and its inhibitors, interleukin-1, interferon

and elastase in patients with adult respiratory distress syndrome after trauma, shock or sepsis. Am Rev Resp Dis 145: 1016–1022
168. Roten R, Markert M, Feihl F, Schaller MD, Tagan MC, Perret C (1991) Plasma levels of tumor necrosis factor in the adult respiratory distress syndrome. Am Rev Resp Dis 143: 590–592
169. Hirano T, Matsuda T, Turner M et al. (1988) Excessive production of interleukin 6/B cell stimulating factor-2 in rheumatoid arthritis. Eur J Immunol 18: 1797–1801
170. Bhardwaj N, Santhanam U, Lau LL et al. (1989) IL-6 in synovial effusions of patients with rheumatoid arthritis and other arthritides. J Immunol 143: 2153–2159
171. McDowell TL (1990) IL-6 production in patients with rheumatoid arthritis and controls. In: Dinarello CA, Kluger MJ, Powanda MC, Oppenheim JJ (eds) The physiological and pathological effects of cytokines. Wiley-Liss, New York, pp 69–74
172. Houssiau FA, Devogelaer JP, van Damme J, DeDeuxchaisne CN, van Snick J (1988) Interleukin 6 in synovial fluid and serum of patients with rheumatoid arthritis and other inflammatory arthritides. Arthritis Rheum 31: 784–789
173. Swaak AJ, van Rooyen A, Nieuwenhuis E, Aarden LA (1988) Interleukin 6 (IL6) in synovial fluid and serum of patients with rheumatic disease. Scand J Rheumatol 17: 469–474
174. Gosset P, Perez T, Lassalle P et al. (1991) Increased TNFα secretion by alveolar macrophages from patients with rheumatoid arthritis. Am Rev Resp Dis 143: 593–597
175. Waage A, Halstensen A, Espevik T (1987) Association between tumor necrosis factor in serum and fatal outcome in patients with meningococcal disease. Lancet 1: 355
176. Waage AP, Brandtzaeg P, Halstensen A, Kierulf P, Espevik T (1989) The complex pattern of cytokines in serum from patients with meningococcal septic shock. J Exp Med 169: 333
177. Mustafa MM, Ramilo O, Olsen KD et al. (1989) Tumor necrosis factor in mediating experimental *Haemophilus influenzae* type B meningitis. J Clin Invest 84: 1253–1259
178. Leist TP, Frei K, Kam-Hansen S, Zinkernagel RM, Fontana A (1990) Tumor necrosis factor α in cerebrospinal fluid during bacterial but not viral meningitis. J Exp Med 167: 1743
179. Helfgott DC, Tatter SB, Santhanam U et al. (1989) Multiple forms of IFN β2/IL6 in serum and body fluids during acute bacterial infection. J Immunol 142: 948–953
180. Waage A, Halstensen A, Shalaby R, Brandtzaeg P, Kierluf P, Espevik T (1989) Local production of tumor necrosis factor α, interleukin 1 and interleukin 6 in meningococcal meningitis. J Exp Med 170: 1859–1867
181. McClain CJ, Cohen D, Ott L, Dinarello CA, Young B (1987) Ventricular fluid interleukin 1 activity in patients with head injury. J Lab Clin Med 110: 48–53
182. Mustafa MM, Ramilo O, Llorens XS, Olsen KD, Mangness RR, McCracken GH (1990) Cerebrospinal fluid prostaglandins, interleukin 1β and tumor necrosis factor in bacterial meningitis. Am J Dis Child 144: 883–887
183. Quaglianello VJ, Long WJ, Scheld WM (1987) Human interleukin 1 modulates blood–brain barrier injury in vivo. Interscience Conference on Antimicrobial Agents and Chemotherapy, abstr 614
184. Wispelwey B, Long WJ, Castracane JM (1988) Activity following intracisternal inoculation of *H. flu* type b lipopolysaccharide into rats. Interscience Conference on Antimicrobial Agents and Chemotherapy, abstr 873
185. Casey L, Simpson S, Balk R et al. (1989) Tumor necrosis factor in patients with septic syndrome. FASEB J 3: A635
186. Casey L, Balk R, Simpson S et al. (1990) Plasma tumor necrosis factor, interleukin 1β and endotoxin in patients with sepsis. In: Dinarello CA, Kluger MJ, Powanda MC, Oppenheim JJ (eds) The physiological and pathological effects of cytokines. Wiley-Liss, New York, pp 37–42
187. Dofferhoff AS, Bom VJJ, De Vries-Hospers HG et al. (1992) Patterns of cytokines, plasma endotoxin, plasminogen activator inhibitor, and acute phase proteins during the treatment of severe sepsis in humans. Crit Care Med 20: 185–192
188. Girardin E, Grau GE, Dayer JM, Roux-Lombard P, J5 Study Group, Lambert PH (1989) Tumor necrosis factor and interleukin-1 in the serum of children with severe infectious purpura. N Engl J Med 319: 397
189. Damas P, Reuter A, Gysen P, Demonty J, Lamy M, Franchimont P (1989) Tumor necrosis factor and interleukin-1 serum levels during severe sepsis in humans. Crit Care Med 17: 975–978
190. Kern P, Hemmer CJ, Gruss HJ, Dietrich M (1989) Elevated tumor necrosis factor α and

interleukin-6 serum levels as markers for complicated *Plasmodium falciparum* malaria. Am J Med 87: 139–143
191. Grau GE, Taylor TE, Molyneux ME et al. (1989) Tumor necrosis factor and disease severity in children with falciparum malaria. N Engl J Med 320: 1586–1591
192. Hack CE, De Groot ER, Felt-Bersma RJ et al. (1989) Increased plasma level of interleukin-6 in sepsis. Blood 74: 1704–1710
193. Callandra T, Baumgartner JD, Grau GE et al. (1990) Prognostic values of tumor necrosis factor/ cachectin, interleukin 1, alpha interferon and gamma interferon in the serum of patients with septic shock. J Infect Dis 161: 982
194. Callandra T, Gerain J, Heumann D, Baumgartner JD, Glauser MP (1991) High circulating levels of interleukin 6 in patients with septic shock: Evolution during sepsis, prognostic value and interplay with other cytokines. Am J Med 91: 23–29
195. Parker MM, Parrillo JE (1983) Septic shock: Hemodynamics and pathogenesis. JAMA 250: 3324–3327
196. Parker MM, Shelhamer JH, Bacharach SL et al. (1984) Profound but reversible myocardial depression in patients with septic shock. Ann Intern Med 100: 483–490
197. Shirmer WJ, Schirmer JM, Fry DE (1989) Recombinant human tumor necrosis factor produces hemodynamic changes characteristic of sepsis and endotoxemia. Arch Surg 124: 445–448
198. Remick DG, Kunkel R, Larrick JW, Kunkel SL (1987), Acute in vivo effects of human recombinant tumor necrosis factor. Lab Invest 56: 583–590
199. Tracey KJ, Beutler B, Lowry SF et al. (1986) Shock and tissue injury induced by recombinant human cachectin. Science 234: 470
200. Tracey KJ, Lowry SF, Fahey TJ et al. (1987) Cachectin/tumor necrosis factor induces lethal shock and stress hormone release in the dog. Surg Gynecol Obstet 164: 415–422
201. Natanson C, Eichenholz PW, Danner RL, Eichacker PQ (1989) Endotoxin and tumor necrosis factor challenges in dogs simulate the cardiovascular profile of human septic shock. J Exp Med 169: 823–832
202. Mathison JC, Wolfson E, Ulevitch RJ (1988) Participation of tumor necrosis factor in the mediation of bacterial lipopolysaccharide-induced injury in rabbits. J Clin Invest 81: 1925–1937
203. Leighton TA, Averbook AW, Klein SR, Bongard FS (1991) Time course of cardiopulmonary effects: tumor necrosis factor and endotoxin are similar. Am Surgeon 57: 836–842
204. Johnson J, Meyrick B, Jesmok G, Brigham KL (1989) Human recombinant tumor necrosis factor α induction mimics endotoxemia in awake sheep. J Appl Physiol 66: 1448–1454
205. Stephens KE, Ishizaka A, Larrick JW, Raffin TA (1988) Tumor necrosis factor causes increased pulmonary permeability and edema. Am Rev Resp Dis 137: 1364–1370
206. Goldblum SE, Sun WL (1990) Tumor necrosis factor-α augments pulmonary arterial transendothelial albumin flux in vitro. Am J Physiol 258: 157–167
207. Goldblum SE, Jay M, Yoneda K, Cohen D, McClain CJ, Gillespie M (1987) Monokine-induced acute lung injury in rabbits. J Appl Physiol 63: 2093–2100
208. Johnson J, Brigham KL, Jesmok G, Meyrick B (1991) Morphologic changes in lungs of anesthetized sheep following intravenous infusion of recombinant tumor necrosis factor α. Am Rev Resp Dis 144: 179–186
209. Wheeler AP, Jesmock G, Brigham KL (1990) Tumor necrosis factor's effects on lung mechanics, gas exchange and airway reactivity in sheep. J Appl Physiol 68: 2542–2549
210. Kips J, Tavernier J, Pauwels RA (1992) Tumor necrosis factor causes bronchial hyperresponsiveness in rats. Am Rev Resp Dis 145: 332–336
211. Redl H, Schlag G, Lamche H (1990) TNF and LPS-induced changes of lung vascular permeability: Studies in unanesthetized sheep. Circ Shock 31: 183–192
212. Kreil EA, Greene E, Fitzgibbon C, Robinson DR, Zapol WM (1989) Effects of recombinant human tumor necrosis factor-alpha, lymphotoxin and *E. coli* lipopolysaccharide on hemodynamics, lung microvascular permeability and eicosanoid synthesis in anesthetized sheep. Circ Res 65: 502–514
213. Evans DA, Jacobs DO, Revhaug A, Wilmore DW (1989) The effects of tumor necrosis factor and their selective inhibition by ibuprofen. Ann Surg 209: 312–321
214. Blick M, Sherwin SA, Rosenblum M, Gutterman J (1987) Phase I study of recombinant tumor necrosis factor in cancer patients. Cancer Res 47: 2986–2989
215. Tracey KJ, Fong JY, Hesse DG et al. (1987) Anti-cachectin/TNFα monoclonal antibodies prevent septic shock during lethal bacteremia. Nature 330: 662

216. Talmadge JE, Bowersox O, Tribble H, Lel SH, Shepard HM, Ligitt D (1987) Toxicity of tumor necrosis factor is synergistic with gamma interferon and can be reduced with cyclooxygenase inhibitors. Am J Pathol 128: 410–414
217. Ohlsson K, Bjork P, Bergenfeldt M, Hageman R, Thompson RC (1990) Interleukin-1 receptor antagonist reduces mortality from endotoxin shock. Nature 343: 550–552
218. Tracey KJ, Lowry SF, Cerami A (1988) Cachectin: A hormone that triggers acute shock and chronic cachexia. J Infect Dis 157: 413–420
219. Grimble RF (1989) Cytokines: Their relevance to nutrition. Eur J Clin Nutr 43: 217–230
220. Morrone G, Ciliberto G, Oliviero S et al. (1988) Recombinant interleukin-6 regulates the transcriptional activation of a set of human acute phase genes. J Biol Chem 263: 12554–12558
221. Mortenesen RF, Shapiro J, Lin BF, Douches S, Neta R (1988) Interaction of recombinant IL-1β and recombinant tumor necrosis factor in the induction of mouse acute phase proteins. J Immunol 140: 2660–2666
222. Perlmutter DH, Dinarello CA, Punsal PI, Colten HR (1986) Cachectin/tumor necrosis factor regulates hepatic acute phase gene expression. J Clin Invest 78: 1349–1354
223. Nijsten MWN, DeGroot ER, TenDuis HJ, Klasen HJ, Hack CE, Aarden LA (1987) Serum levels of interleukin-6 and acute phase responses. Lancet 2: 921
224. van Hisenberg VWM, Kooistra T, van den Berg EA, Princeu HWG, Fiers W, Emeis JJ (1988) Tumor necrosis factor increases the production of plasminogen activator inhibitor in human endothelial cells in vitro and in rats in vivo. Blood 72: 1467–1473
225. Watters JM, Bessey PQ, Dinarello CA, Wolff SM, Wilmore DW (1985) The induction of interleukin-1 in humans and its metabolic effects. Surgery 98: 298–306
226. Smith J, Urba W, Steis R et al. (1990) A phase I trial of interleukin 1 alpha (IL-1α) alone and in combination with indomethacin. Lymphokine Res 9: 568A
227. Beasley D (1990) Interleukin 1 and endotoxin activate soluble guanylate cyclase in vascular smooth muscle. Am J Phys 259: R38–44
228. Smith J, Urba W, Steis R (1990) Interleukin 1 alpha: Results of a phase 1 toxicity and immunomodulatory trial. Am Soc Clin Oncol 9: 717
229. Warren RS, Starnes HF, Gabrilove JL, Oettgen HF, Brennan MF (1987) The acute metabolic effects of tumor necrosis factor administration in humans. Arch Surg 122: 1396–1400
230. Starnes HF, Warren RS, Jeevanandam M, Gabrilove JL, Larchian W, Oettgen HF (1988) Tumor necrosis factor and the acute metabolic response to tissue injury in man. J Clin Invest 82: 1321–1325
231. Chapman PB, Lester TJ, Casper ES et al. (1987) Clinical pharmacology of recombinant human tumor necrosis factor in patients with advanced cancer. J Clin Oncol 5: 1942–1951
232. Michie HR, Spriggs DR, Manouge KR et al. (1988) TNF and endotoxin induce similar metabolic responses in human beings. Surgery 104: 280–286
233. van der Poll T, Buller HR, Ten Cate H et al. (1990) Activation of coagulation after administration of tumor necrosis factor to normal subjects. N Engl J Med 322: 1622–1627
234. Demetri GD, Spriggs DR, Sherman ML, Arthur KA, Imamura K, Kufe DW (1989) A phase I trial of recombinant human tumor necrosis factor and interferon gamma: Effects of combination cytokine administration in vivo. J Clin Oncol 7: 1545–1553
235. Jablons DM, Mule JJ, McIntosh JK et al. (1989) IL-6/IFNβ2 as a circulating hormone: Induction by cytokine administration in humans. J Immunol 142: 1542–1547
236. Ziegler EJ, HA-1A Sepsis Study Group (1991) Treatment of Gram-negative bacteremia and septic shock with HA-1A human monoclonal antibodies against endotoxin: A randomized double blind placebo controlled trial. N Engl J Med 324: 429–436
237. Greenman RL, Schein RM, Martin MA et al. (1991) A controlled clinical trial of E5 murine monoclonal IgM antibody to endotoxin in the treatment of Gram-negative sepsis. JAMA 266: 1097–1102
238. Wheeler AP, Hardie WD, Bernard G (1990) Studies of an anti-endotoxin antibody in preventing the physiologic changes of endotoxemia in awake sheep. Am Rev Resp Dis 142: 775–781
239. Wolff SM (1991) Monoclonal antibodies and the treatment of Gram-negative bacteremia and shock. N Engl J Med 324: 486–488
240. deGroote MA, Martin MA, Densen P, Pfaller MA, Wenzel RP (1989) Plasma tumor

necrosis factor levels in patients with presumed sepsis. Results in those treated with antilipid A antibody vs placebo. JAMA 262: 249–251
241. Beutler B, Milsarek IW, Cerami AC (1985) Passive immunization against cachectin/tumor necrosis factor protects mice from lethal effect of endotoxin. Science 229: 869
242. Grau GE, Vesin C, DeGroote D et al. (1991) Prevention of human TNF-induced cutaneous Shwartzman reaction and acute mortality in mice treated with anti-human TNF monoclonal antibodies. Clin Exp Immunol 84: 411–414
243. Silva AT, Bayston KF, Cohen J (1990) Prophylactic and therapeutic effects of a monoclonal antibody to tumor necrosis factor-alpha in experimental Gram-negative shock. J Infect Dis 162: 421–427
244. Sheehan KCF, Ruddle NH, Schreiber RD (1989) Generation and characterization of hamster monoclonal antibodies that neutralize murine tumor necrosis factor. J Immunol 142: 3884–3893
245. Opal SM, Cross AS, Kelly NM, Sadoff JC, Bodmer MW, Palardy JE (1990) Efficacy of a monoclonal antibody directed against tumor necrosis factor in protecting neutropenic rats from lethal infection with *Pseudomonas aeruginosa*. J Infect Dis 161: 1148–1152
246. Opal SM, Cross AS, Sadoff JC et al. (1991) Efficacy of antilipopolysaccharide and anti-tumor necrosis factor monoclonal antibodies in a neutropenic rat model of *Pseudomonas* sepsis. J Clin Invest 88: 885–890
247. Echtenacher B, Falk W, Mannel DN, Krammer PH (1990) Requirement of endogenous tumor necrosis factor/cachectin for recovery from experimental peritonitis. J Immunol 145: 3762–3766
248. Evans GF, Snyder YM, Butler LD, Zukerman SH (1989) Differential expression of interleukin 1 and tumor necrosis factor in murine septic shock models. Circ Shock 29: 279
249. Sherry BA, Gelin J, Fong Y et al. (1989) Anti-cachectin/tumor necrosis factor antibodies attenuate development of cachexia in tumor models. FASEB J 3: 1956–1962
250. Exley AR, Buurman W, Bodmer M, Bohen J (1989) Monoclonal antibody (Mab) to recombinant human tumor necrosis factor (rhTNF) in the prophylaxis and treatment of endotoxic shock in cynomolgus monkeys (abstr). Clin Sci 76: 50
251. Exley AR, Cohen J, Buurman W et al. (1990) Monoclonal antibodies to TNFα in severe septic shock. Lancet 335: 1275–1277
252. Vincent JL, Bakker J, Marecaux G, Schandene L, Kahn R, Dupont E (1992) Administration of anti-TNF antibody improves left ventricular function in septic shock patients: Results of a pilot study. Chest 101: 810–815
253. Starnes HF, Pearce MK, Rewari A, Yim JH, Zou JC, Abrams JS (1990) Anti-IL-6 monoclonal antibodies protect against lethal *Escherichia coli* infection and lethal tumor necrosis factor α challenge in mice. J Immunol 145: 4185–4191
254. Grau G, Fajardo LF, Piguet PF, Allet B, Lambert PH, Vassalli P (1987) Tumor necrosis factor (cachectin) as an essential mediator in murine cerebral malaria. Science 237: 1210–1212
255. Blanchard DK, Djeu JY, Klein TW, Friedman H, Stewart WE II (1988) Protective effects of tumor necrosis factor in experimental *Legionella pneumophila* infections of mice via activation of PMN function. J Leuk Biol 43: 429–435
256. Nelson S, Summer WR, Bagby GJ (1990) LPS-induced inhibition of lung TNF and host defenses. Prog Leuk Biol 10B: 141–146
257. Seckinger P, Lowenthal JW, Williamson K, Dayer JM, MacDonald HR (1987) A urine inhibitor of interleukin-1 activity that blocks ligand binding. J Immunol 139: 1546–1549
258. Seckinger P, Williamson K, Balavoine JF et al. (1987) A urine inhibitor of interleukin-1 activity affects both interleukin 1α and 1β but not tumor necrosis factor α. J Immunol 138: 1541–1545
259. Arend WP, Welgus HG, Thompson RC, Eisenberg SP (1990) Biological properties of recombinant human monocyte derived interleukin 1 receptor antagonist. J Clin Invest 85: 1694–1699
260. Prieur AM, Kaufman MT, Griscelli C, Dayer JM (1987) Specific interleukin-1 inhibitor in serum and urine of children with systemic juvenile chronic arthritis. Lancet 2: 1240–1242
261. Eisenberg SP, Evans RJ, Arend WP et al. (1990) Primary structure and functional expression from complementary interleukin-1 receptor atagonist. Nature 343: 341–346
262. Carter DB, Deibel MR, Dunn CJ et al. (1990) Purification, cloning, expression and biological characterization of an interleukin-1 receptor antagonist protein. Nature 344: 633–638

263. Hannum CH, Wilcox CJ, Arend WP et al. (1990) Interleukin-1 receptor antagonist activity of a human interleukin-1 inhibitor. Nature 343: 336–342
264. Robb RJ, Kutny RM (1987) Structure–function relationships for the IL-2 receptor system: Analysis of the sequence and ligand-binding properties of soluble Tac protein. J Immunol 139: 855–862
265. Arend WP, Welgus HG, Thompson RC, Eisenberg SP (1990) Biological properties of recombinant human monocyte-derived interleukin 1 receptor antagonist. J Clin Invest 85: 1694–1697
266. Wakabayashi G, Gelfand JA, Burke JF, Thompson RC, Dinarello CA (1991) A specific receptor antagonist for interleukin-1 prevents *Escherichia coli*-induced shock in rabbits. FASEB J 5: 338–343
267. Galve-de Rochemonteix B, Nicod LP, Junod AF, Dayer JM (1990) Characterization of a specific 20–25 kD interleukin 1 inhibitor from cultured human lung macrophages. Am J Resp Cell Mol Biol 3: 355–361
268. Mancilla J, Garcia P, Dinarello CA (1994) Either interleukin-1 or the interleukin-1 receptor antagonist prevents lethal sepsis in newborn rats. Clin Res (in press)
269. Fischer CJ, Slotman GJ, Pribble J et al. (1991) Interleukin-1 receptor antagonist (IL1-ra) reduces mortality in patients with sepsis syndrome. Presentation at the 57th Annual American College of Chest Physicians Meeting, November 1991
270. Cominelli F, Nast CC, Clark BD et al. (1990) Interleukin 1 gene expression synthesis and effect of specific IL-1 receptor blockade in rabbit immune complex colitis. J Clin Invest 86: 972–980
271. Cominelli F, Llerena R, Clark BD, Nast CC, Thompson RC, Dinarello CA (1990) In vivo anti-inflammatory properties of recombinant interleukin 1 receptor antagonist (IL-1ra). Lymphokine Res 9: 597
272. Ramilo O, Saez-Llorens X, Mertsola J et al. (1990) Tumor necrosis factor alpha/cachectin and interleukin 1 beta initiate meningeal inflammation. J Exp Med 172: 497–507
273. Cybulsky ML, Kolditz IG, Movat H (1986) The role of IL-1 in neutrophil leukocyte emigration induced by endotoxin. Am J Pathol 124: 367
274. Giri JG, Newton RC, Horuk R (1990) Identification of soluble interleukin-1 binding protein in cell-free supernatants: Evidence for soluble interleukin-1 receptor. J Biol Chem 265: 17416–17419
275. Gershelwald JE, Fong YM, Fahey TJ (1990) Interleukin 1 receptor blockade attenuates the host inflammatory response. Proc Natl Acad Sci USA 87: 4966–4970
276. Neta R, Vogel SN, Plocinski JM (1990) In vivo modulation with anti-IL-1 receptor (p80) antibody 35f5 of the response to IL-1. Blood 76: 57–62
277. McIntyre KW, Stepan GJ, Kolinsky KD et al. (1991) Inhibitor of interleukin 1 (IL-1) binding and bioactivity in vitro and modulation of acute inflammation in vivo by IL-1 receptor antagonist and anti-IL-1 receptor monoclonal antibody. J Exp Med 173: 931–939
278. Engelman H, Novick D, Wallach D (1990) Two tumor necrosis factor binding proteins purified from human urine. J Biol Chem 170: 1531–1536
279. Porteau F, Nathan C (1990) Shedding of tumor necrosis factor receptors by activated human neutrophils. J Exp Med 172: 599–607
280. Seckinger P, Isaaz S, Dayer JM (1989) Purification and biologic characterization of a specific tumor necrosis factor α inhibitor. J Biol Chemistry 20: 11966–11973
281. Engelmann H, Aderka D, Rubinstein M, Rotman D, Wallach D (1989) A tumor necrosis factor-binding protein purified to homogeneity from human urine protects cells from tumor necrosis factor toxicity. J Biol Chem 20: 11974–11980
282. Novick D, Engelmann H, Wallach D, Rubinstein M (1989) Soluble cytokine receptors are present in normal human urine. J Exp Med 170: 1409–1414

Index

MIX
Papier aus verantwortungsvollen Quellen
Paper from responsible sources
FSC® C105338

If you have any concerns about our products,
you can contact us on
ProductSafety@springernature.com

In case Publisher is established outside the EU,
the EU authorized representative is:
Springer Nature Customer Service Center GmbH
Europaplatz 3, 69115 Heidelberg, Germany

Printed by Libri Plureos GmbH
in Hamburg, Germany